Textb

For Baillière Tindall

Commissioning Editor: Inta Ozols/Jacqueline Curthoys
Project Development Manager: Karen Gilmour
Project Manager: Jane Shanks
Design Direction: George Ajayi

Textbook of Community Children's Nursing

Edited by

Julia Muir
Senior Lecturer in Children's Nursing, School of Healthcare, Oxford Brookes University, John Radcliffe Hospital, Oxford, UK

Anna Sidey
Lecturer/Practitioner in Community Children's Nursing University College Northampton, UK

Foreword by

Elizabeth Fradd
Assistant Chief Nurse – Nursing Practice, Department of Health, London, UK

Baillière Tindall
PUBLISHED IN ASSOCIATION WITH THE RCN
Royal College of Nursing

Edinburgh London New York Philadelphia St Louis Sydney Toronto 2000

BAILLIÈRE TINDALL
An imprint of Harcourt Publishers Limited

First published 2000

0 7020 2622 0

British Library Cataloguing in Publication Data
A catalogue record for this book is available from the British Library

Library of Congress Cataloging in Publication Data
A catalog record for this book is available from the Library of Congress

Note
Medical knowledge is constantly changing. As new information becomes available, changes in treatment, procedures, equipment and the use of drugs become necessary. The editors, contributors and the publishers have, as far as it is possible, taken care to ensure that the information given in this text is accurate and up-to-date. However, readers are strongly advised to confirm that the information, especially with regard to drug usage, complies with the latest legislation and standards of practice.

The publisher's policy is to use **paper manufactured from sustainable forests**

Printed in China

Contents

Section Two: Philosophical Issues Underpinning the Delivery of Community Children's Nursing Practice

Contributors

Clare A Burnett BA(Hons) BAChildren'sNursing
Paediatric Gastroenterology Nurse Specialist, University Department of Paediatrics, John Radcliffe Hospital, Oxford, UK

Sue Burr RSCN RGN RHV RNT MA OBE FRCN
Adviser in Paediatric Nursing, Royal College of Nursing, London, UK

Steve Campbell BNurs PhD RGN RSCN RHV NDNCert FRSH
Head of Division of Children's Nursing and Learning Disabilities Nursing, School of Nursing Studies, University of Northumbria, Newcastle Upon Tyne, UK

Anne Casey RSCN MSc
Editor and Adviser, Royal College of Nursing, London, UK

Imelda Charles-Edwards RSCN RGN RNT MA DipEd
Education Officer, Children's Nursing, English National Board for Nursing Midwifery and Health Visiting, London, UK

Bridgit Dimond MA LLB DSA AHSM Barrister-at-Law
Emeritus Professor of University of Glamorgan, UK

Sue Dryden RGN RSCN DNCert
Senior Nurse Manager, Children's Centre, City Hospital Campus, Nottingham, UK

Sue Facey RGN RSCN DN DipN(Lond) BSc(Hons)
Community Children's Team Leader, Princess Margaret Hospital, Swindon, UK

Kim Gordon RGN RSCN BA(Hons) MSc(pending)
Children's Nurse Practitioner, John Radcliffe Hospital, Oxford, UK

Caroline Gould RGN RSCN DN BSc(Hons) CSP:CCN
Community Children's Nursing Team, Team Leader – Southwark, Community Health South London NHS Trust, London, UK

Julie Hughes RGN RSCN BSc(Hons)CommunityNursing PGCEA
Community Practice Lecturer (Lecturer/Practioner in Community Children's Nursing), Department of Community Studies, University of Reading, UK

Jane A Hunt PhD RSCN RGN DNCert
Senior Nurse for Research and Development, King's Healthcare NHS Trust, King's College Hospital (Dulwich), London, UK

June Hutt RGN RM RSCN DipEd DipNEd RNT MN
Senior Lecturer – Part-time, Oxford Brookes University, UK

Mark Jones MSc BSc(Hons) RN RHV
Primary Care Policy and Practice Adviser, Royal College of Nursing, London, UK

Suzanne Jones RGN RSCN ENB998 MSc PGDAdvancedNursingPractice
Advanced Nurse Practitioner/Team Leader, Diana, Community Children's Nursing Team, Warwickshire, UK

Paulajean Kelly RGN RSCN MSc BSc PGCE
Lecturer Practitioner, City University/Homerton Hospital Trust, St Bartholomew's School of Nursing and Midwifery, London, UK

Peter Kent BA(Hons)
Senior Partner, Helix Partners, London, UK

Andrea Lambert RGN RSCN BSc DNCert
React Community Children's Nurse, Cornwallis House, Oxford, UK

Trish Livsey NNEB RGN RSCN RHV CCN DipCommunityHealth, BA(Hons) PGCE NT
Senior Lecturer in Primary Health Care, St Martin's College, Education Centre, Cumberland Infirmary, Carlisle, UK

Patricia Ludder–Jackson RN MS PNP FAAN
Clinical Professor, Director, Advanced Practice Pediatric Nursing Program, School of Nursing, University of California, San Francisco, USA

Aidan Macfarlane FRCP FRCPCH FFPHM
Doctor, Oxford, UK

Helen Mehaffey RSCN RGN
Directorate Manager, Child Health, North Hampshire Hospital, Basingstoke, UK

Chris Middleton RGN RSCN RCNT RNT DipNEd MA
Nurse Teacher, University of Nottingham, School of Nursing, Queens Medical Centre, Nottingham, UK

Sue Miller RGN RSCN DNCert DipNursing CertEd(FE) MSc BSc(Hons)
Senior Lecturer, Department of Midwifery and Child, University of Hertfordshire, Hatfield, UK

Julia Muir RGN RSCN BA(Hons)
Senior Lecturer in Children's Nursing, School of Healthcare, Oxford Brookes University, John Radcliffe Hospital, Oxford, UK

Sarah J Neill MSc PGDE BSc(Hons) RGN RSCN
Senior Lecturer in Children's Nursing, Centre for Healthcare Education, University College Northampton, UK

Susan Procter PhD BSc(Hons) RN CertEd
Professor of Nursing Research, School of Nursing Studies, University of Northumbria, Newcastle Upon Tyne, UK

Kirsty Read RN LD RNCB BA(Hons)LearningDisabilities BA(Hons)Children'sNursing
Specialist Nurse, Hernes House, Oxford, UK

Phillippa Russell OBE DSc(Soc) BA
Director, Council for Disabled Children, National Children's Bureau, London, UK

Brian Samwell MMedsci BA RGN RSCN PGCE
Community Nurse Manager, Royal Hospital for Sick Children, Edinburgh, UK

Helen Shipton NNEB HPSEB AEB Counc7307 TeachingCert
Community Play Specialist, Paediatric Community Team, Stoke Mandeville Hospital, Aylesbury, UK

Anna Sidey RSCN RGN DN Cert
Lecturer/Practitioner in Community Children's Nursing, University College Northampton, UK

Susan M Spurling MA RGN RSCN RCNT RHV(Dip) RCST RQA
Senior Lecturer/Head of Clinical Development, Letchworth Centre for Healthy Living, Letchworth, UK

Maybelle A Tatman MB BS MSc MRCP FRCPCH
Consultant Community Paediatrician, Child and Family Health, Coventry Healthcare NHS Trust, UK

Saleha Uddin
Link worker, Tower Hamlets Paediatric Home Care Team, Tower Hamlets Trust, London, UK

Lisa S Whiting BA(Hons) RGN RSCN RNT LTCL
Senior Lecturer (Child Studies), University of Hertfordshire, Hatfield, UK

Mark Whiting MSc BNursing PGDip(Ed) RSCN RGN HV DN RNT
Senior Lecturer – Community Children's Nursing, South Bank University, London, UK

Kath Williamson RSCN RGN
Child Family Nurse Therapist, Children and Young People's Clinic, Nottingham City Hospital, UK

Lynn Young RN DN CPT
Community Health Adviser, Royal College of Nursing, London, UK

Acknowledgements

To John, for his unfailing support and patience throughout this whole venture.

To Hendrik, for his inspiration and encouragement.

Foreword

It is a privilege to write the foreword for a textbook which, in my view, is likely to become not only essential reading, but also to act as a significant marker in the history of the further development of community children's nursing.

Many children have, of course, historically always been cared for at home when sick by a range of individuals, notably family members. Their care has frequently been uncoordinated, provided by professionals not skilled in the care of children and services have been patchy and often inadequate. Over recent years however, a new professional group, highly skilled and knowledgeable in the nursing management of children, totally committed to enabling care to take place in the child's own home, whatever their problem, has emerged as a vibrant, creative and competent force.

The struggle to establish community children's nursing teams is reflected in this book. I believe one reason services are now becoming so strong is because the people who have led them and developed them are passionate about the need for appropriate services for children, and also have an abiding commitment to the quality of care for sick children. The contents of these papers reflect this and should therefore be regarded as testimony to their work, as well as to act as an inspiration for all those who still strive to establish or improve services.

The list of contributors, from a range of professional backgrounds and experiences, reflects the quality of the chapter content. Many of the key people who have made a significant contribution to the care of children at home have shared their views and described elements of care delivery.

The book works its way logically through organisational and philosophical issues, to the heart of the book which is about practice. It concludes with a section that encourages the reader to look ahead to new horizons, and new approaches. All the sections within each chapter are well referenced, with identified additional reading lists, as well as a brief summary of the text. This responds well to the need to ensure care delivery is evidence-based, and will greatly assist students or qualified staff new to the field. This is the first time such a comprehensive text has been published about the care of sick children by community children's nurses. My congratulations to all those who have contributed, and particularly to Julia Muir and Anna Sidey, the joint editors.

As health technology advances, the care of children and young people becomes more complex. Children are now being discharged home into the care of a community team, often profoundly sick, or with extremely complex needs. Considerable resources are required, both physical and emotional, to maintain some children and their families. The care is demanding, time-consuming and at times difficult. Equitable services ensure the right of any child to be offered care whatever their circumstances. At times however this too places an additional burden on caregivers, both lay and professional.

Current health policy stresses the importance of partnership working. Nowhere is it more important than in this field where partnership with family members and friends is as essential as partnerships with other professionals, such as the primary care team, Social Services, the voluntary sector, and education.

Nurses working in this field need however to think about other people with whom they should collaborate, for example researchers, in order that we amass 'the evidence' to not only demonstrate the need for such services but to also ensure the effectiveness of the care and services offered. Other important areas of collaborative working include Local Authorities – housing or environment departments, and other professional groups such as those working within complementary therapies, for example as aromatherapist or reflexologist. Community children's nurses are increasingly going to need to be broad in their outlook, open to new ideas and facilitative and flexible in their approaches.

As we move into a new millennium with a new health agenda and new approaches to care such as NHS Direct, we can look forward to the further development of community children's nursing services. But they will need to continue to be child-focused, family-orientated, cost and clinically effective, and of a high quality. Information about them will have to be readily available, and services responsive and equitable as well as capable of demonstrating real health gain. With the focus of care now being away from secondary care, real opportunities exist for children's nurses to be collaborative and innovative, in how they comfort and support sick children and their families. One factor will not change – the children. So listen them, respond to what they say and enjoy working with them.

Nottingham, 2000 Elizabeth Fradd MSc RSCN SCM RN HVCert

Preface

'In the culture I grew up in you did your work and did not put your arm around it to stop other people from looking. You took the earliest possible opportunity to make knowledge available.'

James Black, December 1995
Winner of the Nobel Prize for Medicine

In this first book devoted to community children's nursing, we have actively sought a range of contributors to bring together historical, contemporary and future perspectives on this exciting discipline. We are fortunate to have captured the views and expertise of those practitioners delivering the care, those managing and educating the prospective opinion leaders and those dedicated to developing the art and science of community children's nursing practice through research. We recognise it would be impossible to cover all aspects of this rapidly expanding service, but hope that this book will provide a catalyst for debate and inspire the generation of future texts.

Oxford
Northampton
2000

Julia Muir
Anna Sidey

SECTION

1 ORGANISATIONAL FACETS INFLUENCING THE PROFESSIONAL DEVELOPMENT OF COMMUNITY CHILDREN'S NURSING

This first section considers the many facets that have preceded and influenced the professional development of community children's nursing, alongside the current issues that demand attention. It provides a historical context, outlining the development of nursing, professional bodies and community children's nursing in particular. The realisation of specialist practitioner education is presented through a 100-year account before exploring the current educational agenda. Contemporary issues are also examined, including the dynamic changes in the 'new NHS' and the need for community children's nurses to 'get political'. With the demands for collaborative practice, opportunities for working in partnership with other agencies are described using case studies. The intention here is to offer a foundation to the remaining text.

SECTION CONTENTS

1 A short journey down a long road: the emergence of professional bodies

Chris Middleton

KEY ISSUES

- The late nineteenth century saw nursing achieve respectability, although its definition as 'women's work' meant low status.
- The first professional organisations in nursing disagreed over training, examination and registration of nurses – a split that was to deepen.
- The unionisation of nursing was seen as unethical and contrary to the traditions of vocation and service.
- The division between the unions and the professional bodies allowed others, outside nursing, to dictate policy and development.
- The low status of nursing obstructs its recognition as a true profession.
- By mirroring the development of medicine, nursing has adopted inappropriate medical models in approaches to care.
- The re-emergence of primary health care and the re-discovery by community children's nursing of its roots have provided nursing with a new opportunity to raise its profile and status.
- Recent government policies have recognised the value of nurses and nursing for the contribution they can make to the health of the population.
- Different ways of working and new alliances offer nurses serious opportunities to lead, especially in the field of community care.

INTRODUCTION

Nursing is at once an ancient art and a modern science. Shaped over the last 100 years by external forces and internal weaknesses, nursing is now, as is healthcare, redefined and rediscovered and ready to take up its rightful place in the new National Health Service (NHS). This chapter, while charting the well-known waters of the development of nursing, does so with an eye to the parallels of the emerging status of women in society and developments in medicine.

The delivery of healthcare in the UK has come full circle, with the emphasis now on primary health and the delivery of healthcare in the community rather than secondary care based in hospital. Community children's nursing is, therefore, now ideally placed to, with others, lead the challenges of healthcare provision into the next century.

DEVELOPMENT OF MODERN NURSING

The development of 'modern' nursing can be traced to the mid nineteenth century, although the concept of nursing has much older roots, arising from the care offered to the sick by members of religious orders. Records dating back to 1095 note the practice of nursing as a public service throughout the monastic movement – a service staffed predominantly by men.

With the dissolution of the monasteries in this country in the sixteenth century, the references to nursing as an organised activity all but disappear from the records. It is not until the eighteenth century, with the development of the voluntary hospitals, that nursing starts to re-appear, with any significance, in the history books.

The provisions of the Poor Law Amendment Act 1834 led to the establishment of workhouses and their associated infirmaries. However, it must be remembered that the style of nursing prevalent at the time bears little relation to what we accept as nursing today. Charles Dickens' portrayal of Sarey Gamp in Martin Chuzzlewit (Dickens 1897) reflected the low reputation of nursing at the time. It was commonly regarded as a last resort for people who were unable to gain employment elsewhere.

At this same low point, the winds of change were blowing for nursing. The change movement was catalysed to a large extent by the reforms being implemented by the religious nursing sisterhoods in Europe. In Britain, Florence Nightingale, who was strongly influenced by these sisters of charity, was starting to emerge as an influential agent of nursing reform. In the latter half of the nineteenth century her work and ideas began to have quite a major impact on the future structure and philosophy of nursing.

Nursing history cannot be and should not be viewed in isolation from social history, and it is important to consider the development of the emerging profession in its social and political context. The end of the nineteenth and the beginning of the twentieth centuries saw huge strides being made in the women's suffrage movement. Victorian women were enjoying a previously unknown independence in society. However, this new-found independence for women did not bring with it a new-found status. Victorian society was riven with wide social divisions. Importantly, it was deeply patriarchal, and as nursing became identified as primarily women's work it was inevitably seen as subordinate to that of the man/doctor. Any consideration of the development of and professionalisation of nursing in the UK must also, therefore, review the parallel emergence of the medical profession and the reasons for the dominance of the latter over the former.

Before the discovery of germ theory in the nineteenth century the role of doctors was largely ameliorative, so it was the propagation of this theory that increased their prestige in the public's estimation and this, coupled with the reduction of deaths from infectious diseases at that time, assured their superior position. However, this acclaim is probably based on good 'PR' rather than fact. The reduction in the death rate was due to an understanding of the germ theory and of the cause and spread of disease and its practical application in the area of public health, not as a result of any advance in medical science. The public health model of illness at the time was based on the concept of 'bad air', and one of the most effective strategies to control or eliminate this bad air was the introduction of improved sanitation; it was this relatively simple measure that was actually responsible for the reduction in deaths from infectious diseases.

The medical profession, to protect its dominant status, needed to classify health problems in a way that indicated they were amenable to medical (doctor-led) intervention; the biomechanical model, in which healthcare interventions are based upon the diagnosis and treatment of a specific aetiology, suited the profession's needs perfectly. Medical practice became firmly rooted in 'centres of disease' – hospitals. As hospitals developed, more nurses were needed to staff them, but the requirement was now not just for quantity of nurses but also for quality of nurses. Nightingale, and others of her social class at that time, had prompted an explosion of interest in nursing and had endowed it with an air of respectability:

> 'Nursing's values and culture were expropriated by women of a higher social status and greater wealth than the working-class women who had formed the bulk of the earliest nurses. Self sacrifice, loyalty, obedience and dedication were the key attributes to be instilled into educated young women of "good character".' (Hart 1996)

These educated young women of good character were required to train as nurses to staff the rapidly developing voluntary hospitals. Unfortunately it is these very origins of modern nursing that determined it now as women's work, and in turn this laid the foundations for how nurses were, and to a large extent still are, treated as workers within a patriarchal society.

With the advent of training for nurses the battlelines were drawn for the next fight, which was to establish a register of nurses and also a national final examination at the end of any training course to provide a common benchmark of suitability for registration.

BIRTH OF THE PROFESSIONAL ORGANISATIONS

According to Abel-Smith (1960), the first professional organisation was the British Nurses Association. This group was led by Miss Ethel Manson, who later married Dr Bedford Fenwick. Mrs Bedford Fenwick believed that the only way to ensure the highest possible standard of nursing was to restrict entry to the profession to the daughters of the higher social classes. In 1887, Bedford Fenwick founded the British Nurses Association in direct opposition to the Hospitals' Association, founded by Henry Burdett, a hospital administrator, which had set up a nursing section with its own central registry. Bedford Fenwick's association also set up its own registration system while it pushed for an official national register of nurses.

However, Mrs Bedford Fenwick's ideas for a register of nurses was strongly opposed by Florence Nightingale. Her main objection to the style of registration being proposed was the introduction of an examination to test knowledge. Nightingale herself placed more emphasis on the personal qualities of the person than her intellectual capacity. Other opposition came from Sydney Holland (Abel-Smith 1960 p 3) of the London Hospital where Mrs Bedford Fenwick had worked as a ward sister. He wrote: 'We want to stop nurses thinking themselves anything more than they are, namely, the faithful carriers out of the doctor's orders.'

In contrast to their opposition to nurse registration, the medical profession strongly supported the registration of midwives. Following the creation of the midwifery register under the provisions of the Midwives Act 1902, a select committee was appointed in 1904 to review the issue of registration for nurses. The outcome of their deliberations was in favour of registration. However, it would be some 15 years before Parliament acted on these findings. The requirement for nurses during the First World War brought further impetus for registration and a national standard in training. As a result the College of Nursing was founded. The intention was that the College should become the recognised body for determining the syllabus for nurse training and approving nurse training institutions, and also the registration body for qualified nurses. That was also the desire of the British Nurses Association. After 3 years of bitter wrangling between the two organisations, Parliament decided that the way forward with nurse registration was to form its own General Nursing Council (GNC) with the Nurses' Registration Act 1919. The first state final examination was held in 1925 and the first nurses were admitted to the Register by examination.

The divisions in nursing revealed by the registration debate were mirrored in the attempts by nurses to unionise. Employers and the medical profession obstructed these moves until 1910 when the National Asylum Workers Union (NAWU) was formed. Their priorities were more pay and a shorter working week. The emphasis at the turn of the century on training and registration had produced a shortage of trained nurses. This was exacerbated by the First World War, and by 1918 there was a major shortage of suitable women to train as nurses. According to Hart (1996) the extra burden this placed on existing staff 'had been justified by arguing that increased duties, longer hours and fewer days off were in the interests of good patient care.'

Discontent with pay and working conditions reached a peak in the mid 1930s when many nurses turned to the, by now, widely recognised trade unions for support. However, the College of Nursing, whose articles expressly forbade it becoming a trade union, continued to voice its opposition to the unionisation of nursing and condemned nurses who demanded better working conditions as being unethical, claiming that these demands 'had little in common with the ideals of service which must animate every nurse worthy of her name' (Hart 1996).

In 1939 the Government finally set up a committee to investigate nursing shortages. The committee's recommendation was to meet the unions' demands, an idea that was rejected by the Government at the time. It was not until the formation of the NHS in 1948 that the objectives of nationally negotiated pay and conditions of service were finally achieved.

Within the NHS, the pay and conditions of service of nurses and midwives was to be decided by the Whitley Council. The Council's staff side consisted of union and professional association representatives. The union representation was from the Confederation of Health Service Employees (COHSE), formed from the earlier merger of the National Union of County Officers (NUCO) and NAWU's successor, the Mental Hospital and Institutional Workers' Union. The Royal College of Nursing (RCN) – as the College of Nursing had become – with the support of the other professional associations claimed the largest number of seats of any individual organisation on the Council. With their opposing political and philosophical views, this ensured that nursing was relatively powerless and split.

Twenty years of Whitley Council failure meant that by the 1970s health workers' salaries were out of step and depressed. Nurses, faced with cutbacks in services and resources, became more militant, and both the RCN and

COHSE responded to their concerns with pay campaigns. In 1979 the Conservative Government – with an antinationalised industries, public services and trades unions philosophy – took power. The next 10–15 years saw COHSE and the RCN becoming more and more similar in their demands for nurses' pay and conditions, but still maintaining a distance by disputing how these demands were to be met by the Government. Unfortunately this continued bickering and lack of unity, an echo from the days of the professionalisation debate, allowed the Government further to weaken nursing's influence in healthcare provision by the introduction of general management.

> 'The division between nursing's trade unions and professional associations is almost unique in labour history, indicating nursing's positions somewhere between a skilled trade and a profession. It would be difficult to imagine, for example, doctors or dockers allowing themselves to be so thoroughly split and, consequently, weakened. The differences between them reflect the evolution of nursing's many strands and the people who became nurses.' (Hart 1996)

Hart (1996) makes the very valid point that, although nurses are continually accused of failing to articulate their needs and act in their own best interests, this accusation fails to take account of the fact that they work in and are products of a professionalised service. This has traditionally worked against their interests, denying them choices and exercising power in such a way as to ensure that those issues are never adequately discussed, an opinion perhaps shared by Rafferty (1995) when she said: 'The history of nursing is rarely one of triumph in the face of adversity but of struggle and compromise and often defeat.'

PROFESSIONALISATION OF NURSING

The continuing struggle of nursing to establish itself as an important intellectual force in healthcare delivery and/or reform can be explained in part by its own enduring ability to stab itself in the back. Equally influential, though, are its close but subordinate relationship with medicine and a legacy of populist images that work to undermine public and professional confidence. To overcome these hurdles nursing needs firstly to define itself independently from medicine and secondly to provide with this definition information for itself and the public about its worth, value and status. In a climate of advancing technology in healthcare and a move from a disease focus to a health focus, nurses are in a prime position to establish themselves as a profession on an equal footing with their medical colleagues.

Professionalisation was (and still is) to prove as elusive a quarry as registration had been. Unsurprisingly the issues appear to be the same. Nursing opinion is split between declaring itself a profession by virtue of meeting the necessary criteria to do so, and endlessly debating whether to do so is advantageous. External opinion and activity may serve to hamper the process further. Crouch (1996) argues that weak governing frameworks and organisational marginality within health services hamper the acceptance of nursing as a profession. She goes on to say: 'Health services, professional and organisational bodies, government and in some cases nurses themselves, have allowed nursing to become marginalised, resulting in loss of power for nurses and an increase in bureaucracy.'

Carter (1994) argues that the professionalisation process and debate has been impeded by nursing's failure to confront patriarchal attitudes in the clinical context. The roots of this, Carter believes, lie with Florence Nightingale and her insistence that nurses ask permission from a doctor before carrying out even basic caring tasks – a demand which should not be considered out of the context of the prevailing social attitudes towards women at this time. The ethos of the Victorian age was characterised by an acceptance of male superiority over women.

This doctor–nurse tension is an important consideration in the profession debate. Nurses who perceive professional status as offering them independence, autonomy and empowerment, and therefore a 'way out' of the traditional subservience, see the doctors as an example of how professional status can benefit its members.

'Doctors have money, high social standing and autonomy so why shouldn't we?' (Salvage 1985). However, as Rafferty (1996 p 186) points out, the work of Witz (1992) and Davies (1995) suggests that professions are 'gendered institutions', organised around male patterns of career development and priorities. Nursing, as a female-dominated occupation, does not fit easily into the traditional mould within which the archetypal professions have been cast.

If this situation is to change, it needs to be challenged by both men and women. It is necessary to pit the occupation of the dominant role by men against the hesitancy of women to challenge and their own responsibility for maintaining it.

SPECIALISATION

Although specialisation in name can be traced back to the Nurses Registration Act 1919, Castledine (1998 p 3) argues that:

> 'If specialisation infers a narrowing of the range of work to be done, and an increase in depth of knowledge and skill, then we must take the setting up of the first training school in nursing after the Crimean War by Florence Nightingale as the starting point for specialisation and identification of clinical nursing in the United Kingdom.'

However, he then goes on to distinguish between 'specialisation of nursing', achieved by the introduction of registration and training, and 'specialisation in nursing', which is the issue of concern here. According to Scott (1998), the late 1950s and 1960s in the UK saw an increase in nursing specialisation, particularly in the acute sector. The RCN (1977) saw that this was due in part to a parallel increase in specialisation in medicine; as medical science advances and specialisation increases, suitably prepared nurses must be available to identify the implications of these advances for nursing practice, to prescribe changes in nursing care and to advise on new techniques, in order that the nursing care of patients may reflect these advances.

Developments in the technology of medicine increased the cost of healthcare. To maintain the ideals of the NHS as a service 'free at the point of delivery', hospital administrators had to develop strategies for keeping down the cost of healthcare delivery. One approach was to cluster together high tech/high cost resources into regional centres. This led, naturally, to an increased demand for hospital nurses with specialist knowledge and skills. At this time there was no nationally recognised or regulated system of post-registration education. To meet the demand, therefore, many hospitals set up their own *ad hoc* clinical courses. The GNC was powerless to act to regulate these courses and ensure standards were being maintained, as it had responsibility only for pre-registration education and training.

In 1970, in response to the profession's urgent demands, the Government set up the Joint Board of Clinical Nursing Studies (JBCNS) to monitor and set standards for post-basic courses. NHS reorganisation in the 10 years between the mid 1960s and the mid 1970s had a significant impact on the organisation of nursing. Important among these effects was the Salmon Report (1966) which reorganised the management of nursing, but in doing so, according to Castledine (1998), it also shifted attention from the clinical role of the nurse. The status of the patient care aspect of the nurses' role dropped even further.

The plethora of specialised advanced nursing courses that were produced under the JBCNS appeared to have, at their heart, an increasing emphasis on medical treatment. Castledine (1998) offers the opinion that this was due in part to the 'theory–practice divide' in nursing, leading to a confusion about which way practice should develop.

The specialisation of nurses was not a concept that was universally welcomed. In a report in 1980 (Department of Health and Social Security 1980), the Chief Nursing Officer stated that this would lead to fragmented patient care and would further disintegrate the nursing function. The favoured pathway at the time was that of the general or generalist nurse. This concept is significant as a comment on the internal politics of nursing; however, criticisms of specialisation in nursing are probably not without foundation as early attempts to create specialist nurse roles fell into the trap of following the medical biomechanical model too closely.

By the 1980s there was a backlash. The Merrison Report (1979) had commented on the situation in North America where it had investigated the creation of clinical nurse specialists – nurses whose area of specialisation was clinical nursing. They recognised that a similar model could work in the UK and made specific recommendations about appropriate remuneration for the acquisition and use of advanced nursing skills.

'RE-EMERGENCE' OF PRIMARY HEALTHCARE

The arena for the involvement of nurses in healthcare delivery has never been restricted to that of the acute, secondary sector, although the years since the inception of the NHS have probably focused on its profile in institutions. The existence of primary healthcare – more accurately for the time, public healthcare – can be recognised pre-Nightingale. At the turn of the century Nightingale herself recognised the impact of a person's environment on their health status, and much of her work was directed towards prevention. She also had a significant impact on William Rathbone when he was pioneering district nursing and health visiting services.

It is not until about the 1970s onwards that we start to see primary healthcare being put back under the spotlight. Developments in the technology of medicine had increased the cost of healthcare. Consumers who had grown up with the NHS were becoming more aware of their own health needs and of the shortcomings of the service, and were starting to make their voices heard through patient support groups. The Government set up Community Health Councils in 1974 to provide a consumer's voice in healthcare policy and practice.

During the 1980s surveys were reporting an increasing dissatisfaction among the public with regard to waiting lists, outpatients and the 'inpatient experience'. The Government's response to this was to introduce the ethos of the free market system into the structure and management of the NHS. This was a cost-driven exercise, but the secondary intention was to promote good practice in healthcare delivery at a local level.

In the late 1980s the growth of the primary care sector proceeded apace. Services that had traditionally been the exclusive domain of hospitals were being relocated into the community service, such as minor surgery and specialist outpatient services. Increasingly, what would once have been considered intensive and complex nursing care procedures are being carried out in the community setting; this, of course, has important – and often overlooked – implications for informal carers.

In part, these issues of spiralling acute care costs and growing public protest about the quality of secondary sector care helped to drive the shift of emphasis from institutional to community-based care. Other factors are demographic trends, changing patterns of illness and the development of less invasive medical treatments. The UK was not alone in experiencing this push towards a greater focus on primary healthcare. In 1978 the World Health Organization published 'Health for all by the year 2000', which requested states' parties to place primary care firmly at the centre of their health policies and systems.

The emergence of community children's nursing as a speciality has slightly different roots. The negative impact of hospitalisation on children had been recognised for some time, and in the early 1950s the work of Bowlby (1965) had demonstrated that children were not just small adults: they reacted differently to stressful situations and had special emotional and physical needs that should be met by specialised services. In 1959 the Platt Report (Ministry of Health 1959) strongly recommended the provision of special nursing services for the home care of children, putting an emphasis on avoiding hospitalisation if at all possible and meeting children's health needs in the community.

Unfortunately Platt was largely ignored and developments in community children's nursing were slow and sparse until the early 1990s. Why this should have been so is unclear. But in the last decade the growth of this service has outstripped its adult counterparts. Bradley (1997) offers four factors that may have influenced this rapid growth rate (Box 1.1).

PRESSURES ON THE SYSTEM

'Nurses in the primary health care setting are currently experiencing unprecedented change both from within their working environment and as members of a developing profession' (Bell 1997). According to Coote (1998) there is

BOX 1.1 ***Factors influencing the growth of community children's nursing***

1. **Children's legal rights** – the 1989 United Nations Convention on the Rights of the Child placed a duty on states' parties to incorporate the articles of the Convention into national law. In England the Children Act (Department of Health 1989) had a significant impact on the legal rights of children with regard to issues such as partnership in care and consent.
2. **Professional influences** – a gradual recognition of the potential for care at home with professional support coupled with a move from a paternalistic to an empowerment approach by childcare professionals.
3. **Parental pressure** – the founding, in 1961, of the National Association for the Welfare of Children in Hospital (NAWCH), which was a highly influential parents' action group, now called Action for Sick Children (ASC).
4. **NHS changes** – competition in the NHS 'market' (Department of Health 1993).

expressed public anxiety about health risks, but any action is usually about concerns with the NHS, not health.

> 'This may be because people feel impotent about it. The links between cause and effect are unclear to them. They or we don't know who to blame, or what can be done to make things better.' (Coote 1998)

There is a need to take collective action to improve public health. This is not a new phenomenon, but it is clear that earlier strategies have failed. For example, the Health of the Nation strategy, which was from 1992 to 1997 the central plank of health policy in England, represented the first explicit attempt by government to provide a strategic approach to improving the overall health of the population. In spite of being widely welcomed, it failed to realise its full potential. In 'The Health of the Nation – a policy assessed: the executive summary of two reports into the failings of the HOTN strategy', there are recommendations for future health policy initiatives. Prominent among these is the need to 'make public health part of the core business by embedding it in the organisational culture' (Department of Health 1998a). As Anna Coote says: 'Most activity which makes a difference will come from the bottom up; it will depend on effective, inter-agency working at local level.'

In its White Paper 'The New NHS. Modern, dependable' (Department of Health 1997), the Government made a clear statement about the need to strengthen the contribution made by nursing. Additionally, the Health Services Circular (Department of Health 1998b) 'Better health and better health care' outlines a set of activities to ensure that staff at all levels are enabled to maximise their contribution to health and healthcare through the implementation of 'The new NHS. Modern, dependable' and 'Our healthier nation' (Department of Health 1998c).

Certainly the message that strikes out from 'Our healthier nation' is that everybody has a part to play in improving the health of the population. The Government is committed to producing a national contract for better health under which it will join in partnerships with local communities and individuals to improve health. Action is to be focused in four priority areas:

- coronary heart disease and stroke
- cancers

BOX 1.2 ***Areas covered by Health Improvement Programmes***

- The health needs of the local population and how these are to be met by the NHS and its partners through broader action on public health
- The main healthcare requirements of local people and how local services will be developed to meet these
- The range, location and investment required in local health services

- accidents
- mental health

and the settings for these have been determined as:

- healthy schools (focusing on children)
- workplaces (focusing on adults)
- neighbourhoods (focusing on older people)

What community children's nursing will have to consider is where and how it fits into this strategy. There are some very encouraging messages for nurses and nursing within this strategy document. Health promotion will become a more integral part of healthcare provision than it has in the past. Nurses are in a prime position to take this on board, and have the potential for significant influence in this area. Community nurses will need to develop different approaches and strategies to communicate their health messages.

Different ways of working will need to evolve to focus on specific health issues. This could be an exciting development for community nurses and an opportunity to take the lead in some of the initiatives. This strategy places a new emphasis on children, and will demand a significant input from health visitors and school nurses in terms of programmes of health promotion and in promoting and supporting effective parenting. But there is little mention within the strategy of the role or potential role of the community children's nurse (CCN). However, the Government proposes that the vehicles to improve health and healthcare will be the Health Improvement Programmes (HIPs) (Box 1.2). These HIPs will be developed by health authorities but implemented by Trusts and, in England, Primary Care Groups (PCGs). It is within PCGs that community nurses will have the potential to influence local health provision policy.

THE FUTURE

Bell (1997) noted O'Keefe, Ottewill and Wall's (1992) dire prediction of a pending health crisis which must be taken seriously by community nurses, and the need for them to take full account of key factors that have the potential to underpin the predicament:

- Shift in emphasis from biomedical, curative approaches to preventive approaches
- 'Epidemiological transition' from childhood illnesses to chronic and degenerative disorders
- Iceberg of sickness

- Environmental pollution
- User dissatisfaction
- Widening gap between demand and supply
- Demographic timebomb

We can predict that primary healthcare as a concept and in practice is at, and will remain at, the very heart of healthcare and health service development. This has been stated clearly by recent governmental and international health strategies, and is inevitable if healthcare costs are to be managed.

Recent government initiatives have made it clear that community nurses will be key workers in strategies for improving health:

> 'However it is suggested that community health care nursing requires a radical re-think incorporating the role of the nurse practitioner if it is to remain viable as it moves into the next millennium.' (Bell 1997)

It is, as yet, too soon to consider the impact of the recent review by J M Consulting Ltd (1998) of the regulation of Nursing, Midwifery and Health Visiting and the Nurses, Midwives and Health Visitors Act 1979. However, the report does comment that one of the main weaknesses of the current Act is that it does not reflect the changing structure of the nursing professions, such as the development of community practitioners.

CONCLUSION

In the late nineteenth century modern nursing was born into a deeply patriarchal and socially divided Victorian British society. At its beginning it had in its grasp what we now know to be the root of effective healthcare provision – the public health or primary care. But, as a woman's job, it soon lost any lead it had to the socially and professionally dominant male-dominated medical profession.

In seeking to re-establish itself as a valid force for healthcare assessment and delivery, nursing has faced many battles. Changes have been imposed from outside by forces that have recognised the inherent weakness of a divided group. In the face of such onslaught, nursing has struggled to define itself and its role, but most of the time its biggest enemy has probably been itself.

Fifty years after the creation of the NHS, the social, political and economic wranglings that have been a familiar characteristic of healthcare provision in the UK have finally conspired to produce healthcare policies and strategies that rely on nurses to ensure their success. These, coupled with the establishment of primary care as the very heart of these policies, means that community nurses with their special skills and understanding of communities can and must take up the challenge.

REFERENCES

Abel-Smith B 1960 A history of the nursing profession. Heinemann, London.

Bell R 1997 Towards the next millennium. In: Burley S, Mitchell E E, Melling K, Smith M, Chilton S & Crumplin C (eds) Contemporary community nursing. Arnold, London, p 259

Bowlby J 1965 Child care and the growth of love, 2nd edn. Penguin, Harmondsworth

Bradley S 1997 Better late then never? An evaluation of community nursing services for children in the UK. Journal of Clinical Nursing 6(5): 411–418

Carter H 1994 Confronting patriarchal attitudes in the fight for professional recognition. Journal of Advanced Nursing 19(2):367–372

Castledine G 1998 In: Castledine G & McGee P (eds) Advanced and specialist nursing practice. Blackwell Science, Oxford, Ch 1, p3

Coote A 1998 Cited in: Expert analysis of the new health strategy. From Department of Health online journal, Target. http://www.doh.gov.uk/target/expert2.htm

Crouch S 1996 Professionals – myth or reality? Nursing Management 3(6):12–13

Davies C (1995) Gender and the professional predicament in nursing. Open University Press, Buckingham

Department of Health 1989 The Children Act. HMSO, London

Department of Health 1993 A vision for the future: the nursing, midwifery and health visiting contribution to health and health care. HMSO, London

Department of Health 1997 The new NHS. Modern, dependable. The Stationery Office, London

Department of Health 1998a The Health of the Nation – a policy assessed. The Stationery Office, London

Department of Health 1998b Health Services Circular 1998/021: Better health and better health care – implementing 'The new NHS' and 'Our healthier nation'. The Stationery Office, London

Department of Health 1998c Our healthier nation. The Stationery Office, London

Department of Health and Social Security 1980 Careers in clinical nursing: report of a chief nursing officer's working party. Department of Health and Social Security, London

Dickens C 1897 The life and adventures of Martin Chuzzlewit. Chapman and Hall, London

Hart C 1996 The great divide. International History of Nursing Journal 1(3):5–17

J M Consulting Ltd 1998 The regulation of nurses, midwives and health visitors: report on a review of the Nurses, Midwives and Health Visitors Act 1997. J M Consulting Ltd, Bristol

Merrison Report 1979 Royal commission on the National Health Service. HMSO, London

Ministry of Health 1959 The welfare of children in hospital – a report of the committee (chairman: Sir H Platt). HMSO, London

O'Keefe E, Ottewill R & Wall A 1992 Community health: issues in management. Business Education Publishers, Sunderland

Rafferty A (1995) Unpublished work. Cited in: Kitson A 1997 John Hopkins address: Does nursing have a future? Image – The Journal of Nursing Scholarship 29(2):111–115

Rafferty A 1996 The politics of nursing knowledge. Routledge, London

Royal College of Nursing 1977 Evidence to the Royal Commission on the NHS. Royal College of Nursing, London

Salmon Report 1966 Report of the committee on senior nursing structure. HMSO, London

Salvage J 1985 The politics of nursing. William Heinemann, London

Scott C 1998 Specialist practice: advancing the profession? Journal of Advanced Nursing 28(3):554–562

United Nations Convention 1989 UN Convention on the rights of the child. UNICEF, Geneva

Witz A 1992 Professions and patriarchy. Routledge, London

World Health Organization 1978 Health for all by the year 2000. World Health Organization, Copenhagen

2 1888–1988: 100 years of community children's nursing

Mark Whiting

KEY ISSUES

- Community children's nursing has a complex history dating back to the middle of the last century.
- Much of the history of the provision of formal community children's nursing can be closely linked to the emergence and development of both district nursing and health visiting.
- The rapid growth of community children's nursing in the 1980s and 1990s seems to have occurred more as a result of the pioneering spirit of individual practitioners than as a consequence of identifiable social policy reform.

INTRODUCTION

This chapter is concerned with the historical development of community children's nursing in the UK. Particular attention will be focused upon the emergence, during the closing years of the nineteenth century, of a community nursing service for children based within the Hospital for Sick Children, Great Ormond Street, London. This period is of particular note because it was around the same time that the forebears of the current district nursing and health visiting services were becoming established (Owen 1982, Stocks 1960). Consideration will then be given to the early years of the National Health Service (NHS), focusing on published accounts of service developments in Rotherham, Birmingham, Paddington, Southampton, Edinburgh, Gateshead, Oxford and Brent. An overview of service provision in 1988 will provide a summary of service development up to that date.

The care of the sick child has moved steadily in recent years from being almost exclusively the responsibility of the hospital (Oppé 1971) towards the community (National Health Service Executive 1996). This has been reflected in very significant reductions in the length of time for which children are admitted to hospital, from an average of around 2 weeks at the time of the Platt Report (Ministry of Health 1959) to a little over 2 days by the early 1990s (Audit Commission 1993). As we head into the twenty-first century, inpatient hospital care has been envisioned in the future as being required for only the most acutely or seriously ill members of society and it has been suggested that, in consequence, community healthcare will provide for a much broader range of needs (Department of Health 1997). This is a far cry from the situation that existed in the middle of the nineteenth century, the period to which the opening section of this chapter will now be devoted.

EARLY DAYS

The first children's hospital to be established in the UK was the Hospital for Sick Children, Great Ormond Street, London in 1852 (Kosky & Lunnon 1991, Lomax 1996). However, over 100 years earlier, Thomas Coram had established the Foundling Hospital, also in London. Coram, a retired sea captain, had been appalled at the numbers of dead and dying babies to be found on the streets of London and set about interesting the Government, the Anglican Church and members of the ruling classes in providing financial support for a 'hospital' that was to provide the necessary care for these babies or 'foundlings', many of whom were the illegitimate children of the poor. Coram's attempts to interest the authorities in providing funds for his proposals were largely unsuccessful, and initial funding for the hospital came predominantly from charitable rather than state sources.

The hospital was soon overwhelmed by the demand for admission of 'foundlings' (Lomax 1996). Franklin (1964) reported that, in spite of wealthy patronage, there were insufficient funds to meet the demands of the large numbers of babies who were often abandoned at the hospital entrance. The hospital's governors eventually appealed to the House of Commons for financial support. The Government donated £10 000 to the hospital on the condition that for an initial period of 6 months no infant should be refused admission to the hospital. In the event, unregulated admissions continued for nearly 4 years, often with dire consequences. Of 14 934 babies admitted to the hospital between 1756 and 1760, only 4545 survived (Franklin 1964). Lomax (1996 p 4) suggests that state intervention was, in part, responsible for the discrediting of the hospital, leading to accusations that, by agreeing to accept all children arriving at its doors, it encouraged 'irresponsibility and immorality'.

The Foundling Hospital was concerned primarily with providing protection and education for children rather than with the provision of medical or nursing care. However, in 1852, when Charles West opened the first Hospital for Sick Children in Great Ormond Street, there was a clear recognition of the need specifically to provide both medical and nursing expertise. The establishment of the hospital at Great Ormond Street preceded what can only be described as a tidal wave of activity in the establishment of children's hospitals in the UK. By the turn of the century, there were over 30 children's hospitals and upwards of 50 children's convalescent homes. In addition, many general hospitals had formally dedicated one or more wards exclusively for the care of children (Lomax 1996).

One of the original aims of the Great Ormond Street Hospital for Children was 'to train girls for a few months to enable them to be effective as children's nurses in private families' (Lomax 1996 p 8). However, whilst this may have been the intention of Sir Charles West, it was not until the mid 1870s that formal proposals to develop a private domiciliary nursing service were made to the hospital's management committee.

> 'Some consideration took place on the reference in Dr West's paper to the training of nurses proposed by the Lady Superintendent in visiting hospital out-patients at their own homes, under the regulations suggested by Dr West and coincided in by the Lady Superintendent. The majority of the Medical Officers were in favour of the plan being made trial of for 6 months, but the lay members of the committee were unanimously opposed to the extension of the work of the hospital beyond the walls.' (Hospital for Sick Children 1874)

Despite this initial reticence, by 1880 a scheme to supply trained private nurses was in preparation, and by 1888 a private domiciliary nursing service was operating from the hospital (Hunt & Whiting 1999). In order to treat sick children at home, it was clear that professional supervision was required. Lomax (1996) suggests that many of the early children's hospitals provided a domiciliary visiting service (staffed by the hospital physicians) when they first opened; however, many were forced to abandon this both because of the 'expenses involved and because of opposition from both hospital and general physicians' (p 12). It is unclear how many of the hospitals actually employed nurses to visit children in their own homes, although of the 11 children's hospitals in London by the turn of the century only the Victoria Hospital in Westminster and Great Ormond Street are recorded as so doing (Lomax 1996). In addition, whilst a small number of the provincial children's hospitals had initially provided some home nursing services free of charge, most of these services rapidly became available on a fee-paying basis only – effectively a private outreach nursing service.

For some families, district nurses were available even when the families could not afford to pay for their services. Indeed, it is clear that one of the original intentions of William Rathbone, who had been responsible for the introduction of district nursing in the 1850s, was to provide a nursing service in the community for those (adults and children) who were unable to pay for hospital care. However, Lomax (1996) suggests rather disparagingly that this was 'to some extent at the expense of divorcing institutional practice from domiciliary care' (p 12). A further issue that militated against the development of the outreach nursing service concerned the expenses involved in the training of the nurses, which were incurred within the overall costs of running hospitals. This money was derived largely from donations to the hospitals, and as such it was intended to fund the provision of care for the poor. It was certainly not intended to provide for the training of 'private nurses', available only to those who could pay for their services.

From the outset, the private nursing service based at Great Ormond Street Hospital was staffed by nurses who had been 'trained' in the nursing of children (Wood 1888). Wood (1888 p 507) was very single minded in her insistence that 'sick children require special nursing, and sick children's nurses require special training'.

A register of the nurses providing a private nursing service in patients' homes was commenced in 1888, and included the names of nine nurses – perhaps the earliest recorded team of community children's nurses (Hunt & Whiting 1999). The team of nurses provided for children with a wide range of needs, including those arising from acute infectious disease, chronic nutritional failure and orthopaedic and general surgical problems. Care was ordinarily provided on a 'live-in' basis, and whilst this was often quite short term (for perhaps three to seven days), some children received continuing care from one or more nurses over periods of several months.

The private nursing service was a great success, generating significant sums of money for the hospital and undergoing considerable expansion during the early years of the 20th century. By 1938, thirty nurses were employed, each of whom had been required to be trained by Great Ormond Street Hospital in the care of sick children (Hospital for Sick Children 1936) and each of whom provided full-time nursing care to one single child at a time (with a waiting list of children as soon as one of the nurses became 'free'). However, in 1948, the implementation of the National Health Service Act 1946 brought the Hospital for Children into the 'welfare state' and thus required the dissolution of the private nursing service. On the 14 March 1949, the last remaining member of the nursing staff, who had been caring for a child requiring long-term care, returned to the hospital from duty in the community.

COMMUNITY CHILDREN'S NURSING IN THE EARLY YEARS OF THE NHS

The period from the middle of the nineteenth century up to the inception of the NHS in 1948 was a time of significant expansion and development of both district nursing and health visiting services. In addition to bringing the 'voluntary' and 'municipal' hospitals together under the umbrella of the NHS, the 1946 Act also made arrangements for the statutory provision by health authorities of both district nursing and health visiting services.

A detailed history of the development of health visiting, dating back to the establishment of the Manchester and Salford Sanitary Reform Association in 1852 can be found in the work of Owen (1982). Whilst much of the work of health visitors has always been concerned with the health of children, the provision of 'hands on' nursing care to sick children has never been a significant feature of their work (Clark 1981, While 1985).

The history of district nursing, which has been traced back to the appointment, in 1859, of a single nurse in Liverpool by William Rathbone, has been reviewed in detail by Stocks (1960). The original intentions of the district nursing services were focused in meeting the needs of the 'sick poor', and it is clear that in the latter years of the nineteenth century the care of sick children in their own homes formed a significant part of the nurses' caseload (Rathbone 1890). Baly, Robottom and Clark (1987) suggest that, up to the 1920s, 'much of the district nurse's work was involved in caring for children with infectious diseases' (p 189).

The requirements of the National Health Service Act 1946 for the newly created health authorities to 'secure the attendance of nurses on persons who require nursing in their own homes' (paragraph III section 25) and to 'make provision in their area for the visiting of persons in their homes by visitors to be called health visitors' (part III section 24[1]) represented, in large areas of the UK, little more than the formal realignment of pre-existing services into the new structures of the NHS. However, no specific arrangements were made within the Act for the nursing of children in the community. The extent to which either district nursing or health visiting services were providing care to sick children in the community at the time of the Act is unclear, although it is likely that the number of sick children for whom such services might be provided was very small indeed. Subsequent studies of district nursing (Dunnell & Dobbs 1982) and health visiting (Clark 1981) suggest that this situation remains.

THE CHILDREN'S NURSING UNIT IN ROTHERHAM

The first recorded appointment within the NHS of a nurse involved exclusively in the care of sick children was in Rotherham in 1949 (Gillet 1954). This service was introduced to address concerns relating to a high rate of infant mortality in the preceding winter which was considered to have arisen 'largely due to cross-infection in hospital' (p 684). The service was initially staffed in 1949 by a single Queen's Nursing Sister who had undertaken a 'postgraduate course covering children's diseases' (p 684) and this was supplemented with a second appointment later in the year. Referrals to the service were made by the local general practitioners (GPs) and a major element of the work of the nurses was concerned with the care of children with acute infections. In 1952, for instance, one-third of the referrals to and visits undertaken by the nurses were of this nature (Table 2.1). Gillet confidently asserted that the service contributed significantly to an improvement in the infant mortality rate in the Rotherham district, although no specific evidence to support this claim was provided. He did, however, identify four additional advantages of the services as (Gillet 1954 p 685):

- 'the child remaining at home in familiar surroundings is less likely to fret;
- the danger of cross infection is lessened;

TABLE 2.1 ***Referrals to and visits undertaken by Rotherham Community Children's Nursing Unit in 1952***

Diagnosis	No. of cases	No. of visits
Pneumonia	67	537
Bronchitis	119	990
Gastroenteritis	6	62
Measles	23	197
Measles and pneumonia	9	76
Measles and bronchitis	1	1
Scarlet fever	1	1
Chickenpox	1	7
Pemphigus	3	11
Ophthalmia neonatorum	1	12
Whooping cough	5	56
Whooping cough and pneumonia	1	3
Poliomyelitis	1	3
Total of infectious cases	238	1956
Total of non-infectious cases	475	3881

Source: Gillet (1954).

- the mother is encouraged to help in the nursing of the child and the health teaching to parents and relatives done in these cases is considerable;
- the call on hospital beds for sick children has been reduced.'

A similar list of potential advantages was identified for the domiciliary Nursing Service for Infants and Children in Birmingham and the St Mary's Paediatric Home Care Project in Paddington, London, both of which were established in 1954. No further published reports of the Rotherham service beyond the mid 1950s have been traced, although reference to the service is made in the Report of the Committee on the Welfare of Children in Hospital (Ministry of Health 1959).

THE CHILDREN'S HOME NURSING SERVICE IN BIRMINGHAM

Partly in response to the success of the Children's Nursing Unit in Rotherham, and as a result of a collaborative venture between the Birmingham Health Committee, the House Committee of the Children's Hospital, the Local Medical Committee and the Local Executive Council, a children's home nursing service was established in Birmingham in October 1954. Initially, the service was focused upon 'an area containing a population of about 100 000, around the Children's Hospital and two district nursing centres' (Smellie 1956 p 256). A 'state registered nurse with district training' (Morris 1966) from each of the district nursing centres was appointed specifically to care for children in the community and, before taking up their posts, each nurse spent a week of orientation in the Children's Hospital to familiarize themselves with both current inpatient care and to meet members of the ward and outpatient nursing teams. The nursing staff worked in close collaboration with the local GPs (initially 27 GPs were involved; Howell 1974) and in the first year of their work visited 454 children in their own homes, undertaking a total of 3295 visits. The major focus of the nurse's work was in the management of acute infectious disease. The work was focused largely on the general practice population, but also included a number of children for whom early hospital discharge had been facilitated. Evening visits by the nurses were identified as being the 'most important in allaying the worries and anxieties of the mothers, so that there have been very few emergency calls during the night' (Smellie 1956 p 256).

By 1962 the service expanded to four nurses, and in order to provide a comprehensive service a senior member of the team was seconded to undertake night duty. The team undertook a total of 10 936 visits in 1962. Close collaboration with the general practice population was seen as key to the success of the service, with 39 GPs using the service regularly and 15 occasionally (Howell 1974). In addition, strong links were established with both the health visiting services and with the Birmingham Children's Hospital (Morris 1966). This collaboration is further highlighted in the pattern of referrals to the service reported by Robottom (1969), who noted that, of 1047 referrals made to the service from May 1967 to April 1968, 777 were from GPs, 241 were from hospitals and 29 from health visitors. At the time of Robottom's report, the nurses working in the service were formally identified as 'paediatric nurses', and Robottom herself was certainly a registered sick children's nurse (RSCN). However, in 1974, only three of the five members of the team were RSCNs (Howell 1974).

In 1969, Robottom had noted that only two nurses were working in the service. She recommended that:

> 'for a more effective Children's Home Nursing Unit the first need is an increased paediatric nursing staff. The child population of the city is approximately 257 000: 10 paediatric nurses in addition to the existing two would enable this service in its present form to cover the whole city on a basis of one nurse per 20 000 children.' (Robottom 1969 p 312)

By 1974, four of the five nurses working in the service were 'attached' to one of the four hospitals containing paediatric beds within the Birmingham area (Howell 1974). At this stage there had been a significant shift in the work of the nursing team, away from the care of children with acute problems and towards those with more long-standing nursing needs. This was accompanied by a reduction from 92% referrals by GPs in 1960, to only 43% in 1973.

THE PADDINGTON HOME CARE SCHEME

A 'home care scheme' was introduced in Paddington in April 1954, and was staffed initially by a trained 'paediatrician and three nurses with paediatric training' (Lightwood 1956 p 13). Although the nurses worked closely with the district nursing services, it would appear that none of the original members of the scheme had actually trained as district nurses themselves.

The scheme was initiated because a review undertaken within the paediatric department at St Mary's Hospital had found that:

> 'nearly a quarter of children in hospital during the review period were admitted for conditions which could have been managed at home if the doctors had possessed the facilities and experience required, and that there were other children whose stay in hospital could have been shortened.' (Lightwood et al 1957 p 313).

The establishment of the Home Care Scheme was supported by the Local Medical Committee, the County of London, the Paddington and St Marylebone District Nursing Association, the County Council, the local medical officers of health and the constituent hospitals of the St Mary's Hospital group. It was established with three clear aims (Lightwood 1956):

1. Improving cooperation between hospital staff and family doctors
2. Avoidance of admission to hospital for sick children
3. Cutting the cost of inpatient treatment by providing a cheaper alternative whilst maintaining high standards

The work of the team was very similar to that reported in Rotherham and in the early years of the Birmingham scheme, with a major concentration on the management of symptoms and the care of children with acute febrile illness. Lightwood et al (1957) even described the management in the home (including lumbar puncture) of a 12-week-old infant with meningococcal meningitis.

From the outset and throughout the 45 years of its existence to date, the staff of the scheme has included both RSCNs and registrar or consultant grade paediatricians. It has been argued that the availability of medical staff within the scheme made it very different to those in Birmingham and Rotherham (McClure 1960). However, it is perhaps of rather more than academic interest that, in spite of considerable publicity of the scheme over the years, including multiple publications in reputable medical journals, the model of joint medical and nursing provision developed in Paddington has never been replicated elsewhere in the UK.

The major work of the home care scheme was based, at the outset, upon referrals made by the local GPs and, more often than not, this was followed up by a joint visit between the GP, paediatric registrar and nursing sister. Bergman et al (1965 p 317) suggested: 'Home care is an extramural ward of the hospital', although whether the GPs involved with the scheme shared this view is unclear.

In the first 10 years of operation of the service, 1882 of a total 2923 referrals were made by the family GP. Of these referrals, 2497 children were nursed at home following assessment by the home care registrar, with only 165 children being admitted to hospital (Bergman et al 1965). Table 2.2 shows the diagnostic groups of the children referred to the scheme during the first 10 years, with the five most common medical diagnoses being acute respiratory and infectious problems and accounting for almost two-thirds of all referrals. By the mid 1970s, however, as with the Birmingham service, there had been a definite change in the nature of the workload of the home care team towards children with more chronic problems (Jenkins 1975), a pattern that persists to the present day (Whiting 1994).

TABLE 2.2 ***Diagnostic groups of children referred to the Paddington Home Care Scheme 1954–1964***

Diagnosis	No. of cases
Upper respiratory	594
Lower respiratory	548
Contagious disease	324
Gastroenteritis	233
Otitis media	206
Feeding problems	194
Pulmonary collapse	93
Urinary infection	89
Fever of unknown origin	59
Tuberculosis	52
Postoperative care	44
Congenital heart disease	37
Rheumatic fever	29
Central nervous system disorders	27
Poliomyelitis	13
Skin disease	10
Behaviour disorders	10
Miscellaneous	637

Source: Bergman et al. (1965).

'THE WELFARE OF CHILDREN IN HOSPITAL'

The above-titled report from the Ministry of Health (1959) provided the first official endorsement of the development of community nursing services for sick children. The report recognised the emerging acceptance within the nursing and medical professions of the potential psychological harm that might arise in children as a result of hospitalisation and recommended that 'children should not be admitted to hospital if it can possibly be avoided' (Ministry of Health 1959 para 17). The report further observed 'too few local authorities as yet provide special nursing services for home care of children and the extension of such schemes should be encouraged' (Ministry of Health 1959 para 18).

Whilst it is fair to say that many of the report's recommendations pertaining to the care of children in hospital have been implemented successfully, the proposals for expanding community nursing provision for children fell on very deaf ears indeed. There are no published reports of the establishment of new community children's nursing services until 1969.

AN INITIATIVE IN PAEDIATRIC DAY-CASE SURGERY IN SOUTHAMPTON IN 1969

A paediatric home nursing service was introduced in November 1969 in Southampton (Atwell et al 1973). The service was developed to support the newly established Centre for Paediatric Surgery for the Wessex Region in the Southampton Children's Hospital. In developing the service, there was a clear statement of intent to avoid unnecessary overnight stay in hospital for children, as well as a pragmatic approach to the need to optimise the use of beds and cots in the paediatric unit.

The development of the service was supported jointly by the consultant paediatric surgeon, the senior nursing officer in the community and the local medical officer of health. Initially, two nurses, who held qualifications in both district nursing and sick children's nursing, were appointed to provide follow-up in the community of children who had undergone day surgery. Gow and Atwell (1980) reported that the hospital was providing 10 children's day lists per week (seven general surgical, one dental, one orthopaedic and one medical); however, the service rapidly developed its scope of operation to incorporate follow-up of children requiring inpatient care for medical and surgical problems as well as referrals from GPs, health visitors and social workers (Gow 1976).

A PROGRAMME OF INTEGRATED HOSPITAL AND HOME NURSING CARE FOR CHILDREN IN EDINBURGH

Three distinct, but complementary, children's home nursing initiatives were introduced in Edinburgh between 1969 and 1972 (Hunter 1974, 1977). The first initiative, in 1969, involved the appointment of a paediatric nursing sister within the outpatient department who was responsible for the provision of an outreach service from the Royal Hospital for Sick Children, in order to support the parents of children with 'long-term disability', (including diabetes mellitus or coeliac disease) or congenital abnormality (including cleft lip) (Hunter 1974).

The second service development in Edinburgh involved the secondment to the hospital of a district nursing sister who was already trained as a sick children's nurse. The focus of the nurse's work was in caring for children who had been referred to the hospital either for inpatient care or for outpatient assessment of predominantly acute problems. Hunter (1974) observed that in the month before the nurse's appointment only four children had received care from the district nursing service, but during the first year of the attachment of the district nursing sister to the hospital 2400 visits were paid to children, increasing to 5700 visits in 1972 when a second sister was appointed. A major focus of the nurses' work was in supporting the management of medication regimens, including the administration of drugs by injection. In addition, the management of burn and scald injuries was a significant area of work.

The third element of the Edinburgh scheme initially involved a research project, but rapidly led to the appointment of a nurse working flexibly between the hospital ward, outpatient department and the community, and focused on the care of children with cystic fibrosis.

By 1974, each of these services had developed considerably, and were also supplemented by two further appointments of district nursing sisters covering the north side of Edinburgh and the county of East Lothian (Hunter 1974). I make no apology for quoting the words of the late Muriel Campbell, who was the mainstay of the Edinburgh Children's Home Care Service from its inception and throughout the 1970s and 1980s. In 1986 she wrote: 'We are all very committed to our home care nursing programme and I for one know that in home care I have the best job in the NHS' (Campbell 1986 p 307).

A SCHEME TO PROVIDE HOME NURSING CARE FOR SICK CHILDREN IN THEIR OWN HOMES IN GATESHEAD

A paediatric home nursing scheme was established in Gateshead in 1974, following the appointment of two district nurses who were 'retrained' in the hospital care of children (Hally et al 1977, Jackson 1978), although the nurses working with the scheme retained, as the major focus of their work, an 'adult' patient caseload. It is not altogether clear from these published accounts whether or not the nurses were actually registered as sick children's nurses, although the authors suggest that, in the absence of such qualifications or 'equivalent experience', 'a longer and more formal period of retraining is desirable' (Hally et al 1977 p 764). The Gateshead scheme was very much focused upon children at the interface between hospital and community care, with close involvement of GPs and hospital-based paediatricians. Referrals to the scheme were only accepted on the basis that the children would otherwise have been admitted to hospital or would have required a longer stay in hospital, and consequently the children referred to the scheme were almost exclusively suffering from acute 'paediatric' problems. No further published reference to the scheme beyond 1978 has been found.

A DIABETIC CLINIC FOR CHILDREN IN OXFORD

In 1973, a children's diabetes clinic was established at the John Radcliffe Hospital in Oxford, and the following year a community nursing sister, qualified as both a health visitor and a registered sick children's nurse, was appointed to the team, from the community nursing budget, in order to facilitate the care of children with newly diagnosed diabetes mellitus and to provide ongoing care for children with established diabetes. The nurse was based within the hospital and provided an outreach service exclusively to children with diabetes (Smith et al 1984). This service represented a new development within community children's nursing, that of community outreach nursing within a clearly delineated area of disease specific practice.

BRENT'S INTEGRATED PAEDIATRIC NURSING SERVICE

In 1974, the NHS underwent its most radical reorganisation since its inception. One clear objective of the reorganisation was that, within the newly configured district health authorities, services that had been traditionally described as either 'hospital' or 'community' should be fully integrated. Smith (1977) provides a detailed account of how representatives of three nursing divisions within Brent District Health Authority ('hospital', 'midwifery' and 'community') had each argued that a proposed integrated paediatric unit should be located within their own division. After much deliberation, a decision was finally made to locate the unit within the community nursing division. It was further agreed that this unit would include inpatient and outpatient paediatric facilities, the special care baby unit, school nursing and health visiting.

In 1976, two 'home nurses' and two liaison health visitors were appointed within the newly integrated services (McLetchie 1977). By 1981, the service had expanded to include three sister-grade registered sick children's nurses, and in this year the role of the team was extended to provide a follow-up service for children attending the accident and emergency department (Glucksman et al 1986). In 1982–1983, 556 children who were referred following attendance in the accident and emergency department were visited by the community children's nursing team. The nurses made a total of 1271 visits (average of two visits per child: 351 children (63%) received only one follow-up visit, and the maximum number of visits per child was five). Approximately 40% of the children were referred for follow-up of a minor medical problem, 30% were for removal of sutures and the remaining 30% for soft tissue injuries including burns and scalds (Glucksman et al 1986).

'FIT FOR THE FUTURE'

In 1973, Sir Keith Joseph, Secretary of State for Social Services, brought together, under the chairmanship of Professor Donald Court, a Committee whose terms of reference were: 'To review the provision made for health services for children up to and through school life; to study the use made of these services by children and their parents and to make recommendations' (Department of Health and Social Security 1976 p 397).

The Committee produced its final report in 1976. Amongst its many recommendations, those that are of perhaps greatest interest include the proposal to develop a 'distinct group of nurses called child health visitors, who would combine preventive and curative nursing responsibility for children' (ch 7 recommendation 5), and the suggestion that the child health visitor 'should be assisted in her work in surgeries, health centres and home nursing by a child health nurse who would have paediatric training' (ch 7, recommendation 7). In making these recommendations, the Court Committee was clearly cognisant of earlier developments in the provision of nursing services to sick children in the community. They observed 'nursing support for sick children in the community is currently an underdeveloped area and in terms of its commitment to practical aid and education for parents of sick children, what we are proposing is in many ways a new nursing service' (para 12.16 p 182).

As with many of the recommendations arising from the Court Committee, the responses to these particular proposals were very limited indeed. A policy review group established under the auspices of the National Children's Bureau to review progress in implementing 'Court', observed: 'There has been no lack of committees, reports and studies on these subjects. We have been most unimpressed by the action that has arisen as a result of these studies and deliberations' (National Children's Bureau 1987 p 10).

THE 1980s

Despite the strong endorsements and recommendation of the Court Report, no new community children's nursing services were established for several years. A study of community children's nursing services undertaken by Starbuck in 1981 noted the 'recent establishment' of a home care service for children in Rochdale involving a district nurse and health visitor, but there are no published records of this service, and two subsequent studies received a negative response from the health services in Rochdale when seeking to confirm details of the service (Catchpole 1986, Whiting 1988).

In 1986, Catchpole undertook a survey of community children's nursing service provision in England and suggested that there had been a significant expansion in service provision during the early 1980s. The survey identified 10 new services established between 1983 and 1986 (Table 2.3). Catchpole suggested that one significant feature of the new services was that five out of ten of them were based in hospitals, although most of the long-established services were community based. She also observed that a number of the services that were configured within the community nursing services actually had a base in the hospital paediatric department: 'They all have one common aspect however, which differentiates the service from that of the adult district nursing service and that is they offer an extension of hospital work into the patient's home' (Catchpole 1986 p 23).

In 1988, a national census of community children's nursing provision (Whiting 1988) suggested that the growth in service development described by Catchpole had been sustained. Whiting (1988) identified a total of 24 services

TABLE 2.3 ***Paediatric community nursing services established from 1983 to 1986***

Location	Year established
Swindon	1983
Sutton	1984
Surrey	1984
Nottingham	1984
Manchester (North)	1984
Hartlepool	1984
Blackburn	1985
Northampton	1985
Stockport	1985
Portsmouth	To commence 1986

Source: Catchpole (1986).

BOX 2.1 ***Community children's nursing teams in England in 1988 (Whiting 1988)***

Aylesbury	Basingstoke	Brent
Brighton	Carshalton	Central Birmingham
Doncaster	Ealing	Enfield
Isle of Wight	Kettering	Milton Keynes
Northampton	North Birmingham	North Manchester
North Staffordshire	Nottingham	Oxford
Paddington	Salisbury	Scunthorpe
Southampton	South Birmingham	Stockport

in England in January 1988 (Box 2.1). In addition, 33 districts gave details of plans to establish community children's nursing services; four of these services were actually in the final planning stages and were 'up and running' by April 1988. The research confirmed that the services in Rotherham, Rochdale and Gateshead, referred to above, were no longer operating.

The following summary data are based on responses from the 23 teams that completed the questionnaire within the 1988 study.

Eighteen teams were based in hospital children's wards or departments; five teams were based in community settings. A total of 45 staff were employed as community children's nurses, 44 of whom were registered sick children's nurses (one nurse was an enrolled nurse). Referrals to the teams were predominantly from children's wards in both district general and specialist children's hospitals, but most teams received referrals from a range of hospital and community-based agencies (Table 2.4). All 23 teams provided care both to children with chronic diseases and to those with acute 'medical' problems. Eighteen teams provided care to children with physical handicap and learning disabilities. Nineteen teams followed up children who had undergone non day-case surgery and 11 teams provided day surgery follow-up. Eleven 'teams' comprised only one nurse, five teams had two nurses, and five teams were staffed by three nurses. The largest

TABLE 2.4 ***Major referral sources to 23 community children's nursing teams***

Referral source	No. of teams
General hospital children's ward	22 (96)
Health visitor	21 (91)
General practitioner	19 (83)
Special care baby unit (SCBU)	18 (78)
General hospital outpatients department	17 (74)
Children's hospital children's ward	13 (57)
School nurse	13 (57)
Social worker	11 (48)
General hospital casualty department	10 (43)
Children's hospital outpatients department	9 (39)
Children's hospital casualty	6 (26)

Values in parentheses are percentages. Source: Whiting (1988).

TABLE 2.5 ***Acute and chronic medical conditions forming a 'regular part' of community children's nursing teams, caseloads***

Condition	No. of teams (n = 23)
Respiratory conditions (e.g. asthma)	20 (87)
Children with stomas (e.g. tracheostomy, gastrostomy, ileostomy)	18 (78)
Cancer or leukaemia	17 (74)
Congenital orthopaedic problems	17 (74)
Eczema and other skin disorders	15 (65)
Enuresis or encopresis	15 (65)
Congenital cardiac problems	15 (65)
Acute medical problems (e.g. non-specific infections, gastroenteritis)	14 (61)
Diabetes mellitus	14 (61)
Renal problems (e.g. nephrotic syndrome)	10 (43)
Blood dyscrasias (e.g. haemophilia, thalassaemia, sickle cell disease)	9 (39)

Values in parentheses are percentages. Source: Whiting (1988).

team, in Southampton, was made up of seven nurses, one of whom was a specialist in paediatric diabetes and one was based in a 'special school'. Larger teams were significantly more likely to be involved in the care of children who required post-surgery follow-up. The 11 teams that featured a single nurse provided daytime-only care, usually Monday to Friday, with district nursing colleagues often providing cover at other times. Larger teams were able to provide more extensive cover, although only a small number of teams, with three or more staff, were able to provide a visiting service at weekends. Two services reported that they provided '24-hour care'.

Table 2.5 provides an illustration of the frequency with which each of the 23 community children's nursing services reported their involvement in the care of

TABLE 2.6 ***Activities forming a part of the community children's nursing team's caseload***

Activity	No. of teams (*n* = 23)
Teaching aspects of practical care to parents and children (e.g. giving injections, nasogastric feeding)	23 (100)
Support to families of children dying at home	22 (96)
Teaching of other professional colleagues	22 (96)
Education of children and parents with specific medical problems (e.g. diabetes, asthma)	22 (96)
Postoperative wound care	19 (83)
General health education	19 (83)
Administration or supervision of medication (not intravenous)	19 (83)
Dressings or wound care following trauma (e.g. scalds, lacerations)	18 (78)
Administration of intravenous drugs	12 (52)

Values in parentheses are percentages. Source: Whiting (1988).

children with a range of medical conditions, and Table 2.6 demonstrates the range of nursing activities with which the nurses were involved. Whilst it is evident that, in 1988, there was tremendous diversity in the practice of the community children's nursing services, there was also a core of clinical activity which clearly delineated the care of children in the community from other areas of nursing practice. The formal recognition of this emerging area of practice by the establishment, in 1988, of a Paediatric Community Nurses Forum within the Royal College of Nursing illustrates how far things had progressed from the situation in 1983 when there were only seven services in the whole of England.

CONCLUSION

Community children's nursing has come a long way in the past 100 years. Many models of community children's nursing have developed and many titles have been used to describe those practitioners – registered children's nurses, working in community settings and providing care for children who require the particular skills and knowledge of those nurses if they are to achieve optimal health. There is, however, a central core to that practice, the work of the community children's nurse, which defines and delineates that practice and makes it unique. Although there is much that is still to be achieved, and the concerns expressed by the Health Committee (1997) make it clear that this is the case, we should be rightly proud that we have come a long way on our journey to provide a nationwide community children's nursing service (Whiting 1985).

REFERENCES

Atwell J, Burn J M B, Dewar A K & Freeman N V 1973 Paediatric day case surgery. Lancet ii:895–897

Audit Commission 1993 Children first: a study of hospital services. Audit Commission, London

Baly M E, Robottom B & Clark J M 1987 District nursing, 2nd edn. Heinemann, London

Bergman A B, Shrand H & Oppe T E 1965 A pediatric home care program in London – ten years' experience. Pediatrics 36:314–321

Campbell M 1986 Community nurse – a typical day ... British Journal for Nurses in Child Health 1(10):307

Catchpole A 1986 Community paediatric nursing services in England: 1985. Unpublished results, Oxford Polytechnic

Clark J 1981 What do health visitors do? A review of the research 1960–1980. Royal College of Nursing, London

Department of Health 1997 The new NHS. Modern, dependable. The Stationery Office, London

Department of Health and Social Security 1976 Fit for the future. The report of the Committee on Child Health Services, vol 1. HMSO, London.

Dunnell K & Dobbs J (1982) Nurses working in the community. HMSO, London

Franklin A W 1964 Children's hospitals. in: Poynter F N L (ed) The evolution of hospitals in Britain, p 103. Pitman, London.

Gillet J A 1954 Children's nursing unit. British Medical Journal 684:1954

Glucksman E, Tachakra S S, Piggott S & Lea H 1986 Home care team in accident and emergency. Archives of Diseases in Childhood 61:294–296

Gow M A 1976 Domiciliary paediatric care in Southampton. Queen's Nursing Journal October: 192, 205

Gow M A & Atwell J 1980 The role of the children's nurse in the community. Journal of Pediatric Surgery 15(1):26–30

Hally M A, Holohan A, Jackson R H, Reedy B L E C & Walker J H 1977 Paediatric home nursing scheme in Gateshead. British Medical Journal 1(6063):762–764

Health Committee 1997 House of Commons Select Committee. Health services for children and young people in the community: home and school, 3rd report. The Stationery Office, London

Hospital for Sick Children 1874 Medical Committee minutes, vol 6: Special meeting of the joint committee – March 18. Archives of the Great Ormond Street Hospital NHS Trust, London

Hospital for Sick Children 1936 General rules for the private nursing staff. Archives of the Great Ormond Street Hospital NHS Trust, London

Howell M 1974 Domiciliary care of sick children in Birmingham – its history and development. Presented to the Annual Conference of the National Association for the Welfare of Children in Hospital. NAWCH, London

Hunt J & Whiting M 1999 A re-examination of the history of children's community nursing. Paediatric Nursing 11(4):33–36

Hunter M H S 1974 A programme of integrated hospital and home nursing care for children. Presented to the Annual Conference of the National Association for the Welfare of Children in Hospital. NAWCH, London

Hunter M H S 1977 Paediatric hospital at home care: 1. Integrated programmes. Nursing Times Occasional Papers 10 March: 33–36

Jackson R H 1978 Home care for children. Journal of Maternal and Child Health (March):96,98,100

Jenkins S M 1975 Home care scheme in Paddington. Nursing Mirror 27 February:68–70

Kosky J & Lunnon R J 1991 Great Ormond Street and the story of medicine. Granta Editions London

Lightwood R 1956 The home care of sick children. The Practitioner 177:10–14

Lightwood R, Brimblecombe F S W, Reinhold J D L, Burnard E D & Davis J A 1957 A London trial of home care for sick children. Lancet 9 February: 313–317

Lomax E M R 1996 Small and special: the development of hospitals for children in Victorian Britain. Wellcome Institute for the History of Medicine, London

McClure C R 1960 The St Mary's Hospital home-care for sick children scheme. Public Health 74(8):313–316

McLetchie C 1977 Specialist in home care: paediatric home nurse. Internal report. Brent Health District, London

Ministry of Health 1959 The welfare of children in hospital – report of the committee (chairman, Sir H Platt) HMSO, London

Morris I 1966 Nursing children at home. Nursing Times 16 December:1653–1656

National Children's Bureau 1987 Investing in the future: child health ten years after the Court Report – a report of the Policy and Practice Review Group. National Children's Bureau, London

National Health Service Executive 1996 Child health in the community. A guide to good practice. The Stationery Office, London

Oppe T 1971 Home care for sick children. British Journal of Hospital Medicine 5(1):39–40, 43–44

Owen G M 1982 Health visiting. Cited in: Allen P & Jolley M (eds) Nursing, midwifery and health visiting since 1900. Faber and Faber, London, p 92

Rathbone W 1890 Sketch of the history and progress of district nursing from 1859 to the present date. Macmillan, London

Robottom B 1969 The contribution of the children's nurse to the home care of children. British Journal of Medical Education 3(4):311–312

Smellie J M 1956 Domiciliary nursing service for infants and children. British Medical Journal i:256

Smith J 1977 Brent's integrated paediatric nursing unit. Nursing Mirror 4 August:22–24

Smith M A, Strang S & Baum D 1984 Organisation of a diabetic clinic for children. Practical Diabetes 1(1):8–12

Starbuck C 1981 Nursing care of children in the community. BSc nursing dissertation, University of Manchester

Stocks M 1960 A hundred years of district nursing. Allen and Unwin, London

While A E 1985 Health visiting and health experience of infants in three areas. PhD thesis, University of London

Whiting M 1985 Building a nationwide community paediatric nursing service. Nursing Standard 419:5

Whiting M 1988 Community paediatric nursing in England in 1988. MSc thesis, University of London

Whiting M 1994 40 years on and still a viable product. At Home: The Newsletter for Homecare Therapy Initiatives Caremark, Leyburn, Yorkshire

Wood C J 1888 The training of nurses for sick children. Nursing Record 6 December: 507–510

3 A 'new' National Health Service

Aidan Macfarlane

KEY ISSUES

- Changing priorities within the 'new' NHS
- Major factors influencing service provision for children and young people
- Opportunities for 'getting involved' in changing commissioning priorities

INTRODUCTION

The organisation of the National Health Service (NHS) is undergoing increasingly rapid change and it is unlikely that, in the future, it will ever again be a truly 'static' organisational system.

The art in understanding the structure of the NHS is therefore not to worry about either the detail or the actual names of anyone within the structure, but to try instead to understand the broad concepts as to what the various 'parts' are meant to do and where the power lies. The reason why you need to have an idea as to how the overall structure of the NHS works at a *clinical* level is to understand where to go should you wish to create change in order to improve the delivery of your clinical service.

Resources within the overall NHS are, in terms of money, staff, equipment, etc., absolutely finite and limited, and decisions about what is more or less important in terms of where these limited funds should go is done by setting priorities at all levels. That is, priority setting is done by you as a clinician, by primary care groups, by health authorities, by the NHS Executive, by the Department of Health (DoH) and by the Government.

As a clinical deliverer of clinical services, you must know how to influence these priorities as they will have a profound effect on the services that you personally are delivering both in terms of resources (staff, equipment, environment, etc.) and on the actual type of clinical service, i.e. what effective preventive or treatment interventions you are using on a day-to-day basis (although these latter are also influenced by professional bodies such as the Royal College of Nursing, Royal College of Paediatrics and Child Health, etc.).

MAJOR FACTORS INFLUENCING SERVICE PROVISION FOR CHILDREN AND YOUNG PEOPLE

The four themes central to the new National Health Service

These are given in Box 3.1; although these statements (DoH 1997) may seem like 'political' speak they are broadly important (but do not have to be understood in detail).

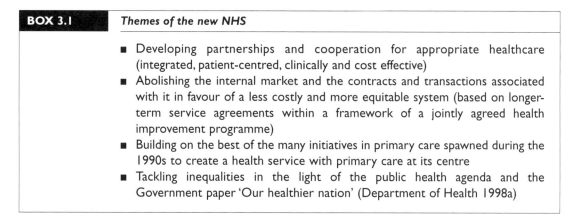

BOX 3.1 *Themes of the new NHS*

- Developing partnerships and cooperation for appropriate healthcare (integrated, patient-centred, clinically and cost effective)
- Abolishing the internal market and the contracts and transactions associated with it in favour of a less costly and more equitable system (based on longer-term service agreements within a framework of a jointly agreed health improvement programme)
- Building on the best of the many initiatives in primary care spawned during the 1990s to create a health service with primary care at its centre
- Tackling inequalities in the light of the public health agenda and the Government paper 'Our healthier nation' (Department of Health 1998a)

Changes in the health of children and young people and society's needs

These include:

- A greater emphasis on as near as possible 100% of children achieving maximum self-esteem and potential by providing them with (1) parents with excellent parenting skills, (2) a good education, (3) the prospect of full employment, and (4) the ability to meet the flexible demands of a rapidly changing society
- A 'health' system which provides the 80% of children who will need virtually no medical 'illness' services with excellent primary and preventive care
- Ensuring that the 15% of children who will need to be treated for illnesses that are straightforward are treated using effective and evidence-based interventions (e.g. children with asthma)
- Ensuring that the 3% of children who have illnesses that are complex and difficult to treat (e.g. cystic fibrosis, cerebral palsy, complex congenital heart disease) have this treatment using appropriate technology combined with the highest standards of humane care
- Opening up debate on the 2% of children with very complex illnesses or disability over the ethical questions as to whether they should be allowed to suffer the consequences of doctor interventions (e.g. complex genetic disorders, severe cerebral palsy)
- Dealing with the much greater parental expectations, especially from those who have greater direct access to medical information using the World Wide Web, but accepting that there will also be a greater gap between the 'haves and have nots' of this information
- The need to ensure a far greater parental (and child, where suitable) input in discussions on management of sick and disabled children

Actual structure of the new National Health Service

Starting at the top of the NHS, and probably of least direct importance to most clinicians in their day-to-day work, is the DoH and the NHS Executive. At the very top is the Secretary of State for Health (Figure 3.1) and four ministers who are responsible for certain related subjects, such as public health, women's health, resources and waiting lists. As can be seen from Figure 3.2 children's services are one part of the NHS Executive. The NHS Executive is responsible for a number of different departments (directorates) as shown in Figure 3.2, only one of which is 'Health Services'. The Health Services Directorate is again broken down into a number of different departments, only one of which is 'Health Services for Young People and Women'. Young people in this case includes children.

The NHS Executive also works out of eight regional offices, which have recently been reorganised, and relate to 100 health authorities in England, 430 NHS Trusts and an unknown number of primary care groups (PCGs) (in England). It is worth noting that in Wales where there are five health authorities, in Scotland where there are 15 health boards and in Northern Ireland where there are four health and social service authorities, there are slightly different health service structures.

Of much more importance to clinicians is the structure of PCGs and how they relate to district health authorities at a local level. Again, there will be variations in the structures and concepts laid out below for Wales, Scotland and Northern Ireland.

Primary care and primary care groups

These are at the heart of the changes in the new NHS and the document 'The New NHS. Modern, dependable' (Department of Health 1997) outlines four possible levels of responsibility for PCGs:

- At minimum they will support the health authority in commissioning care for its population, acting in an advisory capacity
- At a more sophisticated level they will take devolved responsibility for formally managing the budget for healthcare in their area, as part of the health authority
- They may then become established as free-standing bodies accountable to the health authority for commissioning care

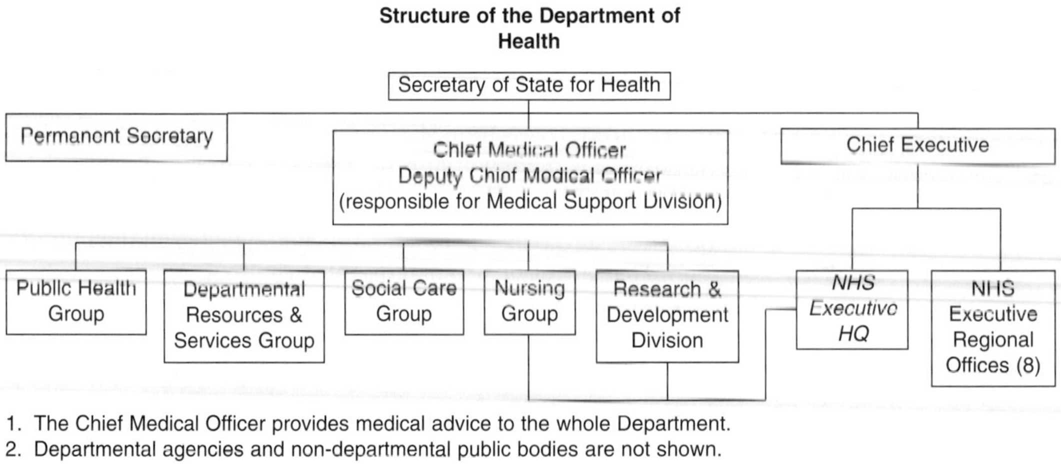

Figure 3.1 Structure of the Department of Health

Chief Executive
Staff: 8
Costs: £0.05m
Programme: n/a

Chief Medical Officer	**Human Resources**	**Nursing**	**Health Services**	**Research & Development**	**Planning**	**Finance & Performance**
	staff 162 *Costs £5.55m* Programme £1406m	*Staff 17* *Costs £0.92m* Programme £0.03m	*Staff 208* *Costs £7.29m* Programme £149m	*Staff 32* *Costs £1.31m* Programme £426m	*Staff 328* *Costs £23.34m* Programme £1225m	*Staff 173* *Costs £5.59m* Programme £3663m
Function Medical Education Unit (Staff costs included in Human Resources)	**Function** NHS Development Unit Pay and Conditions Employment Issues Equal Opportunities Workforce Planning and Education Medical Workforce Planning	**Function** Nursing & Quality	**Function** Health Services (Emergency, General, Women, *Children,* Mental Health, People with Learning Disabilities, Continuing Care) NHS Public Health Development Unit	**Function** NHS Research & Development	**Function** Planning (Strategy, Business Planning, Capital Strategy, Foresight, Secretariat) Analytical Services (EOR & Statistics) Communications Primary Care IM&T (Dental and Optical Services, Pharmacy and Prescribing) Corporate Affairs (Organisational Development, Non-Executive Appointments and Openness, Consumer and Patient Issues, Non-Clinical Support Services)	**Function** Securing & allocating resources Monitoring & analysis of NHS performance Accounting to Parliament & the public Developing the finance function in the NHS

Figure 3.2 NHS Executive structure

- Finally, they could become established as free-standing bodies accountable to the health authority for commissioning care and with added responsibility for the provision of community health services for their population, including the running of community hospitals (i.e. a Primary Care Trust)

Specific points as regards PCGs are outlined in Box 3.2.

BOX 3.2 ***Known specifics about primary care groups***

- They are statutory organisations which at all levels are accountable to health authorities.
- They are geographically 'locality' based, each covering a population of approximately 100 000.
- They include nurse and social services representation as well as general practitioners.
- All GP practices are part of a PCG.
- There should be clear arrangements for public involvement including open meetings.

New key principles to commissioning in the new NHS

- **Promoting partnership** – between health authorities, NHS Trusts and general practitioners via PCGs using an 'open and transparent approach' to sharing financial position and prospects
- **Developing service and financial frameworks** – in consultation with general practitioners, other key professionals and local interests. Health authorities are to collate all commissioning intentions through the production of a framework document for their area
- **Involving the public** – by including local people, including service users and carers, using wide informal consultation on developing services and the financial framework
- **Developing service agreements** – having developed frameworks, attention will be paid to detail of service agreements and include:
  - — what services are provided in terms of scope and activity
  - — setting quality standards
  - — defining the funding
  - — monitoring arrangements
- **Developing longer-term agreements** – building on the partnership approach

Partnerships and teams in commissioning

The discussion document 'Partnership in action' (Department of Health 1998b) proposes legislation to improve strategic planning between health services and social services, to improve joint commissioning and service provision. The DoH proposes to do this by having pooled budgets between health and social services deployed under a lead commissioner for certain areas of common health and social services integrated provision. This will influence enormously the use of resources for supporting many children and their families and will have far-reaching implications.

However, in the area of overall health commissioning and priority setting, there are still a great many complex and unanswered questions which include:

- Who defines needs (e.g. Public Health, management of the local health authority, Trusts, PCGs, government, the public)?
- Who defines appropriate and effective interventions (e.g. Public Health, clinicians, Department of Health)?
- Who defines priorities (e.g. Government, Public Health, executive of the local health authority, clinicians, the public)?
- Who ensures change takes place (e.g. management of the local health authority, management of Trusts, PCGs)?
- Who monitors changes and quality (e.g. management of the local health authority, management of Trusts, Public Health, PCGs)?

Health improvement programmes

Health improvement programmes are a new strategic approach to developing the health of a population at health authority level and are taking over from the contracting process. They cover all age groups and are being drawn up by health authorities (usually under the auspices of Directors of Public Health). They are central to the commissioning process and, from 1999, contracts will have been replaced by service agreements expressed through health improvement programmes. They are a planning process that has to be agreed across all involved parties – health authorities, Trusts, PCGs and local authorities – but health authorities have responsibility for coordinating the commissioning process to action health improvement programmes.

National service frameworks

National Service Frameworks, by which the DoH identifies certain priority areas of work, are responsible for setting national standards and defining service models using evidence-based knowledge. They will define services for a service or care group and will be responsible for putting into place strategies to support their implementation. They should also:

- Establish support performance measures against which progress within an agreed timescale can be measured
- Be supported by the Commission for Health Improvement, which will assure progress through a programme of systematic service reviews
- Take forward the existing frameworks for cancer and paediatric intensive care
- Begin to develop frameworks for mental health (mainly services for adults of working age but will link with children's services in terms of successful mental health promotion strategies) and coronary heart disease (NHS with partner agencies)
- Be developed by an expert reference group of health professionals, service users and carers, health service managers, partner agencies and other advocates

In the future, National Service Frameworks will be chosen by the DoH on a number of grounds, which include:

- Demonstrable relevance to the Government's 'Our healthier nation' agenda
- Important health issues in terms of mortality, morbidity, disability or resource use
- An area of public concern
- Evidence of a shortfall between actual and acceptable practice with real opportunities for improvement (this could provide an opportunity for the development of community children's nursing services)

Although children (particularly the needs of disabled children) and families are also being put forward by many organisations as a National Service Framework for the future, the DoH has not chosen it as a priority area for the immediate future as a number of other areas, including the mental health of adults, are considered to be of higher priority.

High-level performance indicators

There is also an initiative from the NHS Executive to develop a number of 'performance indicators' which are (1) based on information currently available at health authority level, (2) of acceptable quality and (3) available nationally in a reasonably up-to-date form. They are not intended to be comprehensive in covering all aspects of NHS activities but are being chosen to throw light on particularly important health service objectives and activities. The proposed performance indicators under various headings and as they relate to children services are shown in Table 3.1.

TABLE 3.1 ***Performance indicators***

	Indicator	Area
Fair access	Conceptions below the age of 16 years (rate in girls aged 13–15 years)	Access to family planning services
Effective delivery of appropriate healthcare	Percentage of target population vaccinated and percentage of orchidopexies below age 5 years	Health promotion/disease prevention
	Surgical intervention rates for glue ear	Appropriateness of surgery
	Severe ear, nose or throat infection, and kidney and urinary tract infection	Primary care management
	Chronic care management of asthma, diabetes, epilepsy	Primary care management
Efficiency	Day-case rate and length of stay in hospital (case-mix adjusted)	Maximising resource use
	Hospital and community health service unit cost (aggregate measure of cost per patient treatment)	
Patient care experience of the NHS	Patients having to wait more than 2 hrs for emergency admission, and patients with operations cancelled for non-medical reasons	Accessibility
	Outpatients seen within 13 weeks of general practitioner referral and inpatient admission within 3 months of a decision to admit	Waiting times
Health outcomes of NHS care	Decayed, missing and filled teeth in 5-year-olds	NHS success in reducing levels of disease, impairment and complication of treatment
	Avoidable diseases including notification rates of pertussis in children, notification rates for measles, notification rates for tuberculosis	NHS success in reducing the level of disease, impairment and complications of treatment
	Emergency psychiatric readmission rate	NHS success in reducing the level of disease, impairment and complications of treatment

TABLE 3.1 *Continued*

Indicator	Area
Infant deaths – composite indicator consisting of stillbirth rates and infant mortality rates	NHS success in reducing premature deaths
Avoidable deaths – mortality rate from fractured skull and intracranial injury, mortality from asthma, mortality from appendicitis	NHS success in reducing premature deaths
In-hospital premature deaths – 30-day perioperative mortality rate	NHS success in reducing premature deaths

HOW TO BE EFFECTIVE IN CHANGING COMMISSIONING PRIORITIES

General factors

First, one has to accept that most of what has been commissioned in the past will continue to be commissioned in the same way in the future. This is because the overall number of individual activities being commissioned in the field of paediatrics and child health run into hundreds, if not thousands, and the time involved in reviewing the evidence that even one or two of these activities should be increased, decreased, ceased or changed is enormous.

Second, there is the realisation that some decisions about service delivery need to be made nationally. Thus decisions about screening programmes (e.g. for hearing defects in children) should be made nationally because of (a) quality issues, (b) funding issues, (c) equity of access issues, and (d) the science is so complicated. The way to influence these national decisions is to try to get elected on to the relative committee, for example the National Screening Committee.

Third, as already mentioned, priority setting takes place at many different levels of the NHS, and it is likely that, as a clinician, the local priority-setting group or forum (if there is a local one at health authority level) will be the best option if you feel strongly about priority issues. Knowledge about the priority-setting organisations are best found out about via the local director of public health.

Specific ways to influence

Primary care groups need to be informed and influenced by clinicians working in the field so that they:

- Understand and support parents in their role as the primary healthcarers of children
- Support primary prevention initiatives relative to childhood illnesses (e.g. immunisations, 'back to sleep' campaigns)
- Understand and act on the social context of child health in cooperation with local council services

- Use contemporary information relative to effective interventions in the field of child health
- Understand the prevalence of childhood disability, and the community management needed to care for these children
- Have a basic understanding of the 'rights of the child' and child protection issues

Health improvement programmes must include features relative to the health of children and young people. This can be achieved by clinicians:

- Working with the local director of public health to ensure that the needs of children and young people are addressed in the health improvement programme and elsewhere in the health authority's strategic plans
- Working with their local PCGs to ensure that the needs of children and young people are addressed in the health improvement programme and in more local strategic plans

Nationally, by:

- Writing about concerns and priorities to the relative Royal Colleges with copies to other relevant organisations*
- Writing to local members of parliament with copies to other relevant organisations*
- Working with relevant voluntary organisations such as Save the Children Fund to get media coverage*

CONCLUSION

Although the NHS is a huge and complex organisation, its final 'activities' are provided by clinicians at field level, such as community children's nurses, who are preventing ill health and treating illness in the population so as to create a final 'product', which is a healthier nation. In developing health services and setting priorities it is therefore essential that (1) the voice of the whole of society (which pays for the activity and product via taxes) is heard and (2) the voice of the 'worker' who carries out the activity that produces the product is also heard.

To this second end, community children's nurses need to understand where they can be most effective in influencing the priorities given to services for children and young people and the relative health outcomes resulting from these services.

* Under the last Government, Trusts began to put 'gagging clauses' into many NHS workers' contracts. You should check your legal position before 'going public'.

REFERENCES

Department of Health 1997 The new NHS. Modern, dependable. The Stationery Office, London:

Department of Health 1998a Our healthier nation. The Stationery Office, London

Department of Health 1998b Partnership in action. A discussion document. The Stationery Office, London:

4 Role of the community children's nurse in influencing healthcare policies

Sue Burr

KEY ISSUES

To maximise the potential to influence healthcare policies community children's nurses need to:

- Ensure that the needs of children and their families are always the focus of their activities
- Acknowledge an individual responsibility to participate in the formulation and implementation of healthcare policy at local, national and international level
- Identify opportunities and be knowledgeable about the processes available
- Develop a broad vision of children's health and the societal and governmental factors that impinge on health and healthcare provision
- Actively seek to work with others across professional and organisational boundaries
- Have confidence in their knowledge and skills, be informed, actively disseminate good practice, reveal inequalities, be assertive and persistent

INTRODUCTION

Healthcare policy should incorporate the specific needs of different groups within the population, ensuring that the most vulnerable groups receive particular consideration. Children are one of the most vulnerable groups, but in a National Health Service (NHS) focused on the physical health needs of adults the specific needs of children, particularly those with continuing complex health needs, are frequently ignored.

Community children's nurses (CCNs) must ensure that the needs of the children are central to all their activities and take an active role in reminding others of that fact. Management and organisational structures and processes should support the meeting of needs – not the other way round.

Healthcare policy is formulated by the Government of the day at both national and local level. In this complex society a myriad of factors influences the Government's policy making, but first and foremost all nurses need to acknowledge that they have a professional responsibility to influence healthcare policy.

WHY NURSES SHOULD INFLUENCE NATIONAL HEALTHCARE POLICY

Nurses are the healthcare professionals who have both the most intimate and continuous contact with people, whether in the promotion of health, during sickness, rehabilitation or bereavement. They are the largest group of healthcare professionals nationally and internationally. Logically, nurses' influence on healthcare policy should be crucial to its development, but too often nurses neither seek nor have influence.

Nursing organisations have recognised the importance of the nurse's role in policy making. The International Council of Nurses (ICN) (1985) issued a policy statement which included the following:

> 'ICN strongly believes that international organisations and national governments should recognise the expertise of professional nurses and utilise it in policy making and the planning of health services. ICN also believes that active participation of professional nurses in policy making at all levels of health is essential'.

In the mid 1980s Dame Sheila Quinn and Trevor Clay, both vice presidents of the ICN and respectively president and general secretary of the Royal College of Nursing (RCN), continually urged nurses to 'get political' and to utilise their power within the political system. However, political leadership in nursing within the UK and its theory and practice have received little attention and thus remain poorly developed.

In the UK all nurses are required by the United Kingdom Central Council (UKCC) Code of Professional Conduct (UKCC 1992) to protect the public and to provide a good quality of care to patients. To do so, nurses must be involved in both the shaping and implementation of policy. The Code also requires nurses to be advocates for their patients. This is particularly pertinent for nurses caring for the most vulnerable groups in society, of which children are one.

The RCN's Charter (RCN 1916) includes 'promoting the advancement of the science and art of nursing for the benefit of patients'. To do that RCN members have to influence national and local healthcare policy.

Whilst nursing organisations have clearly stated the importance of nurses being involved in shaping healthcare policy, individual nurses have been slow to respond. This gives cause for concern because the reluctance of nurses has resulted in others taking the initiative and nursing issues being marginalised. Interestingly, nurses are increasingly recognising their role in empowering patients/clients but remain reluctant to use the same processes to empower nursing.

NURSES' RELUCTANCE TO PARTICIPATE IN POLICY MAKING

Many factors influence healthcare policy. These include the values of society, its culture, the socioeconomic situation, the political ideology, and the power of professional and consumer groups. The Government's actions will be further influenced by practical considerations such as the size of its majority and the date of the next general election. Several of these factors particularly affect the nursing profession, for example the traditional role of women in a profession where the majority of members are female. The hierarchical culture of nursing has perpetuated the myth that healthcare policy is the responsibility of senior managers, with little acknowledgement by nurses in clinical practice of their responsibility. Traditionally nurses were trained to respond unquestioningly to orders. In addition, nursing was often viewed as being 'above' party politics, which were not considered appropriate for nurses to be involved in. Nurses appear to have some confusion about political acumen, crucial to exerting influence on policy formulation and personal affiliation to a political party.

The power of the male-dominated medical profession and, until recently, nurses' limited educational opportunities have contributed to their reluctance to influence policy, although by the sheer size of numbers, nurses should be able to exert considerable power. Clay (1987) recognised that they have been slow to acknowledge that power, too often expending energy disagreeing amongst themselves.

The radical changes in nursing education should assist all nurses to recognise their responsibility to influence policy and to identify and utilise the opportunities available. The RCN Association of Nursing Students' resolution to RCN Congress in 1997 'that this meeting of RCN Congress supports the introduction of political education as an integral part of pre-registration courses' was passed with a good majority and marks a watershed.

It is important to convince all nurses of their responsibility to influence policy whatever the post held or healthcare setting in which they practise. Nurses at the client/patient interface have as much to contribute as senior managers who, too often, are remote from clinical practice.

CHILDREN, CHILDREN'S NURSES AND HEALTHCARE POLICY

Children's lack of political power, alongside the traditional view that caring for children is suitable employment for women not able to undertake more responsible work, is reflected in the low status and value attributed to children's nursing.

The Health Committee (1997) states:

> 'It would be fair to conclude that until recent years, insufficient attention was paid to the need to train nurses to deal with the specific health needs of children.'

and

> 'Likewise, insufficient effort appears to have been made to capitalise on the skills of qualified children's nurses.'

The Department of Health's response (1997) states:

> 'We acknowledge that past shortages of qualified children's nurses have limited the opportunities for the health service to benefit from their skills. As the number of children's nurses increases their skills can be

> utilised in many more areas of healthcare for children and young people.'

It is important to remember that studies for the Briggs Report (Briggs 1972) on applicants for the child branch of Project 2000 and for community children's nursing educational programmes reveals no shortage of applicants. The restricted opportunities, funding and failure to acknowledge the value of nurses educated to meet the specific needs of children have been very slow to be recognised by those who hold power within the nursing profession. This requires children's nurses to be particularly active in policy formulation and implementation to ensure that the specific needs of children are considered appropriately.

Emotion and rhetoric are commonly applied to issues concerning children, with the media keen to utilise a 'good' child story. Politicians are commonly seen kissing babies at election rallies but it is rare for any political manifesto to refer to children. If the values of society focus on power, possessions and success of the individual, then the least politically powerful and most vulnerable will suffer.

Whilst rhetoric is common, the reality is different. Children and young people comprise almost a quarter of the population yet, as the Chair of the Select Committee on Health noted in introducing the debate on the Committee's Report on 25 March 1998 (House of Commons 1998) following its Inquiry into Services for Children and Young People: 'it is rare for the House of Commons to debate any issue concerning children.' The presence of about 10 members of parliament (MPs) for the debate was a marked contrast to 'standing room only' for a debate on fox hunting a few weeks earlier, and the full House debating through the night of 24 March on whether public schools could retain the right to beat pupils.

Over a decade ago, the Government recognised that women and women's issues needed an advocate within government if equality with men's issues was to be achieved. Children who have no vote are in an even less fortunate position. Children's issues, even those relating to health, are scattered throughout many ministries, often at the bottom end of each department's agenda. Whilst governments proclaim the importance of children's health for the nation's future, it is traditionally the most junior minister of health who is given responsibility for children.

To address the difficulties of fragmentation and lack of advocates, the Health Committee (1997) recommended the setting up of a subcommittee of cabinet for children, similar to that for women. Unfortunately the governmental response (Department of Health 1997) was:

> 'We have no plans to set up a Cabinet Sub-Committee on Children and Young People.'

In 1999 the Government has a subcommittee of cabinet and a designated minister for women in both Houses of Parliament, but no similar mechanisms for promoting children's issues. This is in contrast to Scotland and Wales where, following the 1997 general election, a minister with specific responsibility for children was appointed.

It is an unfortunate fact that many long-recommended changes in services for children have been ignored until a tragedy occurs. It is often claimed that Mrs Thatcher's major reform of the health service was precipitated by parents attempting to sue her because their child's operation was repeatedly cancelled owing to the shortage of paediatric intensive care beds and nurses to staff them. However, little action specific to paediatric intensive care took place until the well-publicised death of a child who had been transported around the north-west of England whilst a paediatric intensive care bed was sought (North West Regional Health Authority 1996).

It took the activities of Beverly Allitt in 1991 and the subsequent Report of the Inquiry (Clothier 1994) for the Government to issue any directive (Department of Health 1994) that its own guidance regarding the employment of registered children's nurses should be implemented. Unfortunately such directives are not mandatory and only some managers have responded. In 1999 the situation remains that many of the health professionals, including nurses, providing care for children have not undertaken any specific education programme in the needs of children.

SPECIFIC DIFFICULTIES FOR COMMUNITY CHILDREN'S NURSES

CCNs have met additional obstacles in their attempts to influence policy. The introductory chapters set the historical context of the specific difficulties that CCNs encounter. The Government's first interest in child health was precipitated by the shock at the major disabilities and general ill health of recruits to the Boer War. This led to the establishment of infant welfare clinics, school health services and school meals, and any political interest has remained focused on these services for children. Health visitors and school nurses have had strong advocates for their services within professional organisations, whereas CCNs have not.

Parents and paediatric healthcare staff have been keen to adapt the pattern of care to meet children's psychological and changing clinical needs and to develop community children's nursing services. Staff in community services for children, traditionally focused on maintaining health, have resisted these developments. Indeed, this was reflected in the research commissioned by the English National Board (Procter et al 1998). The study revealed that some community nurses and health visitors, whilst not having a full understanding of the role of CCNs or wishing to undertake 'hands on' care, did not welcome the establishment of community children's nursing services.

As the Health Committee (1997) in its third report, 'Health services for children and young people in the community: home and school' was able to conclude:

> 'Children's health services at present are too often based on traditional custom and practice or indeed on professional self-interest. Children's health services must be needs-led, not based on historical patterns or the self-interest of provider groups.'

CCNs have lacked a power base within professional organisations, particularly those concerned wholly with community services. Appropriate educational preparation, or the lack of it, has been a major difficulty and still affects commissioning.

In summary, CCNs have encountered difficulties in influencing healthcare policy for children because:

- Children are not politically powerful.
- Children's nurses in general, but specifically CCNs, have lacked a power base within the nursing profession.
- Nurses working in the community and health visitors, for reasons unrelated to improving services for sick children, have not welcomed the development of community children's nursing services.
- Despite repeated Government recommendations that community children's nursing services should be universally established, no strategy has been formulated, no specific model advocated, no research undertaken, no finances allocated, no governmental initiatives undertaken, and no directives regarding the implementation of guidance issued.
- Community children's nursing teams are often small in number with management of the service being the responsibility of those with no practical experience as a CCN.
- Specific education for CCNs has been available only recently and some commissioners of education have little insight into the need for such services.

It is therefore hardly surprising that some 40 years since the Government recommended the rapid expansion of community children's nursing services (Ministry of Health 1959) that almost 50% of the UK is still without a service. As the Health Committee (House of Commons 1997a) concluded: 'For many years there has been such a service for adults, sick children need and deserve no less.'

CHANGING TIMES

In 1963 President Kennedy reminded us that 'Change is the law of life. And those who look only to the past or present are certain to miss the future'. Change is often painful, and for CCNs it seems exceedingly slow. However, change is central to the present Government's activities.

The Labour Government, elected in May 1997, is introducing a mass of legislation affecting healthcare, and nurses have many opportunities to influence these changes – if only they recognise and utilise them. The Government's White Paper for England 'The new NHS. Modern, dependable' (NHS Executive 1998a), and similar documents in the other three countries of the UK, provides a clear impetus for nurses in clinical practice to influence new patterns of organising, providing and evaluating care. A central vision is the direct link between increasing the participation of NHS staff in decision making in relation to the implementation of policy. The change from hierarchy to shared governance is radical, and nurses will need assistance to become informed and active participants.

The term 'shared governance' is coming into more frequent usage and means different things to different people. Professional organisations have provided guidance for their members (Royal College of Nursing 1998). One interpretation is that it is a system of mutual management that attempts to move away from the traditional hierarchy. It aims to increase the formal participation of nurses in the decision-making process. The evaluation of shared governance within healthcare, particularly in the UK, is limited at present.

Whilst the Government is currently proclaiming increased power to localities, a tight central control is maintained. The power of the medical profession remains clear, but the tide is turning with the preliminary stages of nurse prescribing being implemented (Department of Health 1999).

The regulation of healthcare professions has never been debated so publicly. The public inquiry into the deaths of infants following cardiac surgery at Bristol Royal Infirmary will potentially mark a watershed for the accountability of healthcare professionals and general managers. The establishment of a National Institute of Clinical Excellence in England, the work of the Clinical Resource and Audit Group (CRAG) and development of clinical guidelines through the Scottish Intercollegiate Guidelines Network (SIGN) in Scotland, will enable national standards to be formulated and audited. Nurses, particularly CCNs, must be ready for these changes, and identify and embrace the opportunities that will arise.

HOW CAN COMMUNITY CHILDREN'S NURSES INFLUENCE HEALTHCARE POLICY?

Having acknowledged a professional responsibility to influence change, the opportunities to do so must be identified and utilised. Whilst different governments will introduce a range of changes, which will vary in the four countries within the UK, the mechanisms and opportunities for CCNs will continue to be available.

Developing a broad vision

Finding time to develop a vision can be very rewarding and represents a real basis for developing a strategy to take community children's nursing forward. But, first and foremost, CCNs should remember that vision, leadership and influencing skills are not the prerogative of those who hold senior positions. Every individual CCN has a responsibility to accept a role and to fulfil it.

Reflective practice is 'politically correct' terminology and obviously important to professional development, but developing a vision requires some lateral thinking from a range of perspectives. Many community children's nursing services have developed from a handful of very committed nurses who have worked extremely hard, in isolated circumstances, to develop services with little opportunity to reflect on wider health issues. This can result in a somewhat narrow understanding of children's changing health needs and the services needed to meet them. CCNs – indeed all nurses – must develop a broad vision if they are to provide holistic, good-quality and cost-effective standards for their patients/clients.

CCNs, whilst expressing concern at the fragmentation of care received by children and families, have not always been proactive in working with others. The Government has made it clear that multidisciplinary, multiagency working will become the norm. The NHS Executive discussion document, 'Partnership

BOX 4.1 ***Developing a vision***

- Have you ever made time to consider your vision for community children's nursing?
- What aspects of your role excite you?
- Where are the gaps in service? What frustrates you? How could the difficulties be resolved?
- Have you and your team members critically analysed the difficulties and formulated an action plan for resolving them?
- Is poor communication at the root of many of the frustrations?

in action (new opportunities for joint working between health and social services)' (NHS Executive 1998b), is no doubt the first of many similar publications. CCNs must not only become familiar with such publications but incorporate them into their vision of community children's nursing services and thus adapt their practice (Box 4.1).

If you have not formulated a vision for taking community children's nursing forward, both individually and as a member of a team, consider it as a priority when next formulating objectives.

Know the facts

To influence policy it is crucial to be familiar with the facts relevant to the specific aspect of the policy you wish to influence. These should be produced in a clear, concise document which details the advantages and disadvantages of your proposal over the present situation. Cost-effectiveness, efficiency, equity, consumer preference and accessibility must be considered carefully. CCNs are often in the situation of attempting to influence those who have little insight into the specific needs of children and their families and of the role of the CCN. Whilst financial constraints are often given as a reason to reject proposals for change, there is plenty of evidence of a lack of insight into the needs of children and their families: a change of attitude is required rather than finances.

It is helpful if the main arguments are documented in a summary with particular attention paid to the business plan. Knowing the facts must not be confined to a narrow professional perspective. CCNs must acquaint themselves with wider issues such as organisational change and identify who holds the power both directly and indirectly:

- Does your proposal fit the political or local health agenda?
- Has your manager been asked to comment on a consultation document?
- Is change, maybe a reconfiguration of services, being considered?
- Is increased consumer choice evident?
- Does an influential person (e.g. chair of the Trust or local MP, or a group such as the community health council) have a particular interest?

Bristol and District Community Health Council (1997) has produced an excellent report on the need for a community children's nursing service, which CCNs in other parts of the UK assisted with.

If your proposal is controversial, careful consideration of its preparation before presenting a document to management should be given, as this usually pays dividends. Presentation of papers and posters at professional conferences and articles in professional journals disseminate the information that will reinforce your arguments. This will reveal many of the arguments and concerns that may arise and assist in refining your preparation.

When you are ready, seek the appropriate opportunity to present your case. If not successful the first time, don't give up. Reflect on the event, seek assistance in analysing what happened and why you were not successful, then prepare for another attempt. The 'drip, drip' effect applied in a variety of ways can, in the long term, be very effective.

Use the facts

Acquiring the facts is essential but of little use if not used to improve services for children. There are a myriad of formal and informal mechanisms and opportunities available to CCNs, some very familiar, others, such as the parliamentary processes, less so.

The parliamentary process

Whilst the local MP's surgery should be familiar to all nurses, mechanisms such as Early Day motions or the facility to have questions asked in the House may not. RCN parliamentary officers are keen to assist members in familiarising themselves with the opportunities available. Why not give them a ring and discuss the best way to achieve influence?

The 'all parliamentary select committee on health' is an important mechanism, which nurses have been slow to use. Select committees, set up in 1979 to shadow the work of each Government department, undertake inquiries into specific issues, utilising written evidence submitted by interested individuals and groups. The committee then invites a small number of individuals and groups to give oral evidence before the whole committee.

The Health Select Committee's first inquiry into Services for Children and Young People was undertaken in 1996, with four reports published in 1997 (House of Commons 1997b). The RCN's Community Children's Nursing Forum utilised the opportunity by submitting written evidence and being invited to give oral evidence. The Third Report 'Health services for children and young people: home and school' (Health Committee 1997) is a rich source of information for all CCNs as well as providing an excellent example of how practising CCNs can influence national healthcare policy.

Responding to topical issues

Topical issues may not present in a clear way and CCNs, who do not have a strong power base, need to be particularly vigilant and imaginative to identify and utilise opportunities. For example, the Government's invitation to submit proposals to commemorate the life of Diana, Princess of Wales, was not an obvious opportunity for CCNs to raise the profile of the children and their families who would benefit from a community children's nursing service.

CCNs used the House of Commons Select Committee on Health's shock at the paucity of community children's nursing services and the NHS Executive Report 'Evaluation of the pilot project programme for children with life threatening illnesses' (NHS Executive, 1998c) to support the RCN's formal proposal that community children's nursing services would be a fitting tribute to Diana, Princess of Wales. This 'topical issue' enabled the RCN to inform and influence both the decision makers and the general public of the importance of providing community children's nursing services.

Responding to consultation documents and inquiries

Responding to consultation documents is a proven way of influencing policy whether at local or national level. The RCN Community Children's Nursing Forum was shocked that the UKCC consultation document on the future education and practice of community nursing (UKCC 1993) made no reference whatsoever to services for children who required nursing care in the community. The large working group responsible for its preparation did not include a registered children's nurse. The Forum's strong response to the consultation paper, and the publicity achieved, resulted in the definitive document (UKCC 1994), which acknowledged community children's nursing as one of eight distinct specialities of community nursing, open only to registered children's nurses.

Some opportunities to influence policy are not so clear. For example, the Royal Commission on 'long-term care' (Sutherland 1999) has been interpreted by many as concerning only the elderly. Unfortunately, although the Commission planned to include a range of client groups, it had time to report only on services for the elderly. However, the opportunity to submit written evidence regarding children was utilised and thus raised the specific difficulties for children. Clinical advances have resulted in an increasing number of children with complex clinical needs reaching adolescence and adulthood. The trend in care has shifted from institution to the child's own home, placing considerable responsibility, work and expense on families. Services are fragmented with disputes between health and social services, and with the added complication of education authorities. Agreed criteria for continuing care for children is rare and there is considerable evidence that many families receive little assistance, particularly in areas without a community children's nursing service.

The RCN Community Children's Nurses Forum therefore set up a joint working party with the RCN Children with Disabilities Group to focus on specific issues of concern, and submitted evidence to the Royal Commission.

Collaborative working

Whilst Florence Nightingale achieved considerable influence on healthcare policy as an individual, we live in a very different world. Working collaboratively in the interests of a common aim – to achieve more equal, effective and efficient services for children and their families – is the way forward. That aim must be discussed overtly and understood before joint working is attempted. Collaborative working has been common rhetoric for some years, and in 1998 working in partnership became politically correct (NHS Executive 1998b). The reality is that, since the establishment of the NHS until the present time, there has been little evidence of working across traditional boundaries let alone with social services, education or the voluntary sector. Change will not be easy, but is essential if services are to be improved. Working with others is not an option any longer: it is essential.

CCNs do not have a strong power base and therefore it has proved advantageous to work with others, both professional and lay persons. Since its formation in 1988, the RCN Community Children's Nurses Forum has spearheaded the influence on national health policy relating to community children's nursing services. However, the Forum represents a small group of active members within the RCN and has had to be vigilant and vocal to ensure that its views and concerns are considered appropriately. CCNs have been particularly disadvantaged by the traditional split between hospital and community services, with community nursing services focusing on the promotion of health and health education rather than the care of children with health disorders or disabilities.

Support has been received from paediatricians, paediatric surgeons, paediatric sections of the organisations representing the professions allied to medicine, and particularly from consumer groups, which since the 1960s have exerted increasing influence on healthcare policy and will continue to do so. But CCNs have not always recognised or utilised this support or incorporated a broad perspective into their vision.

Much of the evidence submitted to the House of Commons Select Committee, relating to CCNs, and the difficulties encountered by families when a community children's nursing service was not available, was from consumer organisations. This formal and unsolicited support from so many organisations surprised the RCN's Community Children's Nursing Forum and led to it formally co-opting a representative from Action for Sick Children on to its steering group meetings. It also increased links with other consumer groups.

Community children's nursing services need to identify where their allies are, both nationally and locally. Local organisations are particularly important because they vary considerably between localities and usually have excellent local networks, which can be very supportive to families and community children's nursing services.

The Diana, Community Children's Nursing Teams focus on working together, whether that be within health services, or between health, social services, education and the voluntary sector (NHS Executive 1998d). This philosophy is clearly reflected in the Resource Pack entitled 'Sharing the Care' (English National Board & Department of Health 1999). Having defined funding, these teams should be able to cut across the traditional boundaries that prevent continuity and cost-effective, efficient care, which causes so much frustration not only to the children and their families but also to staff and volunteers. Hopefully they will provide a model for the future and, once again, CCNs will have been at the forefront of breaking down unhelpful traditional boundaries and changing practice in order to enhance the care of sick children and their families. This is a good example of CCNs influencing healthcare policies.

CONCLUSIONS

The invisibility of the value of nursing has resulted in nurses having to influence policy by identifying and utilising opportunities, because it is rare for nurses to be presented with clearcut tactical manoeuvring. Children's lack of political power, the small number of CCNs and their lack of a power base have added to the difficulties.

Times are changing, and not only in organisational and clinical issues. Nurses are slowly acknowledging their responsibility to influence healthcare policy, becoming familiar with the mechanisms available and more confident and competent in their actions concerning healthcare policy. CCNs have achieved much, particularly considering their small number and the many obstacles experienced. There remains much to achieve, but change is here. Embrace the opportunities it provides.

The Government's choice of community children's nursing teams, led by registered children's nurses with a community qualification, is a fitting tribute to the life of Diana, Princess of Wales and marks a watershed in the development of community children's nursing. It also provides CCNs with opportunities to influence healthcare policy.

CCNs must look beyond the immediate frustrations of day-to-day clinical practice and resolve, both as individuals and as members of a small group of nurses, to become actively involved in shaping healthcare policy at local, national and international level, to ensure that tomorrow's children and their families will have the benefit of a universally accessible service wherever they live. As Clay (1987) reminded us: 'Participation in the political life of the country is the alternative for individual nurses to the silent frustration of the past or industrial action'.

FURTHER READING

Burr S 1998 Making waves. Nursing Management 5(6):8–11

The potential of the House of Commons Health Select Committee as a powerful mechanism to influence healthcare policy is explored with specific reference to the Inquiry into Services for Children and Young People.

Burr S 1998 Children: picking up the pieces. Nursing Management 5(7):6–10

The main themes of the four Reports of the House of Commons Health Select Committee 'Inquiry into services for children and young people', published in 1997, are summarised and nurses are urged to take action.

REFERENCES

Briggs A 1972 Report on the Committee on Nurse Education. HMSO, London

Bristol and District Community Health Council 1997 Forgotten families, health services for children with severe disabilities. Bristol and District CHC, Bristol

Clay T 1987 Nurses, power and politics. Heinemann, London

Clothier C 1994 The Allitt Inquiry: independent inquiry relating to deaths and injuries on the children's ward at Grantham and Kesteven General Hospital during the period February to April 1991. The Stationery Office, London

Department of Health 1994 The Allitt Inquiry. The Report of the Clothier Committee. HMSO, London

Department of Health 1997 Government response to the Reports of the Health Committee on Health Services for Children and Young People, Session 1996 97: 'The specific health needs of children and young people' (307-I); 'Health services for children & young people in the community, home and school' (314-I); 'Hospital services for children & young people' (128-I); 'Child and adolescent mental health services' (128 I). The Stationery Office, London

Department of Health 1999 Review of prescribing, supply and administration of medicines. Final report. The Stationery Office, London

English National Board for Nursing Midwifery and Health Visiting and Department of Health 1999 Sharing the care. Resource pack for Diana, community children's nursing teams. ENB, London

Health Committee 1997 Third report. Health services for children and young people in the community: home and school. House of Commons session 1996–97, minutes of evidence and appendices. The Stationery Office, London

House of Commons 1997a Health Select Committee. Session 1996–1997. Second report. The specific health needs of children. The Stationery Office, London

House of Commons 1997b Health Select Committee. Session 1996–1997. Children's health. Minutes of evidence vol II, and appendices vol III. The Stationery Office, London

House of Commons 1998 Debate on children's health, 25 March 1998, Hansard. The Stationery Office, London

International Council of Nurses 1985 Policy statement. Nurses' involvement in health care policy. ICN, Geneva

Ministry of Health 1959 The welfare of children in hospital. HMSO, London

National Health Service Executive 1998a The new NHS. Modern, dependable. Department of Health, London

National Health Service Executive 1998b Partnership in action (new opportunities for joint working between health and social services). Department of Health, London

National Health Service Executive 1998c Evaluation of the pilot project programme for children with life threatening illnesses. Department of Health, London

National Health Service Executive 1998d Diana children's community nursing teams. Department of Health, London

North West Regional Health Authority 1996 Inquiry into the care and treatment of Nicholas Geldard (Inquiry chairman, Judge Bill Ashworth). NHS Executive, North West RHA, Warrington

Procter S, Biott C, Campbell S, Edward S, Redpath N & Moran M 1998 Preparation for the developing role of community children's nurse. English National Board for Nursing, Midwifery and Health Visiting, London

Royal College of Nursing of the UK 1916 Royal College of Nursing Charter. RCN, London

Royal College of Nursing 1998 Guidance for nurses on clinical governance. RCN, London

Sutherland S 1999 With respect to old age: long term care, rights & responsibilities. The Stationery Office, London

UK Central Council for Nursing, Midwifery and Health Visiting 1992 Code of Professional Practice. UKCC, London

UK Central Council for Nursing, Midwifery and Health Visiting 1993 Consultation on the Council's proposed standards for post-registration education. UKCC, London

UK Central Council for Nursing, Midwifery and Health Visiting 1994 Future education and practice of community nursing. UKCC, London

5 Improved integration within public and community health

Lynn Young

KEY ISSUES

- The changing Government agenda for integrated services
- Integrated nursing teams
- The development and function of primary care groups
- Health action zones and healthy living centres
- Opportunities for community children's nursing

INTRODUCTION

Mr Blair could easily be described as a prime minister with a mission, leading a Government in a hurry. In the same way that Mrs Thatcher wanted rapidly to change the culture and direction of the UK, so too does Mr Blair. While Mrs Thatcher once stated 'there is no such thing as society', Mr Blair's Government seems determined to put policies in place that have the potential to help improve community health, diminish health inequalities and end social exclusion. Government strategy is aimed, in the longer term, at promoting the regeneration of self-reliant and cohesive communities, particularly in areas that have been blighted by the effects of long-term unemployment and poverty.

During 1998 an enormous amount of energy and enthusiasm was released in the world of health and social care, due mainly to the plethora of the Government's radical and inspirational new policies. The English health reforms, described in the White Paper 'The new NHS. Modern, dependable (Department of Health 1997a) and the equivalent papers for Scotland, Wales and Northern Ireland (Department of Health 1997b, 1997c, 1999) are of particular interest to the nursing profession. As nurses face the millennium, a tidal wave of Government initiatives, aimed at developing improved integrated services, is flooding the National Health Service (NHS) and the community at large.

For many years, debates and discussions have centred around the inability of different care agencies and informal carers to work together, focusing on the problems of the family or the individual rather than on the needs of the service and its employees. It is a salutary lesson to health and social care workers that, when a child is harmed or dies as a result of abuse, the subsequent public enquiry has often revealed that far from being neglected by the public services, a large number of professionals were closely involved. Despite the fact that resources were dedicated to the 'child at risk', preventable tragic death has occurred, often on account of the different agencies failing to communicate effectively.

It is sometimes incredible to members of the public that, when they are in need of a range of services, they can often find themselves in the middle of a wildly complex maze of different rules, budgets, philosophies and professionals who, with the best will in the world, fail to agree with one another.

The unfortunate result of our present system, and the inability of care agencies to cooperate, is that families, despite overwhelming problems, sometimes choose to remain in control and cope alone. Descriptions of fragmented services, and the human misery caused by poor integration, have been well documented by the press, a number of voluntary organisations, individuals and academic institutions.

The Cumberlege Report (Department of Health and Social Security 1986) described examples of stunning and inspirational community nursing services, but also offered constructive recommendations on how practice and primary healthcare services could be improved. The Report called for the development of strong primary healthcare teams which would profile the needs of their populations and agree upon action plans aimed at improving health and health services. While the word 'integration' is not used in the Report, over a decade later it is interesting to note that many of the recommendations, relevant to improving integration, are being implemented.

Present Government policies are a powerful catalyst for further integration. Developing improved integrated services is high on the present health and social care agenda. Government is striving to 'build a system of integrated care, based on partnership' (Department of Health 1998a) by removing false barriers and helping different organisations to work better together in order to improve care for the public. The English discussion document 'Partnership in action' (Department of Health 1998a) makes proposals that, if implemented, will improve the integration of health and social care services and therefore their performance. The Government White Paper 'Modernising social services' (Department of Health 1998b) continues the drive to integrate services including that of education, which further increases the number of proposed changes aimed at improving the health and well-being of children.

It can be both difficult and challenging to achieve improved integration between carers and professionals and the organisations in which they work, but we now have reason to be optimistic. Current policies and initiatives, together with the commitment of those involved, have enormous potential for improving the lives of the most vulnerable members of our communities.

Community nurses have been listened to. Their particular efforts to integrate the different nursing disciplines, as well as to improve integration between the community Trust and general practice, health and social care, and the acute and primary healthcare sectors, is impressive. Working in the community can be complicated and frustrating, especially when there is a failure to coordinate services. Nurses know that, once at home, people do not fit neatly into boxes for the convenience of the services.

Integration is defined by the Concise Oxford Dictionary as 'to complete an imperfect thing by the addition of parts' and 'to bring or come into equal participation'. The community is complex. The responsibility lies with service providers to distance themselves from social and professional tribalism and to concentrate more on what needs to be done and how problems can best be solved.

Long before we had knowledge of the present Government's plans for the NHS, community nurses in a number of areas had been seeking ways to improve primary healthcare through the development of strong and robust integrated nursing teams. Now that we have a better understanding of Government plans for the NHS and social care services, nurses working in integrated teams are in a strong position to take the lead in implementing improved services within their locality. They are well placed to show others, such as general practitioners (GPs) and social service personnel, the way forward in line with the Government aspirations described in 'The new NHS' (Department of Health 1997a) and the discussion document 'Partnership in action' (Department of Health 1998a).

INTEGRATED NURSING TEAMS

> 'Integrated nursing brings together the different skills, knowledge and expertise of a team of nurses so that priority needs can be met and a comprehensive service provided within a community.' (Young & Poulton 1997)

A number of nurses who have helped to develop integrated teams report that success can depend very much on the commitment also shown by GPs and management. When this happens, extraordinary change can be achieved. One powerful key to change is the ability of nurses to shift their attention from caseload-specific activities and traditional titles to the health needs of the local population and ways in which the team can best promote health gain. The following characteristics can help guide nurses through the process of improving integration:

- The team's desire to improve the quality of care and treatment drives motivation.
- Stronger integration brings benefits to nurses in terms of improved job satisfaction and raised morale.

The new primary care groups (PCGs) should have confidence that their primary healthcare services are valued by the population and are effective and affordable. However, professional philosophies need to be examined within PCGs as boundaries in care delivery become more 'blurred'. Clinical leadership is crucial. Entrenched attitudes, professional self-interest and clinical practice have to shift and traditional roles be confronted. Successful leadership often reduces management costs and increases funds for direct patient care. The following examples are offered.

The Birtley Community Nursing Team in Newcastle comprises those who, among a large number of nurses, have successfully developed integrated teams and have documented their experience of providing services to the local population (Birtley Community Nursing Services 1998). One of their projects was to improve the child health clinic by tackling issues such as waiting times, the appointment system, the facilities, and parental involvement and satisfaction. The child health clinic is now run by a GP, health visitor, nursery nurse and two practice nurses, although the GP and health visitor times have now been reduced. The evaluation of this project has demonstrated that the desired outcomes appear to have been achieved by the team. They also developed a 'clinical

BOX 5.1 ***Care of children with life-threatening illnesses***

- Each district should have a senior health service appointment to coordinate services for children with life-threatening illnesses.
- The role of key worker should be made explicit and be enhanced. The key worker should be the first point of contact and be responsible for coordinating services for the family.
- Families need community children's nursing services and these nurses need to be team members in order for them to be supported and for workload and stress to be shared.
- Respite care services and community children's nursing services should be well integrated and under one management structure.
- Social care services should also be integrated with community children's nursing services.

supervision project' for child protection following dissatisfaction expressed by nurses with the existing system. The result of the project is the expansion of the school-nurse role and the model of clinical supervision has moved away from focusing entirely upon child protection and now 'addresses all aspects of children and families in need' (Birtley Community Nursing Services 1998).

The NHS Executive document 'Evaluation of the pilot project programme for children with life threatening illnesses' (NHS Executive 1998) offers much information on a 5-year series of pilot projects into the study of services for children with life-threatening illnesses. The Conservative Government started the programme in 1992 and an evaluation took place in 1997. The main conclusions drawn following the evaluation are shown in Box 5.1.

Many community nurses believe strongly that, once they have put their own house in order, they are then better able to work towards integrating the family of nursing with the wider world of medicine, public health, social care and other significant sectors such as education and employment.

THE NEW NHS: PRIMARY CARE GROUPS

The UK is committed to a new public health programme – a programme that diminishes health inequalities and social exclusion. There is a consensus that improved interagency and professional integration will make a valuable contribution to achieving the programme's aims. While considerable efforts are being made to achieve improved integration, the UK is presently developing four national health services. Political devolution has resulted in each country having its own White Paper on health. 'The new NHS' (Department of Health 1997a) is the English paper, Scotland has 'Designed to care' (Department of Health 1997b), Wales has 'Putting patients first' (Department of Health 1997c) and Northern Ireland's paper is 'Fit for the future' (Department of Health 1999).

While the principles and intentions described in the four White Papers are similar, they differ in language, organisational development and the position of nurses in the new commissioning structures. The English PCGs, in particular, have received an enormous amount of attention and are, without doubt, a tremendous success for nursing. PCGs are the new vehicle for health commissioning. England

BOX 5.2 ***Initial aims of primary care groups***

- Improved health and reduced health inequalities of their population
- Improved primary healthcare and general practice
- Improved integration between health and social care services
- Improved services for the most vulnerable groups in the community
- Meeting the aims and objectives of the health authority's health improvement plan
- Implementing a framework of clinical governance
- Commissioning a range of secondary care services (level 2 PCG)

now has approximately 1000 PCG nurse members who, from 1 April 1999, took on full corporate Board responsibilities and executive functions. PCGs are the bedrock of 'The new NHS' and dramatically restructure the NHS. However, PCGs are more about new behaviour than new structures. They will need different skills and expertise from those used within GP fund-holding and the internal market if they are to help achieve improved public health.

Developing a fully integrated health and social care service should be first and foremost in the minds of new PCG members, regardless of their discipline or employer. PCGs will initially have to look at ways of achieving the aims outlined in Box 5.2.

PCGs have certain topics to tackle. For some, child health is likely to be a popular choice. In this instance a child health focus group will be developed which should include a number of clinical specialists and perhaps a representative from a children's voluntary organisation. The group will need to profile the existing child health services and the health needs of children within their area. It should then present an action plan, aimed at improving the health of the children and the child health services, to the PCG. The focus group will have to work closely with the chief executive of the PCG to ensure that the services are developed in line with the PCG primary care investment plan, the health authority's health improvement plan and significant NHS frameworks. Child health focus groups should obviously include community children's nurses (CCNs).

Community nurses are now alongside their GP colleagues in the driving seat of the NHS. Their experience of developing integrated teams will, without doubt, prove to be a tremendous asset to the PCG Board and act as a catalyst for achieving improved integration across all sectors. Nurses, once again, demonstrate that the success of the health and social care system depends, to a large extent, on them taking the lead in policy, management and organisational developments as well as direct patient care. Nurses have the ability to bring both clinical knowledge and the human experience to the PCG Board. This will result in more effective service development and improved integration in line with the current Government aspirations.

HEALTH ACTION ZONES

'Health Action Zones are partnerships between the NHS, local authorities, community groups and the voluntary and business sectors to develop and implement a health strategy to deliver within their area measurable improvements in public health and in the outcomes and quality of treatment and care.' (Department of Health 1998a)

Health action zones (HAZs) are concerned with developing an integrated approach to tackling certain problems that are adversely affecting a section of the population. The overall aim is for the health of the worst off in our communities to improve at a faster rate than that of the general population. Artificial barriers which impede integration, and therefore standards of care, will be broken down. Action will be taken to prevent ill health, improve health and reduce health inequalities. The 15 areas containing a HAZ began to implement their programmes on 1 April 1999, and a second wave of applicants, which was accepted as a HAZ, commenced on 1 April 2000.

CCNs working within a HAZ should take the opportunity to become involved in new child health projects. A number of areas have explicitly focused part of their HAZ programme on the special health needs of children. CCNs have a significant part to play in HAZ programmes such as this, alongside health visitors, midwives, school nurses and other health professionals, as well as colleagues in social services and education.

HEALTHY LIVING CENTRES

During 1998 the Government announced that National Lottery money could be spent on health, along with other good causes. £300 million has been ring-fenced to fund a number of community projects throughout the UK which will focus on helping people to improve their own health and well-being. As a result the health living centre (HLC) initiative developed. These are concerned with improving the quality of life for individuals by increasing independence and their ability to live with dignity.

HLCs will need the involvement of the community and the cooperation of all stakeholders, private and public, if they are to have a positive impact on the health of individuals. Businesses, schools, local and health authorities, general practices and the voluntary sector will need to build on their existing relationships and, in partnership, develop an integrated approach to tackling health inequalities.

Examples of these HLCs, which provide a blueprint for future developments, include the Bromley by Bow centre in East London, the West End Health Resource Centre in Newcastle, the Neptune Health Park in the West Midlands, and the Brockenhurst Healthy Village near Southampton.

It is important to know that a significant catalyst for the Bromley project was the unfortunate death of a local citizen following a number of service failings due to a complete lack of integration. The belief that health needs to be addressed in a totally holistic way has resulted in Bromley by Bow HLC developing a whole range of integrated activities that help to improve health. The result of this philosophy is that community nurses, GPs, other community disciplines and volunteers share a building where dance and painting classes, community projects, complementary therapies and physical fitness sessions take place. Traditional boxes have been removed and professionals are thinking differently. While specialisms need to continue, the consensus is that 'we need to push the process of integration even deeper into our structures' (Bromley by Bow 1998).

It is expected that areas with a HAZ will receive funding for their own HLC, but in order for them to be successful in their bid they need to demonstrate how they will focus activities on the wider community and not simply a minority group. CCNs working within a HAZ are likely to have a HLC as their work-base rather than the traditional hospital or health centre in the future. There are enormous opportunities for CCNs to participate actively in the drive to develop integrated services for children, and their involvement will certainly make a major contribution to achieving better health for all children.

CONCLUSION

CCNs are pivotal to a number of major Government initiatives concerned with services for children. Ministers are determined to force different agencies to cooperate, in particular health and social care services. National priorities have been set, which include the modernisation of primary healthcare and improving services for children. While health and social services are to share the task of reducing health inequalities, other priorities are led by either the health or local authority.

CCNs will need to straddle health, education and social care settings in the drive to improve the quality of care received by children and their families. The NHS is taking the lead on primary healthcare, and social services has the lead on child welfare. A powerful incentive to develop integrated children's services therefore exists.

Nurses have learnt much from the failings of the past and are forging ahead in the unstoppable drive to develop integrated services. New initiatives, such as those mentioned here, demand a fully integrated approach if they are to be successful. This means that those involved will need to indulge in 'joined up thinking' in the move to improve the public health. CCNs are pivotal to achieving improved healthcare services and long-term health gain for children, and need to be involved in the vast number of developments leading us into the twenty-first century.

REFERENCES

Birtley Community Nursing Services 1998 Birtley community nursing services to people in and around Birtley. Portfolio of evidence. Birtley Community Nursing Services, Birtley

Bromley by Bow Healthy Living Centre 1998 Bromley by Bow Newsletter. Catalyst, issue 1. Bromley by Bow HLC, London

Department of Health 1997a The new NHS. Modern, dependable. The Stationery Office, London

Department of Health 1997b Designed to care. The Stationery Office, London

Department of Health 1997c Putting patients first. The Stationery Office, London

Department of Health 1998a Partnership in action. A discussion document. The Stationery Office, London

Department of Health 1998b Modernising social services. The Stationery Office, London

Department of Health 1999 Fit for the future. The Stationery Office, London

Department of Health and Social Security 1986 Neighbourhood nursing – a focus for care. The Cumberlege Report. HMSO, London

National Health Service Executive 1998 Evaluation of the pilot project programme for children with life threatening illnesses. The Stationery Office, London

Young L & Poulton B 1997 Integrated nursing teams can influence locality commissioning. Primary Health Care 7(10):8–10

6 Working in partnership with the voluntary sector

Peter Kent

KEY ISSUES

- What is the voluntary sector?
- How the voluntary sector is funded and managed
- Services available and how to assess their value
- How to contact the voluntary sector
- How to work alongside or in partnership with voluntary organisations
- The future of the voluntary sector

INTRODUCTION

Community children's nurses (CCNs), along with many other health professionals, will work with voluntary organisations from time to time. This may involve little more than obtaining information on behalf of a family but may equally extend to a close, formal, working relationship where decisions are made collaboratively and responsibility is shared. To get the best from this relationship, a sound understanding of the voluntary sector and how it is organised, managed and funded is required. This chapter provides an overview, rather than a comprehensive historical description, of the voluntary sector in the UK, and gives the reader sufficient understanding to enable good working relationships to be developed that will be of benefit to children and their families. The current relationship with the state, particularly the health service, will be considered, including the implications for joint working in the mixed economy of care. The chapter concludes with a brief consideration of what the future may hold for voluntary–statutory sector partnerships.

THE VOLUNTARY SECTOR

The voluntary sector is not a homogeneous group of like-minded organisations. Nevertheless, it is possible to provide a snapshot of the sector today that will enable effective working relationships to be developed. First, it is important to know that a number of terms are used to refer to organisations belonging to the sector. A voluntary organisation is essentially one that does not owe its existence to some statutory means. No law or Act of Parliament says it must exist; it exists because someone wants it to and has some objective they believe can be achieved by getting together with others and taking collective action. Charities, for example, are voluntary organisations, but not all voluntary organisations are charities. Not-for-profit organisations are often voluntary organisations, too, as are non-governmental organisations (NGOs). However, once again, not all will be charities and, indeed, some will not be voluntary bodies at all and may be private organisations. The size and history of voluntary organisations is, not surprisingly, equally diverse. Some are national bodies with thousands of members, whereas others comprise a small group of local people with a shared interest or need (Kendall & Knapp 1996).

STRUCTURE AND FUNDING OF VOLUNTARY ORGANISATIONS

Given the diversity of the sector, management of voluntary organisations varies. Small local organisations may be run entirely by a committee of volunteers and employ no paid staff. Large national bodies will have sophisticated management structures that reflect their status as multi-million-pound enterprises. Some organisations, too, will rely solely on volunteer staff. Whether or not this is so may, however, have little to do with the size of the organisation. Small organisations are just as likely to have few volunteers as a large national body, and some of the biggest charities have huge numbers of volunteers, for example the St John's Ambulance Brigade or the Red Cross. The number deployed can have as much to do with the nature of the service provided, or the pool of people available as potential volunteers, as with the internal structure of the organisation.

Raising the funds to sustain a voluntary organisation can consume a good deal of time and effort. Much of the income will be from voluntary donations: donations made by the general public and others, from membership subscriptions or as a result of organised events. Organisations that have existed for some time will usually have investment income and income from legacies. The smaller, and newer, the organisation the more likely it will be to rely on voluntary income. The number of people involved in fundraising will depend on a number of factors, not least the size of the organisation. Staff in smaller organisations can find themselves spending a good deal of time fundraising, including having to raise their own salaries.

A major source of income is, of course, the state – primarily central and local government and health authorities. Traditionally funding for the voluntary sector came in the form of grants, either one-off payments or funding spread over a number of years. For organisations working in the field of health and social care, an important source of funding has been the Department of Health's Section 64 programme. This is a general 'power to fund' which is contained in primary health legislation and has been used over the years to support voluntary organisations engaged in activities that are consistent with the government of the day's policy objectives. Not all organisations are eligible for such grants and there have always been more applicants than recipients. In more recent years the practice of grant-making under Section 64 has changed. Rather than funding core expenditure there has been an emphasis on projects, coupled with a reluctance to continue renewing grant aid at the conclusion of each project. Nevertheless, many major national organisations do continue to receive significant funding, which suggests in the final analysis that the decisions can have political considerations (Davis-Smith et al 1995, Palmer & Hoe 1997).

COMMISSIONING AND CONTRACTING

Perhaps the most significant recent development has been the move to contracting and purchasing of services based on a relationship differing very little from similar relationships in the private sector. This method of purchasing or commissioning health and personal care services was initiated by the previous Conservative Government, which wanted to introduce a contract culture to the welfare state and divided the health service into purchasers and providers (Department of Health 1989).

The Labour Government has introduced a new structure based on primary care groups (PCGs), rather than general practitioner (GP) fundholders (Department of Health 1997), and in local government has replaced compulsory competitive tendering with the concept of best value. The Government's intention is to create what is referred to as an economy of mixed care. The welfare state should no longer be the provider of first resort and there should be no automatic assumption that the National Health Service (NHS) or local authorities should provide the majority of healthcare and personal social services. Health authorities will continue to commission services until they are replaced by Primary Care Trusts (in England), which will then assume responsibility for commissioning but remain accountable to the health authority. However, what happens in England will not be replicated throughout the UK. In Wales, there will be 22 'local health groups' which, like English PCGs, will bring together health professionals and representatives of other agencies to advise health authorities on the commissioning of services. In Scotland, there are plans for some seventy 'local healthcare cooperatives', voluntary groupings of GPs that may opt at some future point to hold a budget for commissioning primary and community care. In Northern Ireland, decisions on reform of health structures must wait until the elected assembly has been established.

Local authorities will provide fewer services directly and be seen increasingly as commissioners on behalf of their communities. The Government believes the result will be a more competitive environment governed by measurable standards of value for money and quality of service enshrined in the commissioning criteria. The subsequent contracts and service agreements will also be subject to scrutiny, review and renewal. This should serve both to maintain competition and as a brake on health and social care spending, which the Government seeks to limit without explicit rationing of resources or services. Despite the increasing emphasis on quality of service in the contractual relationship, there are no national quality standards for the voluntary sector, and quality assurance can vary significantly across the sector (George 1997, Levaggi 1996).

WHAT VOLUNTARY ORGANISATIONS DO

In the health sector, voluntary organisations run hospices, ambulances, paramedic services, counselling services, childcare and services for the elderly, provide advice, support and information and employ nurses, physiotherapists, social workers and doctors. Generally speaking the services seek to complement those of the health service. Grant-making trusts and other charities can make grants to individuals in need for equipment, financial hardship or respite care. Most, too, take pride in their professionalism. An organisation that depends on volunteers can deliver a professional service just as well as an organisation employing predominantly salaried staff. The important distinction is the organisational culture and attention to procedures governing selection, training, supervision, confidentiality, monitoring and evaluation. Organisations exist to provide a single service that meets a particular need, usually among a very specific group of people, while others provide a wide range of services for broad categories. There are organisations that exist in one location only and others that are national bodies with local branches or groups enjoying varying degrees of autonomy. Before deciding whether to use an organisation's service it is important to assess its ability to deliver that service in a manner and context that meets appropriate standards of professional practice. This can be carried out in much the same way as assessing the suitability of services within the NHS before making a referral. The most important criterion is to establish that the people running the service or organisation do so in a manner that is broadly consistent with your own, your employer's and your professional body's views of good practice (Harvey & Philpott 1996).

CONTACTING THE VOLUNTARY SECTOR

Most areas will have a Local Council for Voluntary Service (LCVS) or similarly titled body that both represents and supports local voluntary organisations. The National Council for Voluntary Organisations (NCVO) will know the name and contact details of the LCVS in any particular area. NCVO will also have information about national organisations that have local branches or regional offices, and publishes a directory of voluntary organisations (NCVO 1998). Other useful sources of information include the local authority, which may also produce a directory, and the local community health council. Organisations sharing a particular interest or operating in a particular service area often collaborate, forming umbrella groups. Larger umbrella groups also employ their own staff, who can be an invaluable source of information and support. The telephone directory and colleagues may also prove to be invaluable sources, not only for the immediate area but for those working in allied fields or in neighbouring areas. Voluntary organisations, especially small charities, will not always be aware of what is available from the health service, and CCNs can be a valuable link between community and hospital, encouraging dialogue and joint planning. Conversely, CCNs may be unaware of the extent of support available by some organisations, such as the example illustrated in the case study.

CASE STUDY

Jane is a CCN based at the Whittington Hospital in north London. The hospital serves an area of high social need and has faced severe financial pressures owing to an outbreak of influenza during the winter. One of the families on Jane's caseload has a child with cystic fibrosis who needs a course of intravenous antibiotics. The child and family would prefer that this course of treatment take place at home, and the child's mother has been trained to carry out the necessary procedures. However, she is nervous about taking on the responsibility for these for the very first time. She feels that, if she could have someone present while she administers the first few doses, she would gain confidence and soon be able to continue the treatment alone. Jane cannot, unfortunately, commit herself to being present personally because she has a large caseload of ill children and is the only CCN available. She contacts the Cystic Fibrosis Trust for advice and discovers they have a fund to support and encourage home care. The Trust donates a grant, which enables Jane to employ a suitably qualified colleague, who works part-time, to supervise the course of treatment on this occasion.

WORKING WITH THE VOLUNTARY SECTOR

Entering a partnership with a voluntary organisation is in principle much the same as conducting any other relationship. It requires confidence in the partner's ability, trust in their integrity and commitment, and agreement to work together in a manner that is based on an explicit understanding of the rights and responsibilities of the partners. The economic, cultural and political environment in which the organisation exists needs to be understood. The limitations that exist owing to finance or small numbers of trained staff must be recognised. Clearly, some forms of partnership working will be informal and may involve little more than superficial contact from time to time with, for example, an information service or helpline. Other partnerships will require the agreement reached to be confirmed in writing. This can help not only with the management of the relationship but also provides others with a clear picture of what was agreed and with whom responsibility for particular aspects of the partnership lies. Once again, CCNs can perform a valuable role linking the voluntary sector at local level with the health service. There may be formal mechanisms for consultation, such as joint planning committees, but not all small organisations are comfortable with these or can participate. With their combination of hands-on experience and understanding of both children's needs and health service structure, CCNs may be ideally placed to help voluntary organisations talk to and even negotiate with commissioners.

Many organisations will, of course, be very familiar with contracts or service agreements between purchasers and providers, and both operate in and understand the mixed economy of care. They will deliver services according to clearly prescribed criteria and in a manner laid down by the commissioning authority. Their ability to move beyond the boundaries of their contract or agreement may, however, be limited. Their obligations to the purchaser need to be understood in case they compromise the partnership, and the nature of the service can change, or even terminate, if the purchaser negotiates new terms when the contract is reviewed. An informal partnership will be based largely on personal relationships, and requests for support or a service will be negotiated equally informally on a day-to-day or case-by-case basis. Where a contractual basis for the partnership exists, negotiations will be much more formal and may involve intermediaries, such as commissioning managers (Palmer & Hoe 1997).

CASE STUDY

Assisted Living is a local voluntary organisation that provides respite for children with severe disabilities. It receives its income primarily from the local council's social services department, which 'spot purchases' services but has strict criteria that must be met. The health authority makes a grant for support that can enable children to be cared for at home rather than in hospital, and a grant from the National Lottery Charities Board completes the funding. Unfortunately, there is a small number of children who do not meet the council's criteria and are waiting to be discharged from hospital. The CCN and the director of Assisted Living discuss the situation and agree to organise a meeting between the health authority, social services and the families to discuss what can be done. At the meeting it is agreed that health and social services will support an application to the Joint Consultative Committee for a funded project to meet the needs of this group of children.

FUTURE OF THE VOLUNTARY SECTOR

Given the Government's intentions are clear for the foreseeable future, and their term of office may well extend beyond a single term, the economy of mixed care is the environment in which the voluntary–statutory partnership will operate. This does not mean that voluntary organisations will all become contractors on behalf of the state. The majority of charities, for example, carry out their work with little or no money from the state. Nevertheless, organisations that are significant providers of services in the field of health and social care are likely to have contractual relationships with commissioning authorities. They will also be in a competitive environment where they compete not just with other voluntary organisations but the private sector too. The implications for partnership may be profound even though, perhaps somewhat ironically, the Government is equally keen to promote partnerships (Department of Health 1998). Some voluntary organisations fear for their very existence, should they lose a major contract. Others will adapt and prosper. As with most socioeconomic changes, the organisations in the middle may experience the most severe squeeze.

CONCLUSION

The voluntary sector can justifiably be referred to as the third sector of the economy. It employs several hundred thousand people and has an annual turnover of over £1 billion. Voluntary organisations are also significant providers of health and social care services. Indeed, it would be difficult to envisage the NHS without the thousands of voluntary organisations working alongside the statutory sector. To obtain the most appropriate care for children and their families, CCNs need to learn about the organisations working in their field and how their services are made available. They can be powerful agents for change, playing a key role in developing new partnerships and services. This requires working in collaboration. Collaborative working can be a purely informal arrangement between nurse and colleague in a voluntary organisation, or may be based on the contractual arrangement between commissioning authority and voluntary organisation. In many cases there will be a mixture of arrangements, reflecting the mixed economy of care. If CCNs are to ensure that children receive the best possible service they will need to understand this relationship and have an appreciation of the political and financial context within which it is set.

Good practice will be founded on understanding, trust and confidence in each other's ability to work together in the interests of the people that matter most: the children and those who care for them. The voluntary sector is already a major partner in the delivery of health and social care services. However, the relationship between the sector and the health service has changed significantly in the past decade and many voluntary organisations are now contracted to provide services and must negotiate with health and local authorities in much the same way as the private sector. Opportunities for partnership at local, regional and national level exist and are encouraged by central government. Nevertheless, such opportunities require careful preparation and, like all relationships, take time to develop. Once established, however, partnerships can make a lasting contribution to the quality of life enjoyed by children.

FURTHER READING

Clutterbuck D & Dearlove D 1996 The charity as a business: managing in the voluntary organisations. Routledge, London

This book will enable the reader to discover more about how the voluntary sector is having to learn to engage with the private sector and adapt to its way of functioning.

National Council for Voluntary Organisations A map of quality standards: a guide to understanding quality systems for the voluntary sector. Hamilton House Mailings, London

The voluntary sector is attempting to come to terms with 'best value' policy of the Labour Government. A guide to the process of contracting and commissioning, and what is central to the Government's vision in the relationship between commissioners and providers, is provided in this text.

Reading P 1994 Community care and the voluntary sector: the role of voluntary organisations in a changing world. Venture, Birmingham

Community care is a partnership, and this book remains one of the most informative and up-to-date publications on this current debate.

REFERENCES

Davis-Smith J, Rochester C & Hedley R (eds) 1995 An introduction to the voluntary sector. Routledge, London

Department of Health 1989 Working for patients. HMSO, London

Department of Health 1997 The new NHS. Modern, dependable. The Stationery Office, London

Department of Health 1998 Partnership in action. A discussion document. The Stationery Office, London

George M 1997 On the spot. Community Care 1202:23

Harvey C & Philpott T (eds) 1996 Sweet charity: the role and workings of voluntary organisations. Routledge, London

Kendall J & Knapp M 1996 The voluntary sector in the United Kingdom. Manchester University Press, Manchester

Levaggi R 1996 NHS contracts; an agency approach. Health Economics 5(4):342–352

National Council for Voluntary Organisations 1998 Directory of voluntary organisations. NCVO, London

Palmer P & Hoe E (eds) 1997 Voluntary matters: management and good practice in the voluntary sector. Directory of Social Change, London

7 Working in partnership with education

Phillippa Russell

KEY ISSUES

- Current Government policy and new opportunities for partnership between community children's nursing and education services
- The importance of early identification of special educational needs and the connections between social disadvantage and educational difficulties
- Working with children, their families and schools: what community children's nursing services can contribute to the education of children with special health care needs or disabilities
- Recognising the diversity of special healthcare needs which schools and families now endeavour to meet in the community (including the increase in children who are 'technically dependent' with multiple complex healthcare needs)

INTRODUCTION

The House of Commons Health Committee's (1997) report on the specific health needs of children and young people set a new agenda for partnership between the National Health Service (NHS) and education services. The Committee strongly endorsed the role of community children's nurses (CCNs) and envisaged a more diverse role within the education system than that of the current school nursing services (sections 13–15). The same committee also noted the changing pattern of disability and chronic medical conditions in children, with increasing numbers of children with complex needs requiring health-specific nursing advice or care in school settings.

The past 2 years have seen an unprecedented interest by central government in improving standards in education. The key theme of 'excellence for all' acknowledges that schools and education authorities alone cannot make a difference to the life chances of children and young people. As 'Meeting special educational needs: a programme of action' (Department for Education and Employment 1998) clearly states, improved coordination and cooperation between child health services and education are crucial to improve achievement. Such cooperation can function at different levels but will, importantly, offer new opportunities to community nursing services to work in partnership with families and schools.

HEALTH INEQUALITY AND EDUCATIONAL AND SOCIAL DISADVANTAGE

The same years have seen growing concern about health inequality and social and educational disadvantage. Hilary Graham (1999), in her keynote address to the Community Practitioners and Health Visitors Conference, noted that:

> 'Inequalities in health occupy a central place in the history of health visiting and school nursing, with the professions established at the end of the 19th century as part of a wider public health strategy. At the end of the 20th century, health inequalities are again top of the public health agenda.'

Education is important for the future well-being of children and families and 'Our healthier nation' (Department of Health 1998a) cites schools as a key health setting. Whilst health-related education is obviously a key factor, general educational attainment is also fundamental as it opens the door to making healthy choices and raising expectations. As Graham (1999) observed, there is a 'long shadow of disadvantage', which means that children born into poorer circumstances experience more material, psychological and educational risks. The National Child Development Study (Davie et al 1999) clearly demonstrates the cumulative consequences of disadvantage in terms of educational achievement as well as future socioeconomic and health status in adult life. The Government has established a Social Exclusion Unit to endeavour to address the root causes of social, educational and health inequality. But solutions will be complex and they will require partnerships at local level between a wide range of community services.

There is growing interest in early identification and intervention in terms of preventing subsequent educational failure. The Government's 'Surestart Programme', launched in 1999, will target resources at the most disadvantaged communities and envisages a powerful and influential role for health visitors and community nurses working in partnership with education and social services. As the Acheson Report (1998) observes,

> 'Education is a traditional route out of poverty for those living in disadvantage ... education can play an important role in reducing health inequalities by ensuring that children are equipped with the knowledge they need to achieve a healthy life.'

Acheson (1998) envisages community health services (most probably community nurses) and schools working in partnership to address healthy living (and thereby improve educational achievement). Importantly, the Report mirrors the key messages in the Surestart Programme about involving parents (in particular mothers) in contributing to their children's well-being. 'Well-being' is very relevant to educational achievement. The contribution of health visitors to young children's learning through home visiting programmes is validated by Robinson (1999), in a review of the research literature on the effectiveness of domiciliary health visiting. Russell (1999) reviewed the research literature on the connection between disability and disadvantage and the effectiveness of early intervention and home visiting programmes for parents. She drew similar conclusions about the positive role of community nurses as Portage home visitors and parent educators and advisers in helping parents to be active partners in the care and education of children with disabilities or special educational needs.

PARTNERSHIPS BETWEEN COMMUNITY NURSING SERVICES AND EDUCATION: WHAT KINDS OF ROLES?

The Code of Practice on the Identification and Assessment of Children with Special Educational Needs (Department of Education and Employment 1994) and the Education Act 1996 set the scene for a partnership approach to assessing special educational needs. Community nursing services can have an important role to play, not only in clearly identifying any special health needs that will directly affect a child's education, but in working to support parents in helping their own children and in listening to and supporting the children themselves. The involvement of children in assessment and decision making can be very challenging, but it can also be positive. Russell (1998), in a review of policy and practice in involving disabled children in decision making, notes the role of community nurses as 'health advocates' for disabled or sick children and the value of making children active partners in their care and education programmes.

The contribution of community children's nursing services to raising parents' expectations and contributing to their children's educational progress and overall development is illustrated by Cunningham & Davis (1985). They note the potential of health visitors and other community nurses as parent advisers, home visitors and members of Portage home teaching schemes in a study of different frameworks for collaboration between parents and services.

The following three case studies illustrate the impact of a disability or special healthcare need upon children's education and personal growth and development. They also demonstrate the potential for community children's nursing services to contribute to assessment and problem solving in educational settings.

CASE STUDY

Emily is aged 13 and has moderate learning disabilities, diabetes and epilepsy. She attends a mainstream school, with additional support. Emily's mother has long-term mental health problems and has difficulty in Emily's diet and insulin management. Emily has had two petit mal seizures because of failure to take her medication appropriately. Her small size and her irritable behaviour, if her insulin levels fall, have made her a constant target for teasing and minor bullying, and her attendance at school is irregular. There is concern about her relationship with a fellow male pupil because of her immaturity and her need for affection.

Sam's story

Sam is 7. He is 'technically dependent' (the term 'technically dependent' is in general usage and is understood by education and social services as well as child health services) and has a gastrostomy. He has a rare degenerative condition and his mobility has declined in the past 12 months. However, he is still a lively child and anxious to continue to attend school with his friends. He has recently started to have episodes of incontinence, which cause him acute embarrassment. His respite carers feel they can no longer offer him short-term breaks because of a lack of clarity about their legal liability for his care. They are also concerned about carrying out procedures which they feel might lead them to being accused of child abuse because of an absence of local guidance on invasive care.

Kayleigh's story

Kayleigh is 10 and has asthma. She has had five visits to casualty and three admissions to hospital because of accidents over the past 6 months. She and her mother are in short-term accommodation on a run-down inner-city estate. Kayleigh's father is awaiting trial for serious assault on her mother and in theory has no contact with the family. Kayleigh's behaviour is causing increasing concern at school. She has frequent outbursts and has nearly been excluded because of kicking other children. Her general practitioner considers that she and her mother are both probably suffering from clinical depression. The school is worried both about managing Kayleigh's behaviour and the possibility that the behaviour may be due to abuse.

Emily, Sam and Kayleigh have very individual special educational and healthcare needs. They also illustrate the challenges and the opportunities for community nursing services to support vulnerable children in education.

PRACTICAL HELP WITH MANAGING CHILDREN WITH MEDICAL CONDITIONS IN EDUCATIONAL SETTINGS

Emily's poor attention and her behaviour at school have improved significantly because:

- A CCN with special expertise in childhood diabetes has worked with her to give her greater responsibility and confidence in managing her diabetes.
- Liaison with the practice nurse at the family's health centre also ensured that Emily's mother was more vigilant about her daughter's diet and encouraged her to self-inject.
- The practice nurse has also introduced Emily's mother to a local support group for parents of children with special needs and put her in touch with the British Epilepsy Association. Both organisations have given her helpful written information, videos and practical advice. Emily's mother has admitted to feeling that epilepsy is stigmatising and hoping that the seizures were 'just febrile convulsions'. She now feels more confident through seeing other parents coping positively.
- Emily was fond of sweets and sometimes stole sweets and biscuits from her class. This behaviour resulted in much of the teasing, which in turn caused her to drop out of school. The school nurse was able to include diabetes in a 'health awareness' programme at the school and to encourage Emily's class to understand her frustration at the deprivation of sweets, and to give her some support.

Emily's behaviour has improved. Liaison between the school and community children's nursing services has made the school's current Personal Health and Social Education (PHSE) programme more accessible to a child with a learning disability. Emily's relationship with her former 'boyfriend' is now 'friend' only and she is enjoying more social activities with her peer group at school. Most importantly, the community nursing services have worked with the school to give it greater confidence and to ensure that Emily's diabetes as well as her epilepsy is acknowledged within her individual education plan (IEP) and within her Statement of Special Educational Needs. The school has now introduced an anti-bullying policy and this includes explicit reference to children with disabilities or other special needs.

Sam's disability and his need for a high level of personal and nursing care present particular challenges. Initially there was ambivalence in his special school about providing the level of technical support that he required because of issues of legal liability. Sam's mother was frequently requested to come into school to supervise his feeding and personal care. The pressures upon her were so heavy that she was diagnosed as having clinical depression. As noted above, the respite carers were as ambivalent as the school about what procedures they could carry out. The local community children's nursing service resolved the difficulty by:

- Working with the specialist community children's nursing team who supervised Sam's care to agree a protocol for Sam's personal care.
- Agreeing a 'whole school policy' regarding invasive care procedures and specifying Sam's needs within his Statement of Special Educational Needs. The school and the community children's nursing service drew upon guidelines from recent research (Servian et al 1998) in developing agreements for all concerned.
- Providing training and support for Sam's learning support assistant and in drafting her job description. The assistant has nursing experience and can in turn advise and support on the day-to-day management issues of other children with special care needs.

As a consequence:

- The health authority has agreed that, because of Sam's special needs, the school will have regular support from a CCN who will work closely with teachers, parents and others to ensure that there is a carefully integrated programme.
- Because Sam's education and home care can be planned together, the difficulties with the respite carers have been resolved and Sam now spends two nights a week with his link family. He enjoys sharing their family life and his mother's health has improved because she has additional time to share with her other children. The integrated management approach also ensures that the right equipment is available at home, school and the respite carers.

Children like Sam, with complex disabilities, are becoming more common in community services. Commentators outline the challenges they present to services, whilst emphasising that good-quality community nursing support can enable children to participate actively in educational and other activities (Servian et al 1998, Townsley & Robinson 1999). The Social Services Inspectorate (1998) notes the impact on all services of the increasing number of children with complex disabilities and medical needs. This publication commends the role of nurses in training and supporting a range of carers in schools and community services, and cites a training programme at the St Helens and Knowsley Hospitals as a useful example.

Kayleigh comes from a family under stress. Her asthma is exacerbated by the damp poor housing she is living in and by her mother's smoking. Her mother attributes her multiple accidents to falls on uneven stairs and poor lighting (together with glass in the children's outside play area). However, there are concerns about possible physical abuse. Kayleigh's quality of care has been improved by:

- Support from a community mental health nurse for her mother, to encourage her to use local community services and to think through her present situation.
- Support from the health visitor who is able to give practical advice on the management of Kayleigh's asthma, to make certain that Kayleigh attends outpatient appointments at the local hospital and to discuss home safety with the family.
- Encouragement and reassurance from the school nurse about using an inhaler. Kayleigh had been 'hiding' her inhaler because she did not wish to look 'different' to other pupils. Kayleigh has been encouraged to talk about her behaviour and her kicking out. She admits she is angry about her father and the loss of her former home, and 'just takes it out on people'. She sees the school nurse regularly and has now been encouraged to participate more actively in her IEP and to set herself targets for her school work and behaviour.
- The community children's nursing service has also been involved in making recommendations to the local housing department about the importance of the family being rehoused in warm and dry accommodation.
- Some issues about Kayleigh's quality of care still remain. A community nurse attached to the local child protection team has been asked to monitor the situation. She is able to offer Kayleigh's mother support in a local parent group, which provides support and parent education for vulnerable families.

A year on, Kayleigh's asthma and her behaviour have improved. The family has been rehoused. Her mother is having treatment for her mental health problems and is attending the support group regularly. She has admitted that she has sometimes pushed Kayleigh in the past, but there have been no further admissions to casualty or hospital.

CONCLUSION: THE NHS AND EDUCATION – MESSAGES FOR THE FUTURE

The debate about inequality and educational achievement highlights the growing importance of community nursing services working with parents and children in schools. The evidence about the value of early intervention creates a range of opportunities for health visitors and other community nurses in developing their skills in supporting and educating parents, and in ensuring that the growing number of children with complex disabilities and special needs are properly supported by community services. The special contribution of CCNs relates to their ability to:

- Work directly with children and families in their local communities (which is of particular importance for 'hard to reach' families who seldom attend hospital or other appointments)
- Develop good working relationships with other local professionals in health, education and social services, which facilitates partnership approaches when children and families have multiple needs
- Offer a non-stigmatising and acceptable service
- Provide practical advice and offer solutions to day-to-day problems (many schools in particular say that they often need advice on very practical difficulties relating to the care or management of a child, for which they would prefer a 'named person' in the locality)

As the Government response to the House of Commons Health Committee (Department of Health 1998b) noted:

> 'We strongly support the development of community children's nursing services, which offer an increased quality of care to children and their carers. Paediatric community nursing services are particularly helpful for children who have a disability or chronic illness in order to prevent admission to hospital and to support both their care and their education and development'.

And, as a parent said to me at a recent conference:

> 'When you have a disabled child, you collect a 'Noah's ark' of professionals. Your whole life is taken over. My life was saved by my health visitor, the school nurse and a learning disability community nurse. They visited me at home. They enjoyed a good laugh (well, we would have cried if we hadn't laughed!). And they really helped John's teachers to understand why he was sometimes so difficult, how they could meet his care needs. It was such practical sensible help. It made us feel we had a future. You need a good friend if you have a disabled child. We got three!'

FURTHER READING

Servian R, Jones V & Lenehan C 1998 Towards a healthy future: multi-agency working in the management of invasive and life-saving procedures for children in family based services. Norah Fry Research Centre, Bristol

Gives practical advice on the management of children with complex health care needs in the community. These guidelines are particularly useful because they offer a model for interagency working and address the needs of children who are increasingly using local community services but require careful support and management.

Department for Education & Employment 1998 Meeting special educational needs: a programme of action. DfEE, London

Sets out a new agenda for children with disabilities and special educational needs. The programme of action acknowledges the important role of a range of community health services in supporting children with special educational needs and outlines a range of other relevant Government initiatives.

Health Committee 1997 The House of Commons Health Select Committee. Health services for children and young people in the community: home and school. Third Report. The Stationery Office, London

Department of Health 1998 Government response to the reports of the Health Committee on health services for children and young people. The Stationery Office, London

These two publications offer invaluable information both on current child health policy and practice and on future directions in developing community children's nursing services.

Department for Education & Employment 1994 Code of practice on the identification and assessment of special educational needs. DfEE, London

To be revised in 1999, this publication sets out the current arrangements for the identification and assessment of special educational needs, including the contribution of community child health and nursing services to assessment and reviews.

Russell P 1998 Having a say? Partnership in decision-making with disabled children. National Children's Bureau, London

This was commissioned by the Department of Health and looks at positive partnerships between a range of healthcare and other professionals and children and young people with disabilities and special healthcare needs. The report gives practical examples of involving children (and families) in decision making and treatment.

REFERENCES

Acheson D 1998 Independent inquiry into inequalities in health. The Stationery Office, London

Cunningham C & Davis H 1985 Working with parents: frameworks for collaboration. Open University Press, Milton Keynes

Davie R, Butler N & Goldstein H 1972 From birth to seven: a report of the National Child Development Study in association with the National Children's Bureau. Longmans, London

Department for Education & Employment 1994 Code of practice on the identification and assessment of special educational needs. DfEE, London

Department for Education & Employment 1998 Meeting special educational needs: a programme of action. DfEE, London

Department of Health 1998a Our healthier nation. The Stationery Office, London

Department of Health 1998b Government response to the reports of the Health Committee on health services for children and young people. The Stationery Office, London

Graham H 1999 Inequalities in health: patterns, pathways and policy. Community Practitioner 72(2)

Health Committee 1997 The House of Commons Health Select Committee. Health services for children and young people in the community: home and school. Third Report. The Stationery Office, London

Robinson J 1999 Domiciliary health visiting: a systematic review. Community Practitioner 72(2)

Russell P 1998 Having a Say? Partnership in decision-making with disabled children. National Children's Bureau, London

Russell P 1999 Disability and inequality. Council for Disabled Children, London

Servian R, Jones V & Lenehan C 1998 Towards a healthy future: multi-agency working in the management of invasive and life-saving procedures for children in family based services. Norah Fry Research Centre, Bristol

Social Services Inspectorate Council for Disabled Children 1998 Disabled children: directions for their future care. Social Services Inspectorate/Department of Health Publications, London

Townsley R & Robinson C 1999 What rights for disabled children? Home enteral tube feeding in the community. Children and Society 13(1):48–60

8 Educating community children's nurses: a historical perspective

Mark Whiting

KEY ISSUES

- As the locus of care for children moves inexorably from hospital to community, it is essential that registered children's nurses undergo appropriate preparation for their role in community care.
- The history of education of community nurses dates back over a 100 years.
- It is only in the very recent past that the specific learning needs of registered children's nurses have been recognised.

INTRODUCTION

During the late 1980s, this author undertook a research study in which the focus was the development of community children's nursing services in England (Whiting 1988). The research involved a national census survey by questionnaire which was followed by interviews with representatives of every community children's nursing team in England. One of the most significant issues to emerge from that research was the concern amongst many community children's nurses (CCNs) regarding the educational preparation for their new role in caring for children in community settings.

The questionnaire stage attracted a response rate of 97.9% (186 questionnaires were returned from a total of 190 English district health authorities). Twenty three community children's nursing teams were identified within the research; one further team was known to exist at the time of the research, but due to staffing problems within the team at that time the questionnaire was not returned. Team leaders in the 23 teams completed questionnaires in which they were asked to provided biographical details of the members of their teams.

The 23 teams were staffed by 45 CCNs, 44 of whom (97.8%) were registered sick children's nurses (RSCNs) and the one nurse who was not qualified as a children's nurse was a district enrolled nurse. Twenty five of the nurses (55.6%) had completed a programme of educational preparation in community nursing (22 were district nurses; two were health visitors; one nurse held both district nurse and health visitor qualifications). The team leaders were asked to give some indication of the educational qualifications that they considered to be a requirement for nurses working within their teams. Although there was strong support for all nurses to hold registration in children's nursing, only 11 team leaders (47.8%) regarded possession of a community nursing qualification as a prerequisite to practise. Ten team leaders considered the district nursing qualification to be a necessity and one team leader argued that the district nursing and health visitor qualifications were of equal value. Three of these respondents suggested that a specific qualification in community children's nursing would be beneficial. Those respondents who were themselves qualified as community nurses were significantly more likely to support the undertaking of community education programmes.

The issue of education was explored in further detail at the interview stage. Semi-structured interviews were undertaken on-site in the team work-base for each of the teams and, whenever possible, the interviews involved all members of the staff who were on duty on that particular day. In addition to the 23 teams involved at the questionnaire stage, the one additional team who had not completed a questionnaire and two 'new' teams established during the spring of 1988 were interviewed (26 teams in total). A total of 39 nurses including all 26 team leaders participated in the interviews. Comments made within the interviews were not attributed to individual participants and it was therefore not possible to link the data obtained within the interviews to the biographical profiles of individual CCNs.

Nurses in 17 teams (65.4%) commented positively on the need for community education. Members of six teams specifically stated that the district nursing course was of value. Three CCNs stated that the education institutions in which they had undertaken their own district nursing course had developed imaginative approaches to their programmes in order to facilitate the students' specific self-declared learning needs (i.e. these institutions had both encouraged the students to take opportunities to gain practice experiences with child patients and had granted permission for the students to undertake some written course work with a focus on children). However, nurses in 10 teams raised particular concerns about the course, the most frequent of which was related to the age of the patients being visited by the district nurses. An extensive study of district nurse caseloads undertaken by Dunnell and Dobbs in the early 1980s (Office of Population Censuses and Surveys 1982) found that 74% of patients were over the age of 65 years. Smaller-scale studies undertaken by Watts (1976) and Ellis et al (1985) had reported an even higher percentage of the district nurse caseloads to be elderly. This was clearly a major issue. Three CCNs reported that in order to gain a place on the district nursing course they had been specifically required to gain 'adult' nursing experience in hospital even though they had considerable experience in paediatrics and were intending to practise as CCNs and not as district nurses upon completion of the course. Nurses in five teams made specific comments about the low number of children with whom they had come into contact whilst undertaking the district nursing course.

Despite these concerns, there was considerable support of the need for a community training. In particular, anxiety was expressed at what was perceived to be an increasing tendency to appoint CCNs who had received no formal community training before appointment. As one participant observed: 'district nurses fought very hard for the mandatory training, it would be wrong to sacrifice it' (Whiting 1988 p 107). In addition to the focus on district nursing education, a number of interviewees explored the relevance of health visitor education programmes in meeting the needs of prospective CCNs. Several nurses who had recently completed their district nursing courses commented favourably on the joint sessions held with health visitors during the common-core elements of the courses. Two nurses, who had themselves completed health visitor education programmes, suggested that 'child development' and 'developmental psychology' represented key content areas which might be usefully accessed by prospective CCNs.

It would be appropriate at this point to reflect back on the wider context of the provision of community nursing education and to consider the historical development of education provision in both district nursing and health visiting.

DISTRICT NURSING EDUCATION

The history of district nursing has been traced back to the visionary work of William Rathbone in Liverpool in the 1850s (Stocks 1960). Rathbone recognised from the outset the value of nurse training, and he was not alone in seeking Florence Nightingale's advice on how to secure the services of trained nurses. Nor was he alone in receiving Miss Nightingale's cursory advice. If you want nurses then 'train them yourself' (Stocks 1960 p 25). And so he did. With considerable support and advice from Miss Nightingale, William Rathbone established a training school in Liverpool and by May 1863 'six women had been trained as district nurses' (Stocks 1960 p 31).

In 1868, Rathbone became a member of parliament in Liverpool. As a politician, he spent part of his time in London where, during the mid 1870s, he was actively involved in the establishment of the Metropolitan and National Nursing Association for the Provision of Trained Nurses for the Sick Poor (Baly et al 1987, Stocks 1960), which rapidly established the requirement for a training in district nursing of 6 months' duration.

In 1887, a donation of over £70 000 from Queen Victoria's Silver Jubilee appeal was made to extend the work of district nurses through the UK, and led to the establishment of the Queen Victoria's Silver Jubilee Institute for Nurses. Through a process of affiliation of a number of the existing training organisations, each of which had been established in different areas of the UK by this stage, the Queen's Nursing Institute, as it is now known, rapidly became the national benchmark for district nursing education.

The introduction of state registration for all nurses by the Nurses Registration Act 1919 meant that registration with the new General Nursing Council became a prerequisite for entry to district nursing education. At the time of the Act, however, and in order to facilitate initial establishment of the nurses' Register, it was not a requirement for registrants to have completed a formal training as a nurse (Abel-Smith 1960). This required only the production of:

> 'Evidence to the satisfaction of the Council that they are of good character, are of the prescribed age, are persons who were for at least three years before the first day of November 1919 *bona fide* engaged in practice as nurses in attendance of the sick under conditions which appear to the Council to be satisfactory for the purposes of this provision and have adequate knowledge and experience of the nursing of the sick.' (Nurses Registration Act 1919 ch 94 section 3(2)(c))

Before the Act, the number of district nurses had grown considerably. Many had received no formal training either in general nursing or in district nursing. As a result of the Act these individuals were not only able to register as nurses, but the absence of any statutory requirement for training in district nursing meant that they were also able to continue to describe themselves as 'district nurses'. This situation persisted beyond the time of the establishment of the NHS in 1948. However, during the 1950s, increasing concerns about the number of 'untrained' district nurses led to the establishment of the 'Working party on the training of district nurses' (Ministry of Health, 1955), which reported in 1955 that less than half of the 9203 district nurses then in employment were 'Queen's trained' (Baly et al 1987). In response to this finding, the panel of Assessors for District Nurse Training was established in 1959.

In 1968, the Panel took over from the Queen's Nursing Institute the responsibility for training of district nurses at a national level. One of the Panel's key functions was to advise the Ministry of Health (and subsequently the Department of Health) on matters pertaining to the education of district nurses. One of its first actions was to approve a reduction in the length of training of the district nursing certificate from 6 to 4 months. Whilst there was a widespread acceptance within the profession of the need to increase the proportion of 'trained' district nurses, Baly et al (1987) were amongst a number of commentators who perceived this as a retrograde step: 'the emphasis was on the numbers rather than the need to meet the future health needs of the community' (Baly et al 1987 p 338).

Indeed, the Panel of Assessors themselves saw this as only a short-term solution to the issue of training, and in 1976 the Panel's 'Report on the education and training of district nurses' recommended that a nationally approved district nurse training should consist of a 6-month programme of which two-thirds should be theoretical training and one-third practical experience, to be followed by 3 months' supervised practice. Although the 6-month training was accepted in 1978, the supervised practice component was not introduced until 1982. A new curriculum for district nurse training was introduced in 1978 (Department of Health and Social Security 1978), and in 1981 the district nursing certificate became a mandatory requirement to practise (Kratz 1982).

HEALTH VISITOR EDUCATION

In the 1850s, the original sanitary visitors in Manchester were not required to undertake any specific preparation for their role, but by 1880 a short course of lectures was introduced for new visitors and by 1882 all the women attending the course were required to pass an examination set by a local doctor (Dowling 1973). A requirement for nurses to have previously undertaken nurse training was introduced in Manchester in 1981, at the same time that the title health visitor was first used (Owen 1983).

Owen (1983) observed that, in 1909, London was the first authority to demand a professional qualification for health visitors. In 1919, with the publication of a circular by the recently established Ministry of Health, this standard become generally accepted throughout the country. The Ministry of Health decreed that, by 1928, all health visitors should hold the certificate of the Royal Sanitary Institute (later the Royal Society of Health), the official examining body. At this time, for registered nurses (who were also required to be qualified as midwives), a course of study of 6 months' duration was required to train as a health visitor, although 'direct entry' into health visiting was achievable by completion of a 2-year programme. In 1938, midwifery training was separated into two elements (formally identified as Part 1 and Part 2), and possession of Part 1 only was required for prospective health visitors (Owen 1982, 1983), a requirement that remained in place until 1989.

The formal educational requirements were reinforced in the National Health Service Act 1946 and in the NHS (Qualifications of Health Visitors and Tuberculosis Visitors) Regulations 1948, which reiterated the requirement for possession of the health visitor qualification for all practitioners. The School Health Service (Handicapped Pupils) Regulations 1945 outlined the responsibilities of the health visitor within the school health services in line with the Education Act 1945.

Owen (1982) reported that, by 1950, 32 institutions were involved in the training of around 700 student health visitors per year. Despite this, there was a significant shortage of health visitors (Hale et al 1968) and, to address this, a working party was established with Sir Wilson Jameson as chair. The report of the working party (Ministry of Health 1956) led directly to the publication of the Health Visiting and Social Work Training Act 1962, and ultimately to the establishment of a new training body for health visitors, the Council for the Education and Training of Health Visitors (CETHV) (Wilkie 1979). In terms of this particular chapter, perhaps the most important work of the CETHV related to developments in the syllabus of training for health visitors and the incremental introduction during the 1960s and early 1970s of a full 1-year programme of training to include a minimum of 3 months of supervised practice.

NURSES, MIDWIVES AND HEALTH VISITORS ACT 1979 AND THE NEW STATUTORY BODIES

The Nurses, Midwives and Health Visitors Act 1979 led to the dissolution of both the Panel of Assessors in District Nursing and the CETHV. Their responsibilities for training provision were taken over by the new statutory bodies, the United Kingdom Central Council for Nursing, Midwifery and Health Visiting (UKCC) and the four National Boards. In England, a key element of the English National Board's (ENB) work focused on its responsibilities within the Act to 'have proper regard for the interests of all groups within the profession including those with minority representation' (Nurses, Midwives and Health Visitors Act 1979, section 2(2)). In fulfilling this responsibility, the Board established two key committees: the District Nursing Joint Committee and the Health Visiting Joint Committee (both of which worked closely with colleagues in the other three National Boards). One of the primary functions of the Board related to its responsibilities, inherited from the Panel of Assessors and the CETHV, for the approval and reapproval of education courses (Nurses, Midwives and Health Visitors Act 1979, section 6(1)(a) and (b)).

As early as 1983, the District Nursing Joint Committee recommended to the Board that, where institutions offered both the district nursing and health visiting courses, approval visits should be undertaken on a joint basis; however, at this stage the Health Visiting Joint Committee considered that such changes should be 'implemented slowly' (ENB 1983). This reticence was short lived, and within 4 years 'increasing numbers of joint course approval visits being made by members of the HV and DN joint committees' (ENB 1987 p 21). By this stage, it was clear that in many education institutions there was an increasing tendency towards the closer alignment of health visitor and district nurse courses in terms of an emerging 'common core' of content and in respect of the overall structure and length of the programmes.

TOWARDS A QUALIFICATION IN COMMUNITY CHILDREN'S NURSING

In the autumn of 1987, a small group of nurses came together and established a special interest group for paediatric community nurses within the Royal College of Nursing (RCN). Within a year the group was formally recognised as a professional 'forum' within the RCN. One of the first issues to which the group turned its attention was that of educational provision for prospective (and in some instances already practising) CCNs. Contact was made with the ENB and in its annual report of 1988–1989, the District Nursing Joint Committee noted that 'the issue of community nursing services for sick children, highlighted as an area requiring attention, is being discussed by the Committee as a matter of urgency' (ENB 1989 p 10). In April 1989, a working group was established within the ENB consisting of members of the General and Paediatric Committee and the District Nursing Joint Committee in order to address 'how the longer term needs of paediatric community nurses might be met' (Langlands 1990 p 8).

In 1990, the District Nursing Joint Committee forwarded a paper to the Education Advisory Policy Committee of the UKCC in which it outlined a number of issues that it was hoped the UKCC might consider within its ongoing deliberations on post-registration education. In addition, and in order to provide a short-term solution to the problems outlined in the opening section of this chapter, the ENB produced and circulated to all institutions offering the district nursing course, 'Modified Regulations and Guidelines' for what was described as the 'District nurse and paediatric community nursing course' (ENB 1990). These regulations provided a framework within which registered children's nurses (who must also be registered as a general nurse) might gain a period of experience of 'between four and six weeks caring for the sick/handicapped child' (ENB 1990 p 98) during the supervised practice element of the course and might also undertake some of the examined elements of the course with a focus upon the child.

A number of institutions, including the Combined Buckinghamshire College (Whiting et al 1994), Southampton University (Gastrell 1993) and South Bank Polytechnic, sought formal approval from the ENB to provide these modified programmes during the early 1990s. In spite of the imaginative approaches to curriculum development within these programmes, it remained a fact that the qualification gained upon successful completion of the course was that of district nurse. As Godman observed: 'the time that was "wasted" in both academic and practical preparation of a paediatric nurse to care for adults in the community seems to be an inappropriate use of scarce resources' (in Whiting et al 1994).

To provide further opportunities for registered children's nurses, the ENB also agreed to approve 'programmes generated by institutions specifically to prepare RSCNs and RNs (Child)' and leading to 'recordable qualifications on the UKCC professional register' relating to the community nursing care of children (Langlands and McDonagh 1995). Two institutions, the Oxford Brookes University and the Manchester Metropolitan University, gained approval for such courses in 'Paediatric community nursing/Diploma of Higher Education in Community Health Care for Nurses on Part 8 or 15 of the Professional Register (A50)'.

In 1991, the UKCC published the 'Report on proposals for the future of community education and practice'. This consultation document formally introduced the concept of 'community health care nursing'. In addition, it included a strong endorsement for the emerging 'modular approach to education, which gives flexibility and offers scope for multi-disciplinary and interdisciplinary working' (UKCC 1991 para 26). The report clearly identified a range of nursing needs in the community; however, it completely failed to recognise the specific needs of sick children and made no mention of the rapidly expanding discipline of community children's nursing. These concerns were voiced in a formal written response to the consultation report by the Royal College of Nursing, Action for Sick Children (ASC), the Association for British Paediatric Nurses (ABPN), the British Association for Community Child Health (BACCH), the Joint Committee of Professional Nursing, Midwifery and Health Visiting Associations (England) and the English National Board (UKCC 1992).

The development of proposals by the UKCC for the reform of community nursing education was a major part of the Council's broader work within the Post-Registration Education and Practice Project (PREPP) (UKCC 1990). In 1993, the Council formally incorporated its work on community nursing education into PREPP in a consultation document (UKCC 1993), which commenced by stating that 'The Council has now concluded its work on the proposals arising from the Post Registration Education and Practice Project and the Report on Proposals for the future of Community Education and Practice' (p 1). Within this final consultation document the UKCC proposed six areas of practice in community nursing including, somewhat inexplicably, the 'general nursing care of children which relates to the practice of school nursing and paediatric nursing' (UKCC 1993 annexe 3 p 1). This proposal was greeted with understandable concern by both school nurses and community children's nurses and, in 1994, when the final proposals for the reform of community nursing education were published (UKCC 1994), the two discrete disciplines of school nursing and community children's nursing were formally recognised as separate strands of the new discipline of 'specialist community health nursing'. CCNs would become one of a new breed of 'specialist practitioners' in community nursing.

For many CCNs who had been involved in extensive lobbying of the ENB and UKCC, in particular during the previous 4 years, a collective sigh of relief could now be breathed. The final proposals (UKCC 1994) created a route to specialist professional practice for CCNs within the framework of an equivalent educational pathway to each of the other seven community nursing disciplines, details of which are set out in Box 8.1. Early in 1995, the ENB published updated

BOX 8.1 ***Areas of community health care nursing practice (UKCC 1994)***

General practice nursing
Community mental health nursing
Community mental handicap nursing
Community children's nursing
Public health nursing – health visiting
Occupational health nursing
Nursing in the home – district nursing
School nursing

regulations and guidelines to educational institutions to allow implementation of the UKCC proposals (ENB 1995).

A major problem, however, still remained. By the time the UKCC published its final proposals, there were over 250 nurses employed within community children's nursing teams in the UK (Whiting & RCN 1994). At this time, these nurses were employed in community children's nursing teams within over 80 NHS Trusts and health districts. Many of these nurses had previously gained qualifications in health visiting or district nursing; however, this was far from universal. A survey at the end of 1995 in the Thames Regions found that over 70% of the 139 CCNs employed within 31 teams possessed no community qualification at all (Whiting 1997). This was not a problem that was unique to community children's nursing. As an example of this, the field of practice nursing was predominantly made up of nurses who did not possess a community qualification at all, and practice nurse numbers had grown in the 10 years from 1984 to 1994 from 1920 to 9100 whole-time equivalent staff (National Health Services Executive 1996).

The UKCC recognised that this was a significant concern and, in order to address this, a series of 'transitional arrangements' was proposed to facilitate nurses in the attainment of 'specialist practitioner' status (UKCC 1994 section 10, UKCC 1996). These arrangements provided a series of pathways through which CCNs might gain accreditation of previous learning and experience (Langlands and McDonagh 1995, Myles 1997) in order to allow CCNs to become eligible to use the 'specialist practitioner' title. The 'transitional arrangements' expired in October 1998.

CONCLUSION

This chapter has sought to review the historical development of educational provision for CCNs, including an examination of a range of community nursing educational programmes dating back to the 1860s. There can be little doubt, however, that the rapid growth in the number of community children's nursing services within the UK during the late 1980s and 1990s has been the single greatest influence upon educational development. Whilst district nursing and, to a lesser extent, health visiting educational programmes offered a 'stop-gap' solution to the expressed educational needs of the growing number of registered children's nurses wishing to work in the community, such a solution was clearly unsustainable in the long term. As the number of CCNs grew, so did the need to provide an appropriate educational framework. This chapter has provided a historical review of the background to the introduction of a range of new education programmes and to the development of the specialist practitioner programme in community children's nursing.

REFERENCES

Abel-Smith B 1960 A history of the nursing profession. Heinemann, London

Baly M E, Robottom B & Clark J M 1987 District nursing, 2nd edn. Heinemann, London

Department of Health and Social Security: Panel of Assessors for District Nurse Training 1976 Report on the education and training of district nurses (SRN/RCN). HMSO, London.

Department of Health and Social Security: Panel of Assessors for District Nurse Training 1978 Curriculum in district nursing for State Registered Nurses and Registered General Nurses. HMSO, London

Dowling W C 1973 Health visiting – expansion. Health Visitor 46(11):371–372

Ellis J M, Battle S & Salter B 1985 Day in the life of a DN. Nursing Times Community Outlook 8 November: 11

English National Board for Nursing, Midwifery and Health Visiting 1983 Annual report – 1983 ENB, London

English National Board for Nursing, Midwifery and Health Visiting 1987 Annual report – 1986/1987. ENB, London

English National Board for Nursing, Midwifery and Health Visiting 1989 Annual report – 1988/1989. ENB, London

English National Board for Nursing, Midwifery and Health Visiting 1990 Regulations and guidelines for the approval of institutions and courses 1990. ENB, London

English National Board for Nursing, Midwifery and Health Visiting 1995 Regulations and guidelines relating to programmes of education leading to the qualification of specialist practitioner. Circular 1995/04/RLV. ENB, London

Gastrell P 1993 Diploma courses for PDNs. Paediatric Nursing 5(10):13–14

Hale R, Loveland M K & Owen G M 1968 The principles and practice of health visiting. Pergamon Press, London

Kratz C R 1982 District nursing. Cited in: Allen P & Jolley M (eds) Nursing midwifery and health visiting since 1900. Faber and Faber, London, p 80

Langlands T 1990 Meeting future needs. Paediatric Nursing 2(3):8–9

Langlands T & McDonagh M 1995 The pathways to a specialism. Paediatric Nursing 7(8):6–7

Ministry of Health 1955 Report of the working party on the training of district nurses. HMSO, London

Ministry of Health 1956 An enquiry into health visiting: report of the working party on the field of work, training and recruitment of health visitors (chair, Sir W Jameson) HMSO, London

Myles A 1997 Desperately seeking 'specialist practitioner'? Paediatric Nursing 9(10):14

National Health Services Executive 1996 Primary care: the future. The Stationery Office, London

Office of Population Censuses and Surveys 1982 Nurses working in the community. HMSO, London

Owen G M 1982 Health visiting. In: Allen P & Jolley M (eds) Nursing midwifery and health visiting since 1900. Faber and Faber, London, p92

Owen G M 1983 The development of health visiting as a profession. In: Owen G M (ed) Health visiting, 2nd edn. Baillière Tindall, Eastbourne, p 1

Stocks M 1960 A hundred years of district nursing. Allen and Unwin, London

UK Central Council for Nursing, Midwifery and Health Visiting 1990 The report of the Post-Registration Education and Practice Project (PREPP). UKCC, London

UK Central Council for Nursing, Midwifery and Health Visiting 1991 Report on proposals for the future of community education and practice. UKCC, London

UK Central Council for Nursing, Midwifery and Health Visiting 1992 Report on responses on the 'Report on proposals for the future of community education and practice'. UKCC, London

UK Central Council for Nursing, Midwifery and Health Visiting 1993 Consultation on the Council's proposed standards for post-registration education. UKCC, London

UK Central Council for Nursing, Midwifery and Health Visiting 1994 The future of professional practice – the Council's standards for education and practice following registration. UKCC, London

UK Central Council for Nursing, Midwifery and Health Visiting 1996 The Council's standards for education and practice following registration (PREP) transitional arrangements – specialist practitioner title/specialist qualification. Registrar's Letter 15/1996. UKCC, London

Watts D E 1976 District nurses in East Birmingham Health District 2. Nursing Times Occasional Papers November: 161–164

Whiting M 1988 Community paediatric nursing in England in 1988. MSc thesis, University of London

Whiting M 1997 Community children's nursing: a bright future. Paediatric Nursing 9(4):6–8

Whiting M & Royal College of Nursing 1994 Directory of paediatric community nursing. RCN, London

Whiting M, Godman, L & Manly S 1994 Meeting needs: RSCNs in the community. Paediatric Nursing 6(1):9–11

Wilkie E 1979 The history of the CETHV. Allen and Unwin, London

9 Setting the agenda for education

Patricia Livsey

KEY ISSUES

- Community specialist practitioner
- Diverse student needs
- Availability and range of community experience
- Educational standards

INTRODUCTION

As previous chapters have recognised, community children's nursing has been on the periphery of both children's nursing and community nursing for some time. In March 1994 the United Kingdom Central Council (UKCC) published standards for education and practice following registration, which include standards for post-registration education programmes leading to the specialist practitioner qualification. Eight areas of specialist practice in the community were recognised:

1. Community children's nursing
2. Public health nursing – health visiting
3. School nursing
4. Community nursing in the home – district nursing
5. Community mental handicap nursing – learning disabilities nursing
6. General practice nursing
7. Occupational health nursing
8. Community mental health nursing

With this publication (UKCC 1994), community children's nursing has now been established as a discrete community specialist practitioner qualification. This has provided the opportunity to advance the development of children's nursing for, not only does it recognise that the needs of children must be provided by a discrete community specialist, it also recognises that to be a children's nurse it is not enough to practise outside the hospital setting. By virtue of its development the UKCC (1994) acknowledges the complexity of community children's nursing and the need for specialist nurses who are skilled and knowledgeable children's nurses, who not only have the clinical expertise to care for children but also have the ability to translate their experience within the complex and changing environment that we know as the community.

Educationalists in higher education institutions have since been working with their practice colleagues to produce courses that not only fit the variable needs for community children's nurses (CCNs) locally but also address the wider national context within the framework of the UKCC's requirements. Given that the notion of the role of the CCN has not yet reached maturity or consensus, this has been a difficult task (Procter et al 1998). This is further complicated by the fact that over 50% of the country still does not have a community children's nursing service (Royal College of Nursing 1996). The chapter will identify ways of developing educational provision to address the current diversity within practice and will explore the educational needs of the community specialist practitioner (CCN). The wider areas of child health will be discussed and consideration for future developments will be made.

DEVELOPMENT IN EDUCATIONAL PROVISION

In the past there were mandatory qualifications only for district nurses and health visitors and so, historically, CCNs have either undertaken health visiting or district nursing courses in order to achieve a community qualification (Whiting 1988). However, the relevance of health visiting and district nursing to community children's nursing has always been questionable as district nurse training is focused primarily on the adult population and health visiting develops the students' skills to appreciate the health issues of the population. Hence the UKCC (1994) set standards for specialist nursing practice, which includes community children's nursing. With the community specialist practitioner programme came a recordable qualification and professional recognition. The community specialist practitioner status gives recognition of the unique educational needs of community children's nursing and clearly identifies the importance of this role to other healthcare professionals.

DEVELOPMENT OF THE SPECIALIST PRACTITIONER

Each community nursing specialism constitutes a separate and distinct professional group, yet there are some common elements that run through all the groups. Hyde (1995) explains how this has led to some confusion and often tensions in understanding and appreciating the uniqueness of new areas of practice. The UKCC recognises that some commonality exists between the specialisms and stipulates that common core areas must occupy a minimum of one-third and a maximum of two-thirds of the total community specialist practitioner programme. These similarities and differences can be categorised into three types (Hyde 1995):

1. Areas that are common to all specialisms
2. Areas that are common to some specialisms but not to others
3. Areas that are unique to one specialism

Areas common to all specialisms include subjects such as health promotion, primary healthcare policy, research, caseload management, teamwork and collaboration, leadership, scope of professional practice, quality assurance and audit. Subjects such as child protection and child health are not significant to

TABLE 9.1 ***Examples of similarities within course content***

Specialism	Course content
All specialisms	Health promotion, policy, clinical governance, child protection, etc.
Health visitors and school nurses	Child development, working with families
Community children's nurses, school nurses and health visitors	Mental and emotional health issues, child-specific health promotion, eczema management, constipation management

occupational health nurses but are of paramount importance to health visitors, school nurses, learning disabilities nurses and CCNs. Hyde (1995) further believes that all the specialist pathways have more common areas than they have differences. By comparing the subject areas it is evident that the scope of the CCN runs close to areas within other community specialisms (Table 9.1). None the less, the uniqueness of the specialism must not be undervalued.

Within the classroom the opportunity of sharing knowledge and experience can be advantageous as this setting provides a forum for discussion and debate where the students from the various community specialisms can begin to appreciate their new professional roles. The potential problems lie within practice, as it is essential that students gain the most appropriate experience to ensure the development of a competent and confident CCN who has the skills and knowledge required to move practice forward in a creative, flexible and innovative way (Fradd 1994). The changing dynamics of child health have sought to blur professional boundaries (Porter 1996), providing an opportunity for the student and the educationalist to identify varied practice experiences which will help to prepare the student for the discrete role of CCN within a placement that reflects the belief and values of the service.

The framework for the community specialist practitioner (community children's nursing) experience must embrace a holistic approach to the care of sick children through a family-centred approach (Porter 1996) and must equip students with the appropriate knowledge and skills to undertake their complex and challenging role (Procter et al 1998, Whyte 1992). The experience must recognise that, unlike children in the hospital setting who are recipients of care in an artificially controlled environment, children in the community are in a setting well known to themselves and over which they and their family usually have some control. This sense of control and involvement in the care process must be fostered so that the child and family and the nurse work together.

The uniqueness of each child and family must be recognised and accepted as fundamental to the provision of nursing care. It is therefore important that the preparation of CCNs ensures that students value their individuality within the context of the home environment.

With the recognition that community care expands beyond the boundaries of nursing to overlap with the work of other caring agencies (Newbury et al 1997, Richardson 1996), the student must be encouraged to recognise and embrace the valuable contribution of other workers and professionals in the health and

BOX 9.1 ***English National Board statement of fitness for purpose: community specialist practitioner***

Practitioners who are skilled to meet changing healthcare needs should be (English National Board 1995):

- Innovative in their practice
- Responsive to changing demand
- Resourceful in their methods of working
- Able to share good practice and knowledge
- Adaptable to changing healthcare needs
- Challenging and creative in their practice
- Self-reliant in their way of working
- Responsible and accountable for their work

This includes the identification and integration of:

1. The existing knowledge and skills of the prospective student
2. The knowledge and skills required by the potential practice
3. The learning outcomes identified by the UKCC
4. The experiences available locally and identification of the potential alternative experiences available to complement the learning experience

social care field, and to explore ways in which collaborative partnerships can be developed. This approach should form the basis of teaching, learning and assessment in the practice environment, and is clearly illustrated by the English National Board (1995) (see Box 9.1).

To qualify as a specialist practitioner, the student must undertake a programme of study that meets the requirements set out by the UKCC. Programmes of specialist education should contain four broad areas of practice:

- Clinical practice
- Care and programme management
- Clinical practice development
- Clinical practice leadership

For the CCN, specific learning outcomes also include (UKCC 1994):

- **Clinical nursing practice** – assess, plan, provide and evaluate specialist clinical nursing care to meet care needs of acutely and chronically ill children at home
- **Care and programme management** –
  - initiate and contribute to strategies designed to promote and improve health and prevent disease in children, their families and the wider community
  - initiate action to identify and minimise risk to children and ensure child protection and safety
  - initiate management of potential and actual physical and psychological abuse of children and potentially violent situations and settings

These areas of practice must be translated into practice competencies which the student has to achieve to gain professional recognition from the UKCC

BOX 9.2 ***Range of potential students (Muir 1995)***

- Experienced CCNs with no community qualification
- Traditionally trained hospital-based paediatric nurses
- DipHE/RN(Child) nurses

within their area of specialist community practice. The specialist practitioner programme must be:

- At first degree level
- Include common core, not less than one-third and more than two-thirds of the total programme
- Flexible and modular
- Minimum of 1 year in length
- 50% theory and 50% practice

Entry requirements for the community children's nursing pathway are found in parts 8 and 15 of UKCC register (UKCC 1994). These criteria set the agenda for educationalists to develop courses that meet the requirements of the UKCC. For community children's nursing there is the added challenge of developing courses that address the many interpretations within practice delivery. This is further complicated by the fact that there are so few individuals who have the appropriate qualifications to provide the course. Given the infancy of this specialist education and the limited number of specifically qualified practitioners, this is understandable although problematic. Muir (1995) also identifies the potential challenge of addressing the possible diversity of students who may come from a wide variety of clinical backgrounds, all of whom have completely different individual learning needs (see Box 9.2). This requires careful consideration to ensure that all students have their learning needs met so that they can gain the most appropriate experience and achieve the professional competencies required to gain the community specialist practitioner (community children's nursing) qualification.

It is recognised that all students need to acquire new skills and knowledge in order to fulfil the generic role of community specialist practitioner (Porter 1996). Although students will enter the programme with a wide range of experience, their status on entry must be considered as that of a relative novice, in that they are being prepared for a new role within the community which brings new responsibilities and a higher level of decision making. Benner (1984) describes a model of levels of learning from novice to expert professional practitioner which is concerned with levels of professional activity on theory and practice (Table 9.2).

The ability to reflect upon performance is an essential feature, particularly relevant in the search for new knowledge to push forward the boundaries of professional knowledge, skills and attitudes (Porter 1996). The transition from novice to expert should be facilitated through reflective practice, the art of reflection being viewed as a central process in bridging the theory–practice gap in nursing. S Reveley (unpublished work, 1997) identified the skills required at community specialist practitioner level (Box 9.3). These skills are linked directly to the UKCC learning outcomes for the community specialist practitioner, which the student must achieve through the competence profile.

TABLE 9.2 ***Levels of learning: Benner's model (1984)***

Level	Description	Professional activity
Certificate	Novice	Competent professional practitioner who participates in professional activities safely and can discuss with confidence the theory and research that informs practice
Diploma	Competent	Proficient professional practitioner who responds flexibly to the needs of the individual, demonstrating the ability to analyse and evaluate quality of care critically
Degree	Proficient	Expert advanced professional practitioner who demonstrates expertise in a particular clinical or community setting by responding flexibly and creatively to situations in order to provide a quality personal service for clients and co-workers

BOX 9.3 ***The community specialist practitioner (S Reveley, unpublished work, 1997)***

- Acts as a team leader
- Manages resources effectively
- Manages a caseload
- Manages and supervises others
- Liaises and collaborates with other agencies
- Is an accountable decision maker
- Initiates and monitors patient/client care
- Uses evidence-based practice
- Develops and monitors standards of practice
- Develops clinical practice through research and experience
- Responds to clients' and carers' needs
- Promotes health where possible
- Empowers clients and carers
- Has highly developed clinical skills and uses these in an innovative manner

EDUCATION PROVISION

Pre-registration education is designed to equip practitioners with the knowledge, skills and attitudes needed to provide safe and effective care to children. However, pre-registration education alone does not prepare these practitioners adequately to meet the additional needs of specialist practice. Some practitioners are required to exercise higher levels of judgement, and higher levels of clinical decision making in practice, and will need to monitor and improve standards of care through supervising others. This will include undertaking clinical audit, skilled professional leadership and the development of practice through research, teaching and professional support of colleagues (UKCC 1994).

The course must recognise that community healthcare nurses are reflective practitioners, independent in attending to their learning needs, flexible in applying core principles to complex practical issues, and able to design solutions appropriate to meet individual needs. Through the learning process it is important that students contribute not only to their individual learning needs but also to the learning of others. Each student will bring to the course a variety of experiences, which in being shared, will both contribute to the learning that takes place and help shape the specific experience of the course for each student.

THE STUDENT

It is essential that each student can achieve all the UKCC learning outcomes and so be deemed competent within practice. As each student will be entering the pathway with a variety of experiences, the development of a personal profile enables students to reflect clearly on their own strengths and identify specific areas for development. For example, experienced hospital-based paediatric nurses may identify their specific needs as being the transfer of highly developed skills into the community setting, whereas the experienced community-based children's nurses may gain more by focusing on developing knowledge and skills by working with other members of the primary healthcare team.

To ensure that each student's needs are met within the educational standards of the specialist practitioner programme, it is important that the pathway leader meets with the student and identifies:

- Past nursing experience
- Individual learning needs
- The learning opportunities available within the district

The individual characteristics of each student must be taken into consideration in the placement selection process. A flexible approach is needed which takes into account the combination of (1) no single recognised model within practice and (2) the potential variety of student experience on entering the programme. The overall course experience must be developed to facilitate the diverse needs of each student. The educationalist must therefore negotiate with students to maintain a balance of recognising the individual needs of the student whilst incorporating the overall philosophy of community specialist practitioner education. It is essential that the integrity of the total educational experience is maintained. This further ensures that the student can gain the relevant experience to achieve the community specialist practitioner competencies for community children's nursing.

The experience for each student must be recognised as individual and dynamic. It is therefore essential that each student should identify their initial learning needs. The student and pathway leader will then be able to work together to plan the most appropriate clinical placement. At this point it is important that the needs of the service are borne in mind. It is expected that service managers will be involved in this discussion.

The initial needs assessment should result in an action plan. The student then maintains an ongoing personal 'needs analysis' (Neill & Muir 1997), a process that can be facilitated through the development of a personal profile (UKCC 1994). Students will demonstrate their needs and how these have been met through a learning contract, which will incorporate an action plan and evidence of how objectives have been achieved. As Neill & Muir (1997) explain, the learning experience is a dynamic process: the student's needs will develop and change. To facilitate this process, students maintain a reflective diary to help them identify their learning needs and specific areas of personal development.

BOX 9.4 *Skills and qualities required by community specialist practitioners*

- Reflective
- Independent in attending learning needs
- Flexible in applying core principles to complex practical issues
- Able to design solutions appropriate to meet individual needs

Learning contracts are a useful method of quantifying individual learning needs and can be used to inform the ongoing dialogue between student, pathway leader and community practice teacher, and will facilitate the development of community specialist practitioner skills (see Box 9.4).

DEVELOPING EDUCATION PROVISION IN THE CLINICAL SETTING

Two key challenges that relate to the process of establishing and running a community children's specialist practitioner pathway are placements and supervision.

The placement

Placements can be a particularly challenging issue, especially where no community children's nursing service exists. Even where services do exist, the provision can be focused on a specialist area such as cystic fibrosis, diabetes or asthma. Equally the service may be very limited in the provision offered. To move forward it is essential that a flexible, creative and responsive approach is taken which allows the student to play an integral part in the whole experience.

Students may identify their own areas for development that are not available to them within their current practice experience. Comparative practice can be utilised as a means of addressing these deficits. The length and type of experience will be dependent on the student's individual need. Trust managers must also be involved as students are guaranteed practical placements under the supervision of a community practice teacher. The placement will form part of a tripartite agreement between employer, student and the educational institution. The seconding manager is deemed to be someone who is in a position to guarantee placements, and their involvement is essential. Planning between the course tutor and the student is therefore a crucial component.

The supervision

The UKCC (1995) recognises the need for flexibility. In its position statement the UKCC stated that it 'does not advocate either statutory or prescriptive approach' nor a 'single model approach'. It also recognises that in some areas 'a colleague from another clinical profession may act as a clinical supervisor'. Some would argue that students should be supervised in practice only by a CCN, but situations dictate the need for alternative approaches. Muir (1995)

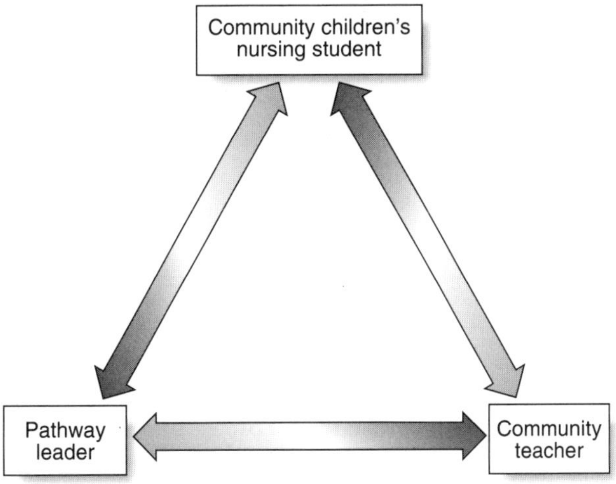

Figure 9.1 The tripartite model.

describes this as the 'chicken and egg' scenario whereby specialist students require supervision on courses in areas with no existing community children's nursing service. These students will become the future supervisors in practice. An innovative approach to the practice experience must therefore be adopted by all involved.

COMMUNITY PRACTICE TEACHERS

It is recognised and accepted that community practice teachers will vary in their experience to meet the individual learning needs of students. However, it is important that the experience is facilitated by a skilled practitioner to ensure that:

1. Concepts and principles of practice examined within the classroom are then applied in practice
2. The student is developing competently in their practice

The tripartite model has emerged to address the development of a more theory and practice-based experience (Neill & Muir 1997) (Figure 9.1). This model serves the student well as it allows for the diverse dynamics within practice, yet maintains the integrity of community children's nursing. The individual needs of students can be addressed as the student, pathway leader and community practice teacher are brought together to explore and develop the learning needs of each student.

For this approach to work it is essential that pathway leaders have a clear understanding of community children's nursing practice. Ideally they should hold the community children's nursing specialist practitioner qualification; however, as community children's nursing is relatively new for many areas this may be unrealistic. It is therefore essential that pathway leaders have at least a children's nursing qualification and a community nursing qualification. They play the pivotal role of linking theory and practice whilst maintaining the focus of community children's nursing practice between the student and the community practice teacher (Neill & Muir 1997). Without this appreciation there is a danger that the student will emerge as some form of quasi-community nurse who has an interest in the care of sick children.

As Neill & Muir (1997) explain, the role of the pathway leader is thus 'essential for the immediate development of future practitioners and the longer-term development or extension of the service'. My own experience as a pathway leader for the BSc(Hons) degree in community specialist practitioner (community children's nursing) provides an example of one possible approach to address the diverse issues faced in practice.

CASE STUDY

A local community Trust had recognised the need to develop a generic community children's nursing service. The College was asked by the Trust to provide an educational programme for a hospital-based children's nurse. To develop the programme there were a number of issues that needed to be considered. First, to meet the educational requirements and competency outcomes of the BSc(Hons) community specialist practitioner (community children's nursing) programme, it was essential that the student gain the necessary practice experience. The practice experience sought to equip the student with knowledge and skills that would not only meet local child health needs but would also provide expertise enabling the student to transfer her knowledge and skills to work within any community children's nursing practice throughout the country. Second, the educational needs of the student had to be taken into account. The student and pathway leader met to consider the following points:

- The student's past experience as a paediatric nurse
- The student's individual learning needs
- Preferred learning opportunities within the local area

The student had gained the DipHE/RN(Child) and worked within the hospital setting. She had previous experience within the community as a student nurse but had no post-registration experience within the community. After discussions with the community manager, a placement was arranged that provided the student with the experience of working within a primary healthcare team alongside a community practice teacher who was an experienced health visitor and community tutor. The rationale for this choice was to:

- Provide an insight into the role of all members of the primary healthcare team
- Appreciate the complexities of community care
- Gain a broader perspective of child health
- Enable a greater appreciation of the role of the health visitor

The placement was considered as a foundation from which the student could develop the knowledge and skills to work within a community setting. It was agreed with the community manager that, from this foundation, the student would develop a small community children's nursing caseload.

To ensure the student's individual learning needs were met, a 'tripartite' approach was taken. This involved the student, community practice teacher and pathway leader meeting three times per term to reflect on 'critical incidents' that arose in clinical practice. The tripartite arrangement addressed the practice dynamics (Figure 9.2).

As there was no generic community children's nursing service available, the experience of developing a community-based children's caseload as part of the practice development provided a unique opportunity to explore the real issues that would directly illustrate the theory–practice links. In addition, opportunities to visit and

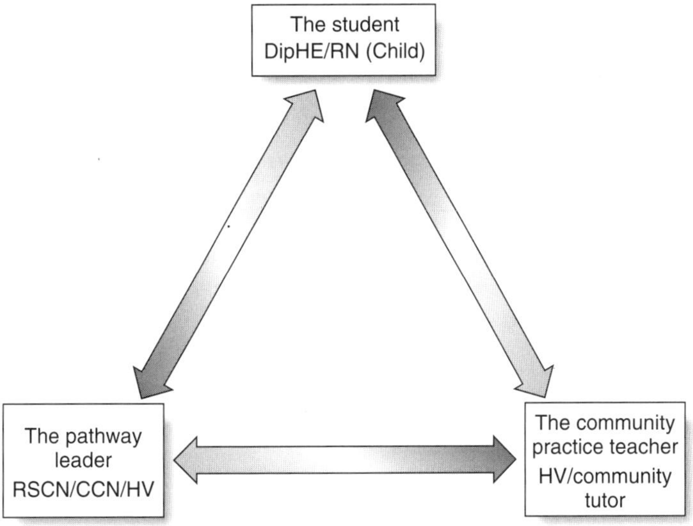

Figure 9.2 Tripartite approach used for community children's nursing students. CCN, community children's nurse; HV, health visitor; RSCN, registered sick children's nurse.

work with other community children's nursing teams around the country, and to visit local statutory and voluntary organisations, were arranged. The student gained valuable practice experience in three ways:

1. The student developed a community children's nursing caseload with the support of her pathway leader.
2. The student was assigned to a health visitor who was an experienced community tutor.
3. The student gained alternative experience in a variety of community children's nursing services throughout the country.

The practice experiences were structured around the student's learning contract. The student explored her learning needs and the development of competencies with the community practice teacher and pathway leader. These were discussed and negotiated within the tripartite meetings, which provided opportunities for the sharing of knowledge and allowed each professional perspective to be explored and debated. The practice developed as the student gained the necessary experience (see Box 9.5).

The caseload

This programme served the student's learning needs and enabled her to achieve the UKCC learning outcomes which were confirmed within the student's competence profile and evidenced within her portfolio of evidence. However, there were concerns pertaining to the potential practice caseload as there was no guarantee that the service would continue after the course ended. It was important to consider what would happen to the children and families on completion of the course. This could have posed an ethical dilemma if the service was withdrawn. This was addressed in two ways:

BOX 9.5 ***Development of the student's clinical practice***

Term 1 September–December	Term 2 January–March	Term 3 April–June	Term 4 July–September
The community	*Nursing in the community*	*Identifying areas for further development*	*Development of specialist role*
Understanding the child and family in context	Gaining alternative experiences	Developing a community children's nursing caseload	Consolidation

Development of caseload

Overall aims
Hospital children's nurse to community specialist practitioner
Transfer of skills from hospital to community

Overall outcomes
Understand community
Understand the broader concepts of child health
Understand the professional role within community practice

1. Through close liaison with the children's ward at the local district hospital and the consultant paediatrician in the selection of children cared for by the student during the course.
2. Through working closely with the health visitor so that she was able to offer continued support in the instances where children had been delegated for the student from the health visitor's caseload.

Consequently no problems arose. None the less, it could be argued that the 'caseload' did not reflect the realities of community children's nursing. Indeed, the size of the caseload did not, but the opportunity to focus on the complex issues of child health needs enabled the student to appreciate such issues as discharge planning and the uniqueness of each child's health needs, and to develop the protocols necessary to offer an effective service.

The placement sought to develop the student's appreciation of community practice *per se*. The experience also enabled the student to gain a greater understanding of the changing role of the health visitor and encouraged her to consider possible developments in collaborative working with other members of the primary healthcare team.

The challenge of developing a caseload within the community setting provided a valuable opportunity to explore the political context of child-focused provision and to consider how theories debated in the classroom can be directly applied in practice. In addition, the student visited other community children's nursing teams around the country and worked with other community practitioners within the area.

It was decided that the caseload would evolve as the student's educational needs were identified. Regular consultations with the consultant paediatrician and the nurses on the children's ward provided an opportunity to identify potential children who could benefit from the community children's nursing service.

There were some constraints that further restricted the service that the student could offer to children and their families:

1. **The limited time available to develop the service** – as the student had a specific number of practice hours to complete for the course, these were divided approximately into 2 days per week. Within this time the student also had to gain experience in other established practices.
2. **Uncertainty as to whether the service would continue after the course ended** – there were ethical considerations that had to be acknowledged. It was therefore decided that only children with short-term nursing needs and those who could be guaranteed continued care would be considered for the caseload.
3. **The student's own level of competence** – the student had to be aware of her own professional limitations and adhere to the UKCC Code of Professional Practice (1992).
4. **Potential resistance to change in established practice** – although the development of a community children's nursing service received support from many clinicians, some reservations and reluctance to accept alternative nursing care provision was experienced. However, there was overall support and enthusiasm which provided a healthy environment to develop the service.

This case study illustrates the principles necessary to devise educational experiences which meet the needs of individual students. A flexible approach is essential to facilitate the development of CCNs as Community Specialist Practitioners.

THE FUTURE

Community healthcare nursing is developing within a rapidly evolving health service alongside the changing pattern of child health. Children's nursing must be willing to embrace these changes. CCNs are strategically placed to develop services through their ability to be flexible, confident and competent in defining the needs of children and their families, and structuring their work to meet those needs. Although children's nurses have always striven to assert their role as advocates of children and their families, with ever-increasing demands and responsibilities being placed on families to care for their children, the need for intelligent, informed advocates for children and their families has never been stronger (Lock 1996). The community specialist practitioner programme provides the opportunity for education and practice to come together and inform the development of future practitioners to meet the challenges ahead.

FUNDING FOR COMMUNITY CHILDREN'S NURSING EDUCATION

Community children's nursing is a relatively young discipline. The work heralds the beginning of a new pattern of healthcare for sick children within the community. Problems lie in how the developments are recognised and valued within the various Trusts. This has a direct influence on how funding is made available for the educational development of nurses who seek to gain the community specialist qualification (CCN). Further problems arise with competition for funding between the traditional community nurses and the new areas of specialist practice. The allocation and arrangements for educational funding for community nurse education is decided at consortia level. Trusts are required to produce evidence to the consortia of workforce planning to support their applications for educational funding, which directly influences the maintenance and development of nursing services. These issues emphasise the need for educationalists and practitioners to work collaboratively with local Trust managers to raise awareness of the need to develop services for sick children within the community. Awareness needs to be raised at both a local and national level, clearly identifying and articulating the potential contribution of community children's nursing services to care for sick children at home (Neill & Muir 1997).

The Health Committee (1997) report acknowledged these problems and recommended that CCN education should be commissioned on the same basis as health visiting and district nursing education. The need for workforce planning is therefore central to the development. This requires evidence through detailed needs assessment. The Trusts, together with the newly emerging primary care groups (in England), need to identify clearly from this process the service that is required to address the health needs of children.

CONCLUSION

This chapter has explored a range of issues that affect the educational provision for community specialist practitioners (community children's nursing). As noted, the situation is characterised by the changes in child health provision, which is responding to the changing patterns of child health. The transfer of skills from hospital-based provision to community-focused care has led to the development of community children's nursing, which seeks to serve the needs of children and their families within their home and community. The service is still relatively young, with no single model of provision identified. It is therefore challenging for educationalists to develop community specialist practitioner courses that embrace the varied needs of potential students and practice. Innovative and flexible approaches, which include collaboration with professional colleagues, have allowed developments to move forward.

Within education provision, the task is set to continue to embrace the ever-changing needs in practice within a framework that provides a flexible approach but does not compromise the maintenance and development of clinical excellence.

FURTHER READING

Booth K & Luker K A (eds) 1999 A practical handbook for community health nurses. Blackwell Science, London

This book brings together the available evidence on a range of issues central to community nurses in their work with children and their families. The aim of the book is to provide an up-to-date reference source.

Cain P, Hyde V & Howkins E (eds) 1995 Community nursing: dimensions and dilemmas. Arnold, London

This book recognises that community nurses are at the sharp end of heathcare, needing to make decisions regarding problems for which there is never a single 'right' answer. The authors offer a rich mixture of ideas, arguments and information which explores and challenges the traditional values within the community healthcare system.

Gastrell P & Edwards J (eds) 1996 Community health nursing: framework for practice. Baillière Tindall, London

This broad-based text provides a stimulating resource to support the work and developments within community nursing practice. The book has taken a 'framework' approach to educational and professional development, which demonstrates the links between theoretical concepts and practice application. A useful book for students, community teachers and educators.

Robinson J & Elkan R 1996 Health needs assessment: theory and practice. Churchill Livingstone, London

This book was developed to assist community nurses to deal with the complex context of current issues surrounding the process of needs assessment so that they can contribute to the debates and develop their practice appropriately. The book addresses both the practical and theoretical perspectives.

REFERENCES

Benner P 1984 From novice to expert: excellence and power in clinical nursing practice. Addison-Wesley, Menlo Park, California

English National Board for Nursing, Midwifery and Health Visiting 1995 Creating lifelong learners. ENB, London

Fradd E 1994 A broader scope of practice. Professional development in paediatric nursing. Child Health, April/May:233–238

Health Committee 1997 House of Commons Select Committee. Health services for children & young people in the community: home and school. Third report. The Stationery Office, London

Hyde V 1995 Community nursing: a unified discipline? In: Cain P, Hyde V & Howkins E (eds) Community nursing: dimensions and dilemmas. Arnold, London: p 17

Lock K 1996 The changing organization of health care: setting the scene. In: Twinn S, Roberts B & Andrews S (eds) Community health care nursing. Principles and practice. Butterworth–Heinemann, Oxford, p 40

Muir J 1995 Community: the student perspective. Paediatric Nursing 7(8):8–10

Neill S J & Muir J 1997 Educating the new community children's nurses: challenges and opportunities. Nurse Education Today 17:7–15

Newbury J, Clarridge A & Skinner J 1997 Collaboration for care. In: Burley S, Mitchell E E, Melling K, Smith M, Chilton S & Cromplin C (eds) Contemporary community nursing. Arnold, London, p 77

Porter E 1996 The child. In: Twinn S, Roberts B & Andrews S (eds) Community health care nursing: principles for practice. Butterworth–Heinemann, Oxford, p 320

Procter S, Biott C, Campbell S, Edward S, Redpath N & Moran M 1998 Preparation for the developing role of the community children's nurse. English National Board, London

Richardson J 1996 Shifting boundaries in paediatric community nursing. In: Gastrell P & Edwards J (eds) Community health nursing: framework for practice. Baillière Tindall, London, p 286

Royal College of Nursing 1996 Community health care nurses: challenging the present, improving the future. Royal College of Nursing, London

UK Central Council 1992 The code of professional conduct. UKCC, London

UK Central Council 1994 The future of professional practice – the Council's standards for education and practice following registration. UKCC, London

UK Central Council 1995 Position statement on clinical supervision for nursing and health visiting. UKCC, London

Whiting M 1988 Community paediatric nursing in England in 1988. MSc thesis, University of London

Whyte D A 1992 A family nursing approach to the care of the child with chronic illness. Journal of Advanced Nursing 17:326–327

SECTION

2 PHILOSOPHICAL ISSUES UNDERPINNING THE DELIVERY OF COMMUNITY CHILDREN'S NURSING PRACTICE

Philosophical principles should permeate practice and require careful consideration. Legal and ethical frameworks are examined alongside more pervasive factors such as the need to deliver culturally sensitive care. This section also explores the everyday challenges of creating and maintaining the many complex relationships that develop in practice, including those between community children's nurses, children, their families and other professionals.

SECTION CONTENTS

10 Nursing the family and supporting the nurse: exploring the nurse–patient relationship in community children's nursing

Brian Samwell

KEY ISSUES

- Value and dangers of intense relationships between the community children's nurse and clients in the context of chronic childhood illness
- Family-centred care
- Key factors in managing intense relationships with children and families, on both an individual and a team level

INTRODUCTION

What is special about community children's nursing? As nurses we can focus on the increasing range of technical and practical care options that we can create in the community. As healthcare activists we can claim our role in redefining the nature of healthcare for children, moving the focus from hospital to community care. Yet many community children's nurses agree that their speciality is defined by the nature of the relationship they have with children and families. This chapter explores some aspects of that relationship and, in doing so, tries to define what is uniquely satisfying but also uniquely dangerous about the community children's nursing role. To do this, it focuses on the times when that relationship is most intense – when care is given to a child with a chronic or life-threatening illness or condition.

CARE OF THE CHILD WITH A CHRONIC ILLNESS

Care of the child with a chronic or serious illness presents a particular nursing challenge. While illness at any age is characterised by crisis and adaptation, in childhood this is superimposed on rapid physical, psychological and social growth. As the child grows, the manifestation and impact of the illness alters, and the psychological and social effects evolve. Such changes carry a potential for distress and psychological damage, often as great as the physical condition itself. This is highlighted by the fact that ill children show a higher incidence of behavioural problems and emotional difficulties than well children (Davis 1993).

The diagnosis of a serious childhood illness is also a crisis for parents. The illness threatens parents' ability to care for and protect their child and so becomes an attack on their own psychological integrity. They may grieve for the child and the anticipated future they have lost. Subsequent developments in diagnosis, condition or disability may compound and renew this sense of loss (Eiser 1993). Amidst this wholesale change in child and family expectations there is a demand to learn new skills: in nursing, in seeking information, and in dealing with a host of professional helpers. Family stress is inevitable, and both physical and psychological morbidity are a common consequence (Cairns 1992).

For the community children's nurse (CCN) to work effectively with these children and their carers, an understanding is needed of the problems and issues peculiar to care in this context. The nurse also needs a model of working which can sustain and make sense of a long-term supportive relationship rather than brief acute interventions. As Phil Madden has noted in the context of learning disability: 'Parents are at the start of a life long journey they did not bargain for. They need to know professionals are going to be with them' (Madden 1995 p 91). A supportive relationship with the child and family, which engages with problems as defined and experienced by them, is a central part of the CCN's role (Procter et al 1998). It is also the medium through which long-term therapeutic goals of child and family health, self-efficacy and empowerment might be attained. CCNs need both to understand and to work with this relationship.

FAMILY-CENTRED CARE

The most commonly used conception of the relationship between nurse and client is that of family-centred care. It is a phrase that has become the touchstone for children's nursing practice in the UK. Indeed, community children's nursing owes its origins to a belief in the benefits of nursing children in the safe and familiar home environment (Royal College of Nursing 1994). The needs of the child are considered within the context of the family unit, where family members are seen as the primary carers, and effective care depends on negotiation and partnership. However, the reality of social life stands in sharp contrast to any simple stereotype of the nuclear family. To work effectively within complex and varied family relationships can require quite exceptional insight and interpersonal skill (Whyte 1992). The range of these skills is suggested in Shelton et al's (1987) framework for family-centred care (Box 10.1).

While family-centred care gives a welcome emphasis to the nursing relationship, in practice it has shortcomings. First, it tends to be stated as a service philosophy with little exploration of the very difficult professional, ethical and political issues raised by a comprehensive definition such as Shelton's. Second, it does not deal with the mutual effects of creating a relationship. CCNs often

BOX 10.1 *A framework for family-centred care (Shelton et al 1987)*

- Recognition that the family is the constant in the child's life, whereas the service systems and personnel within those systems fluctuate
- Facilitation of parent–professional collaboration at all levels of healthcare
- Sharing of unbiased and complete information with parents about their child's care on an ongoing basis in an appropriate and supportive manner
- Implementation of appropriate policies and programmes that are comprehensive and provide emotional and financial support to meet families' needs
- Recognition of family strengths and individuality, and respect for different methods of coping
- Understanding and incorporating the developmental and emotional needs of infants, children and adolescents, and their families into healthcare delivery systems
- Encouragement and facilitation of parent to child support
- Assurance that the design of healthcare delivery systems is flexible, accessible and responsive to family need

work in isolation within exceptionally difficult situations. A nurse may need to work with 30 to 50 families, many of whom will be suffering extreme physical and emotional turmoil. The personal and practical implications of such care are the concern of the remainder of this chapter.

This chapter draws on the results of a pilot study which used the qualitative methodology of naturalistic inquiry to investigate the ways in which CCNs experience and manage long-term, intense relationships with families (Samwell 1999). The study involved interviews with four practising nurses drawn from community children's teams in northern England. Their accounts were analysed to map out the phenomenon of their involvement with families. To make the accounts more personal yet maintain confidentiality, fictitious names have been given to the four nurses.

REWARDS AND DANGERS OF THE NURSE–CLIENT RELATIONSHIP

Like many healthcare workers, CCNs see their relationships with clients as one of the most satisfying parts of their work. All of the nurses in the study reported that their relationship with children and parents was intensely rewarding, often giving them a reason to 'keep going' in a difficult and demanding job. They found the relationships to be more intense and more productive than those experienced in hospital, so much so that two of the nurses said they would never consider moving out of community nursing.

While the client relationship in community children's nursing can give a uniquely rewarding work experience, it can also draw nurses into an ever closer involvement with the families. Care in the home does not have the same inhibitions on involvement and intimacy as care in the busy hospital ward (May 1995, Totka 1996). Since most CCNs can ensure the continuity of their care, there is a greater potential to form personal bonds. Added to this, the nurse may identify closely with the family and the care situation, and find her nursing role confused by her personal roles of parent or protector (McAliley et al 1996). As a nurse in this study commented:

> 'You know how it feels not to have slept for the majority of the night and then to look after someone during the day, who is even more demanding than a normal healthy child. And how lucky I am to have two healthy kids really.'

In some circumstances close identification can lead the nurse to become a family friend or even to be seen as a part of the extended family. Yet such apparently simple human gestures can have dramatic personal effects. Participants described how their private time and emotional energy were absorbed by their personal commitment to families. As an example, the act of giving a home phone number could mean that the nurse was in effect never off duty:

> 'when I was at home I never felt as if I was off duty unless we went away. You couldn't have a drink, or I didn't feel I could have a drink at night just in case someone rang.'

Other examples of commitment included babysitting, visiting and socialising with families outside work hours, the giving of gifts, and helping families with all manner of personal favours. Jane described the temptation to try to organise everything for a family – to become a 'supernurse':

> 'You try to fill in all the forms for them [laughs], you know, sort the prescriptions out, take out the supplies and things like that, rather than sometimes saying 'Look! This is how you go about it ...'

The participants described not just their own emotional difficulties in moving on from close relationships, but also the potential hurt for the family when the attachment was broken. Dependency could become both a professional and a personal problem, as Mary found:

> 'They know all about me and how do I separate, extricate myself from this?'

The challenge of managing this boundary between a personal and a professional involvement became the focus for this study. What follows are just two of the significant themes that summarise the experiences and concerns of this group of nurses. The themes highlight aspects of practice that either help or hinder the nurse who is struggling to maintain balance in her relationships with clients.

BEING FRIENDLY AND PROFESSIONAL

For nurses, conscious of the power and danger that lie within their relationships with families, there was a need consciously to regulate self-presentation, so as to prioritise their professional responsibilities. Sarah described this regulation as 'being friendly and professional'. While there was the potential to be seen as a friend, the nurses saw the inequality in that friendship: 'they see you as a friend but you don't necessarily see them as a friend'. Honesty in the relationship required the drawing of a line between being friendly and being a friend.

Being friendly was the use of interpersonal skills to communicate an interest and commitment: 'You give the smiles, you laugh and you might give some information away about your personal life'. It included being attentive to the needs of child and family, and pacing communication so as to establish confidence and trust. But it also required a certain distance and objectivity. As Jane described, when wrestling with this dilemma:

> 'I think ... just a minute, it isn't acceptable to be there. I can't be objective. I can't be what I need to be for them if I'm too close, even though they want me to be that close.'

For Jane this objectivity was a necessary part of her professional standing: an ability to step back from the complexity of the family's problems in order to help them in their decision making, and to empower them rather than create dependence. The participants drew on their assessment skills and their experience in order to judge the fine line between commitment and over-involvement. Sarah described some of the guidelines she used:

> 'If I get drawn into conversations where families will say ... "if you want to pop round for a drink or whatever?" ... I will be quite firm about it and say no. I've learned to say now I don't mix business with pleasure really, which is not always easy.'
> 'Now one thing a colleague said to me ... if she finds that she is getting into a situation where this is happening (becoming over-involved) she actually will mentally say to herself 'Who are you doing this for?' ... if you at any point say you are not doing it for the family you're doing it for yourself, then you have gone too far.'

Such management requires sensitivity and skill. Jane noted the subtle signals that she might unwittingly give to a family by offering too much information about her personal life. The exchange of information had to be managed gently but firmly, so as to avoid signalling that a more personal friendship was possible or desirable. Such management required personal insight whereby the nurse could see the effect of her own needs, perhaps for affection or a 'need to be needed', which might drive her into a more intimate relationship.

THE LEARNING AND SHARING TEAM

The sharing of concern and commitment between nurse, child and family is clearly an aspect of personal practice. Yet the respondents in this study indicated the links between their personal practice and the wider world of team and health service organisation. Lack of resources was a key factor in forcing these nurses to over-commit themselves. Many families simply did not have the resources or continuity of support they needed, so, driven by compassion and a sense of duty, the nurse was forced to give her personal time and commitment.

The history of community children's nursing has been marked by piecemeal investment, with teams struggling to improve the quality and accessibility of their services (Health Committee 1997, Whiting 1997). All the respondents had experienced the danger and demoralisation of working in isolation, either as a 'team' of one, or within teams that had found no way of sharing the burdens of care. Yet these nurses also described how their teams had learned to respond to the private and personal demands of community children's nursing practice. These responses could be placed in two broad categories.

Creating a trusting and collaborative work environment

The ability of the team to share concerns and experiences was crucial. This did not mean that the team had to be a team of personal friends, but rather that communication within the team was actively prioritised and managed. Such communication took place on many levels, from the basic sharing of information so that all the team had some awareness of the work and concerns of individuals, to a sharing of feelings and a sensitivity to the pressures on colleagues. Ann and Jane could seek help from team members when they found they had got themselves into difficult situations with particular families. Their trust in colleagues meant that they did not always have to be seen to be coping with the demands of the job, but could ask for and expect both practical and emotional support.

All four nurses held their own caseloads, yet their teams had found ways to overcome the natural territoriality that comes with deep involvement. They were able to share knowledge of children and families and, on occasions, share the practical involvement. Jane felt that this sharing gave her 'breathing space' in intense relationships, which could at times seem unrelenting. For both Sarah and Jane it reduced dependence on them as individuals. The family could also benefit from the involvement of other team members who were less tied to the history and emotions in a situation. In addition, it gave the family access to the breadth of expertise of the whole nursing team. Such sharing could be powerful and enlightening:

> 'Well you just seem to be plodding along [with a care problem] and then, all of a sudden, it takes somebody else just to say "Perhaps you should have tried this".'

Team organisation

The participants had recognised the dangers of working in isolation and had developed practical ways of working collaboratively. Measures included a very basic commitment to sharing:

> 'Every day we go through all the patients that we have seen that morning and we discuss all the patients we have seen.'
> 'Not all the members of the team know all the children but as long ... as two or three members of the team know the child then that way we do get some continuity for sickness, annual leave and all these sort of things.'

Team meetings were given a high priority, and there was a willingness to discuss the interpersonal as well as the clinical dimensions of care. Ways were found for caseloads to be shared so that all the team members had some knowledge of the children on other caseloads. For one team it was a matter of principle that the named nurse would take the lead in establishing the relationship with a family but would then, over a period of weeks or months, gradually introduce the family to other team members. Families could come to see that care was not being delivered by one individual but by the whole team. For these nurses such very basic working practice was fundamental in helping them to cope with the stresses of their work. Perhaps such organisation appears exceptional only for nurses who had experienced the effect of its absence.

CONCLUSION

What does this exploratory study tell us about community children's nursing practice? First, it confirms the findings of studies by While (1991), Procter et al (1998) and others that the creation and maintenance of a supportive relationship with child and parent is an essential part of the CCN's role. Technical skills and clinical activity are vital but they do not define the work. Clearly a competence in interpersonal communication deserves much stronger emphasis in both the recruitment and training of CCNs. The management of relationships and relationship boundaries needs to be placed firmly on the educational agenda.

However, relationships are not determined solely by the ability or needs of the individual nurse. A nurse's skill or 'need to be needed' sit alongside other variables which may dictate the course of the relationship, such as the family's lack of resources or the nurse's want of practical and emotional support. Managers, planners and politicians must share responsibility for the personal consequences of under-resourced services. We need to ensure that effective, responsive care can be provided without sacrificing the personal time and resources of individual nurses. Similarly, community children's nursing teams have to examine the effect of their team organisation on individual team members, recognising situations where territoriality or individualised working are unhealthy or indeed dangerous.

This study demonstrated that the creation and management of working relationships is complex and demanding. CCNs do have difficulty in identifying the boundaries between their personal and their professional involvement with families. These participants gave examples of crossing the line, of becoming too deeply involved, which were very similar to the behaviours described by Totka and others (Coffman 1995, Totka 1996). However, the study did not find any simple list of rules that might serve to define or limit the nursing relationship. As Sarah found, she had personal guidelines, gleaned from many years of experience, but these were not written in stone and did not give a recipe for managing her relationships with children and families. Complex situations demand flexible responses.

The participants in this pilot study revealed just the tip of an iceberg of 'situational knowledge' or 'know-how' which they had acquired over time as expert practitioners in their field (Rolfe 1997). The nature of such learning presents both personal and professional challenges to CCNs. We have to find ways to uncover and share experience and expertise. Reflective practice might help to translate this personal experience into the public knowledge necessary to inform the next generation of CCNs. Clinical supervision has an important role in opening up and sharing the personal aspects of work relationships. Clearly there is also an urgent need to continue an exploration of the theoretical basis of community children's nursing practice.

Managing relationships with other people is central to the human experience. For CCNs it is also a crucial factor in effective therapeutic interventions with families exposed to the devastating effects of childhood illness and disability. Through exploring the nature of our relationships we can hope both to increase the power and influence of community children's nursing and to reduce the quite exceptional demands made on the nurses who give that care.

FURTHER READING

Dale N 1996 Working with families of children with special needs: partnership and practice. Routledge, London

An in-depth exploration of the relationship between family and professional which focuses on a partnership approach. Considers important issues such as consent, confidentiality and breaking the news of a diagnosis.

Morse J 1991 Negotiating commitment and involvement in the nurse–patient relationship. Journal of Advanced Nursing 16:455–468

An important piece of research which uses grounded theory methodology to explore the relationship between nurse and patient. Morse found different types of relationship characterised by different levels of interaction, commitment and trust.

REFERENCES

Cairns I 1992 The health of mothers and fathers of a child with a disability. Health Visitor 65(7):238–239

Coffman S 1995 Crossing lines: parents' experiences with paediatric nurses in the home. Rehabilitation Nursing Research 4(4): 136–143

Davis H 1993 Counselling parents of children with chronic illness and disability. British Psychological Society, Leicester

Eiser C 1993 Growing up with a chronic disease. Kingsley, London

Health Committee 1997 House of Commons Health Select Committee. Health services for children and young people in the community: home and school. Third report. The Stationery Office, London

McAliley L, Ashenberg M, Lambert S & Dull S 1996 Therapeutic relations decision making: the Rainbow framework. Pediatric Nursing 22(3):199–203

Madden P 1995 Why parents: how parents. British Journal of Learning Disabilities 23:90–93

May C 1995 Patient autonomy and the politics of professional relationships. Journal of Advanced Nursing 21:83–87

Procter S, Biott C, Campbell S, Edward S, Redpath N & Moran M 1998 Preparation for the developing role of the community children's nurse. English National Board, London

Rolfe G 1997 Beyond expertise: theory, practice and the reflexive practitioner. Journal of Clinical Nursing 6:93–97

Royal College of Nursing 1994 Wise decisions: developing paediatric home care teams. Royal College of Nursing, Paediatric Community Nurses Forum, London

Samwell B 1999 Relationship boundaries in community children's nursing. MA dissertation, University of Sheffield

Shelton T, Jepson E & Johnson B 1987 Family centred care of children with special health care needs. Association for the Care of Children's Health, Washington, DC

Totka J 1996 Exploring the boundaries of paediatric practice: nurse stories related to relationships. Pediatric Nursing 22(3):191–196

While A 1991 An evaluation of a paediatric home care scheme. Journal of Advanced Nursing 16:1413–1421

Whiting M 1997 Community children's nursing: a bright future? Paediatric Nursing 9(4):6–8

Whyte D 1992 A family nursing approach to the care of a child with a chronic illness. Journal of Advanced Nursing 17:326–327

11 Relationships between outreach nurses and primary healthcare professionals

Jane Hunt

KEY ISSUES

- The degree of 'hands-on' nursing care provided by outreach nurses influences the type of relationship they develop with primary healthcare professionals.
- 'Empowerment' is an enriching experience for primary healthcare professionals.
- 'Partnership' evolves through communication with primary healthcare professionals at an early stage in a child's illness trajectory.
- 'Disempowerment' may result as a consequence of outreach nurses providing a predominantly 'hands on' type of care.
- 'Disempowerment' arises through poor communication and may be professionally unfulfilling for some primary healthcare professionals.

INTRODUCTION

This chapter addresses professional relationships between children's nurses whose work extends into the community and primary healthcare professionals. Drawing on the findings from a study which examined relationships between paediatric oncology outreach nurse specialists (POONSs) and other healthcare professionals (Hunt 1996, 1998a, 1998b), three approaches to professional relationships are described: 'empowerment', 'partnership' and 'disempowerment'. These findings may be applied to most children's nurses working across acute hospital and community settings, particularly when providing care to chronically sick children with rare conditions, such as malignant disease and some renal, hepatic, neurological and gastrointestinal disorders, who have been previously well. The term 'outreach nurse' is therefore used to refer to POONSs and to other children's nurses whose work extends from hospitals into the community. 'Primary healthcare professionals' collectively refers to district nurses, health visitors and general practitioners (GPs).

SETTING THE SCENE

'Shared care' is particularly well developed in the care of children with malignant disease (Curnick 1990, Gibson & Williams 1997, Goldman 1990, Greener 1998, Hooker & Williams 1996, Hunt 1991, 1998a, Hulley & Hyne 1993, Patel et al 1997) and has been enhanced through the development of outreach nursing services (Bignold et al 1995, Hunt 1998a, 1998b). The term may be applied when patient care is shared between primary and tertiary settings, between primary and secondary care, or between primary, secondary and tertiary carers (Hunt 1998a). Such practices have been recognised in the care of sick children with a variety of medical conditions since the 1980s (Bacon 1989).

Outreach nursing services, provided from either secondary or tertiary healthcare settings, are of particular importance to primary healthcare professionals who share the care of children with rare medical conditions with acute hospital providers. When such children are registered with a GP practice or health centre, relationships developed with outreach nurses can have a lasting impact not only on relationships formed between primary healthcare professionals and outreach nurses but also on relationships maintained between primary healthcare professionals and families in their care (Hunt 1998a, 1998b).

THE RESEARCH

This chapter draws on qualitative interview data from the second stage of a large two-part study which explored the impact of different funding arrangements on the professional relationships between POONSs and other healthcare professionals (Hunt 1996, 1998a). The first stage was designed to understand better the structure, organisation and working practices of POONSs. Interviews were conducted with all POONSs in post in the UK and the Republic of Ireland during 1993, using a semi-structured interview schedule (n = 43). Findings from the first stage of the study have been reported elsewhere (Hunt 1994a, 1994b, 1995, 1996, 1998a).

The second stage was designed to examine the perceptions and experiences of healthcare professionals working with POONSs. It comprised case studies at three locations, which have been given pseudonyms to maintain their anonymity: Southern Regional, Northern City Children's and Westlands District. The case studies comprised focused in-depth interviews with a broad cross-section of community and hospital-based healthcare professionals including: senior and junior medical and nursing staff, specialist social workers, GPs, health visitors and district nurses. Sixty-five interviews took place between October 1994 and April 1995, 46 of which were conducted with primary healthcare professionals. Participants from the primary healthcare settings are summarised in Table 11.1. Four major themes emerged from the data: team work, relationships between POONSs and other nurses, relationships between POONSs and doctors, and specialist knowledge.

AN 'EMPOWERMENT' RELATIONSHIP

Rare childhood diseases, such as malignancy, and the anxieties that these invariably create (Faulkner et al 1994, Hunt 1998a, 1998b, Peace et al 1994) mean

TABLE 11.1 *Interviews conducted at case study sites*

Primary healthcare interviewees	Southern Regional area	Westlands District area	Northern City area
GP (newly diagnosed patients)	5 (I)	4* (I)	4 (I)
GP (terminal care)	4 (I)	3* (I)	4 (I)
Health visitor (depending on age of child)	4 (1G, 3I)	3 (2I, 1G)	1 (I)
District nurse (depending on disease status of child)	6 (2G, 4I)	3 (I)	6 (I)
Total no. of interviews	19 (16I, 3G)	12* (11*I, 1G)	15 (15I)

*One GP was included twice as interviewed in connection with both a newly diagnosed child and a terminally ill child. I, individual interviews; G, group interviews (two to four interviewees).

BOX 11.1 *Summary of 'partnership', 'empowerment' and 'disempowerment' relationships*

Empowerment
- Primary healthcare professionals taught clinical skills
- District nurses more involved in decision-making processes during child's terminal care
- 'Moderate' levels of communication, facilitated by 'on-call'

Partnership
- Health visitors visited by outreach nurses to develop professional relationships
- District nurses given access to newly diagnosed children
- Greater contact generally between health visitors and outreach nurses
- GPs offered visits to discuss newly diagnosed children

Disempowerment
- Fewer district nurses involved in patient care
- Poorer relationships developed between district nurses and families
- Fewer visits or phone calls to all primary healthcare professionals
- Inconsistent contact with GPs at outset of illness
- No participation of GPs to plan terminal care
- Less face-to-face contact with district nurses and GPs
- Crisis intervention contact with health visitors
- Health visitors and district nurses 'intrude' on relationships established between outreach nurses and families

that primary healthcare professionals can provide specialised care to children at home only if 'empowered' to do so. POONSs who predominantly provide 'hands off' nursing care demonstrated their abilities to empower primary healthcare professionals in this study in a number of ways (Hunt 1996, 1998a, 1998b). Features of 'empowerment' are summarised in Box 11.1.

Teaching and learning 'specialist' skills

A major feature of 'empowerment' involves primary healthcare professionals acquiring 'specialist' skills. In this study, those most commonly referred to are gaining confidence in managing central venous access devices (usually Hickman lines) and gaining knowledge about symptom control during terminal care. Being taught clinical skills enhances primary healthcare professionals' abilities to become decision makers.

Becoming decision makers during terminal care

When the focus of a child's care switches from the hospital to the community, such as during terminal care, primary healthcare professionals, and more particularly district nurses, may be 'empowered' to become decision makers. District nurses in this study considered that POONSs made major decisions about changing drugs or dosages. 'Empowerment' was achieved when district nurses were 'empowered' to provide the daily care required to make small modifications to drug dosages and change syringes of morphine for intravenous administration. As one district nurse said: 'towards the end [the POONS] wasn't actually involved as much with us once we got him pain controlled' (DN4, Northern City area).

Communication within an 'empowerment' relationship

'Empowerment' results in handing over components of care once 'specialist' skills have been learnt by primary healthcare professionals. It follows, therefore, that a feature of 'empowerment' concerns the degree of communication between outreach nurses and primary healthcare professionals: the necessity for outreach nurses to continue contact with primary healthcare professionals, once empowered, may be maintained at 'moderate' levels (Hunt 1996, 1998a, 1998b).

'Empowerment' is further achieved when communication is enhanced by the provision of an on-call service. Although most POONSs in this study provided on-call services, the ways in which these services operated varied (Hunt 1996, 1998a, 1998b). 'Empowerment' is accomplished through the provision of a 24-hr on-call service to primary healthcare professionals during a child's terminal illness. This enables primary healthcare professionals to make immediate contact with outreach nurses should they be contacted by parents or encounter a situation with which they are unfamiliar. They then gain the information and confidence on which to act and are thus 'empowered' to provide that care. As one district nurse in this study commented:

> 'I knew that I could get hold of [the POONS] if I'd got a problem in the last couple or three weeks and by that time I had got to know her well enough to sort of phone her and say, 'I can't cope with this, can you sort of come out', so I had as much contact with her as I felt I needed.'
> (DN3, Northern City area)

Effects of empowerment on primary healthcare professionals

'Empowerment' is an enriching experience for primary healthcare professionals. Whilst many interviewed during the course of this study started off feeling anxious about caring for dying children, those who developed an 'empowerment' relationship with POONSs experienced a sense of satisfaction through their own achievements. It enabled them to solve problems and to gain a sense of control in the care being provided. They were also rewarded by their close relationships developed with families. One district nurse who had had a particularly difficult time, working with a family unable to accept the impending death of their child, summed up her experiences thus:

> 'the experience ... was not a pleasant one except I'm really pleased I got the opportunity to work with [a POONS] ... and, who knows, maybe we'll work together in the future.' (DN5, Northern City area)

A 'PARTNERSHIP' RELATIONSHIP

A 'partnership' relationship differs from 'empowerment' in that some components of care are retained by outreach nurses rather than handed over to primary healthcare professionals. Furthermore, 'partnerships' evolve at an early stage of a child's 'journey' through chronic illness. 'Partnership' relationships exist between primary healthcare professionals and outreach nurses when a 'mixed' type of nursing is practised where both 'hands on' and 'hands off' nursing care may be provided by outreach nurses. 'Partnership' relationships were demonstrated in a number of ways in this study and features of 'partnership' are summarised in Box 11.1.

Communication in 'partnership'

A mixed 'hands on' and 'hands off' approach to care, particularly during a child's terminal illness, facilitates primary healthcare professionals in providing some care to patients whilst the majority is retained by outreach nurses (Hunt 1996, 1998a). It follows, therefore, that there are features of communication between outreach nurses and primary healthcare professionals, in 'partnership', which differ from 'empowerment'. Here, frequent communication between outreach nurses and primary healthcare professionals is necessary so that both parties know who is doing what. 'Partnership' relationships consequently involve 'high' levels of communication between outreach nurses and primary healthcare professionals. In this study, these 'high' levels of communication were maintained by POONSs making large numbers of telephone calls and visits to health centres and from their conducting joint home visits with district nurses (Hunt 1996, 1998a). This latter means of communication enhances opportunities for face-to-face contact, which is much valued by primary healthcare professionals (Hunt 1998a).

Forging relationships at the outset of the 'journey'

A key characteristic of 'partnership', which is closely linked to communication, concerns the establishment of professional relationships with primary healthcare professionals at the outset of a child's 'journey' through chronic illness.

Here, visits to health centres are provided by outreach nurses once treatment has been initiated. These visits allow for a mutual exchange of information and recognise that GPs and health visitors have often had long-standing relationships with families before a child's diagnosis is made.

Relationships between GPs and families, in particular, are often well established before a child's diagnosis. GPs in this study had frequently been contacted by POONSs at the outset of a child's disease and, regardless of the type of relationship formed, most valued telephone calls from POONSs. Without face-to-face contact, however, some GPs had difficulty remembering the information they had been given, with many recognising that POONSs had made little impact on their practice. As one GP explained: 'remembering the existence of these people ... and registering change is something that the human brain has difficulty with' (GP12, Northern City area). In this study, a 'partnership' developed only when outreach nurses offered to visit GPs at their surgeries, establishing face-to-face contact.

In this study, district nurses were generally referred children who were terminally ill, often for specific task-related purposes. However, where a 'partnership' was established, access to families was negotiated for district nurses by outreach nurses at the outset of a child's illness trajectory rather than at the onset of terminal care. Early referrals to district nurses were appreciated by them as a building block on which to develop future working relationships: 'this was just an introduction to build ships on' (DN15, Southern Regional area).

A 'DISEMPOWERMENT' RELATIONSHIP

If the notion of 'empowerment' is implicit through a 'hands off' approach to nursing, then it follows that 'disempowerment' may be a consequence of a 'hands on' type of care being provided by outreach nurses. Some of the characteristics that contribute to 'disempowerment' are highlighted here and are outlined in Box 11.1.

Unplanned referrals

One feature of 'disempowerment' concerns a lack of forward planning and involvement of primary healthcare professionals at key stages of a child's chronic illness 'journey'. An example of this was demonstrated in this study by GPs whose contact with POONSs at the outset of a child's 'cancer journey' was 'hit and miss'. Some GPs said they had not been contacted at all by the POONS in their locality whilst others in the same area reported several discussions with a POONS.

A second example of unplanned referrals in this study includes contact with GPs at the onset of a child's terminal illness. In one of the study areas no GPs had been contacted at the outset of a child's terminal care, and any contact between themselves and the POONS they worked with was often more by chance than planned. For example one GP commented: 'I met [a POONS] ... a couple of times by accident because she happened to be in the house' (GP7, Westlands District area).

In 'disempowerment' relationships, referrals to district nurses are similarly unplanned, with access to patients being provided by 'gatekeepers' other than outreach nurses. In one of the areas studied few district nurses were involved in a child's terminal care (Hunt 1998a, 1998b), and those who were had not been notified by the local POONS service but by other healthcare professionals. For example, one district nurse gained access to a terminally ill child through her close working relationship with a GP, whilst another (unaware of a POONS's involvement) was requested by the intensive care unit at the local hospital to care for an adolescent patient with a Hickman line. The referral was late in the patient's care and, like others, was unplanned and un-coordinated:

> 'in my view I met him too late because at this stage he was receiving treatment through a central venous line ... considering we had an awful lot of nursing care to give at the end it would've been nice to have been involved at an early stage.' (DN7, Westlands District area)

Communication in a 'disempowerment' approach

'Disempowerment' occurs when outreach nurses establish only 'minimal' communication between themselves and primary healthcare professionals. In this study, 'minimal' communication was particularly manifested by those POONSs who made limited numbers of telephone calls and visits to district nurses (Hunt 1996, 1998a). When terminal care lacks coordination, and initial contact between outreach nurses and primary healthcare professionals is erratic, continuing communication is likely to remain poor. Whilst some GPs in this study considered their lack of contact with a POONS, and consequent exclusion from care, to be in the best interest of families, others reflected on the detrimental long-term implications this had had on their professional relationships both with the families concerned and, on occasions, with their colleagues. Two GPs in particular considered their lack of contact with a POONS resulted in families perceiving that they were uninterested and uncaring. These families consequently withdrew from the practices following the death of their child.

Without the establishment of face-to-face contact, poor communication was augmented, compounding 'disempowerment'. This point is illustrated by one district nurse who commented: 'we could have had more face-to-face contact [making] liaison a little easier perhaps' (DN8, Westlands District area).

In a 'disempowerment' relationship, attempts at two-way communication may also be hampered if community staff have difficulty in making contact with outreach nurses. This point is illustrated again by the district nurse in this study who was referred an adolescent patient from the intensive care unit. She commented:

> 'it was also very difficult to get hold of [the POONS] ... it was difficult to track her down, to contact her ... so the arrangement was a message left up on the children's ward and it didn't always work out that we contacted one another.' (DN7, Westlands District area)

The consequence of diminished communication between outreach nurses and primary healthcare professionals is that poor working relationships ensue.

Although poor communication between some POONSs and GPs was apparent in this study, both at the outset of a child's disease and during terminal care, it was particularly explicit through the poor relationships developed between POONSs and district nurses.

Displacing primary healthcare professionals

In 'disempowerment' relationships, displacement of healthcare professionals sometimes occurs. In this study, health visitors were more commonly displaced than other primary healthcare professionals, sometimes being prevented from fulfilling their roles. Health visitors felt that contact with outreach nurses was limited, occurring primarily as a result of 'crisis intervention'. These points are best summed up thus:

> 'I would've been, perhaps been, a more regular visitor if [the POONS] hadn't been involved, so that would've put more onus on me as a support worker.' (HV8, Westlands District area)

> 'I think in some ways maybe I was only contacted because of the, the difficulties in getting this diagnosed and there was a little bit of ill feeling between, I think, the relationships between some of the professionals and I think this is why I was brought in, not to pour oil on troubled waters but there was obviously a lot of unhappiness there.' (HV9, Westlands District area)

Intruding upon established relationships

Many of those interviewed during the course of this research talked of the particularly close relationships that develop between POONSs and families. These close relationships, it was believed, arose through the POONS's abilities to 'boundary hop' between the hospital and the community (Hunt 1998a, 1998b). However, this can contribute to 'disempowerment' when primary healthcare professionals consider they 'intrude' upon these relationships. In this study, this occurred most commonly when district nurses were not provided with direct access to patients by outreach nurses, which resulted in uncertainty about their roles. However some health visitors also considered they were intruding upon relationships between families and POONSs despite having long-established relationships with families themselves. This 'intrusion' is best illustrated by a health visitor who commented:

> 'you find sometimes when a family has a very close bond with a particular professional you almost feel that you're intruding' (HV9, Westlands District area).

Effects of 'disempowerment'

This study found one of the adverse consequences of disempowerment relationships to be that little is learnt by primary healthcare professionals about the disease processes and management of the particular illness. Hence, an air of mysticism about the disease remained. In addition, district nurses and health visitors did not feel professionally fulfilled by this type of relationship and some were left questioning their role. This is epitomised by one district nurse who said:

> 'I didn't know who was in control of the patient's care because she was involved ... so I didn't really know who was in control of the situation ... in the end I took control of the situation when he became bedridden and wasn't able to go to the hospital ... so we were two separate bodies giving what we thought was the right care but nothing was co-ordinated.' (DN7, Westlands District area)

CONCLUSION

This chapter has discussed three approaches to professional relationships: 'empowerment', 'partnership' and 'disempowerment'. Whilst these approaches were identified through a study that examined the professional relationships between POONSs and primary healthcare professionals, implications for all children's outreach nurses have been drawn.

'Empowerment' occurs when outreach nurses work with primary healthcare professionals, teaching and thereby enabling them to participate actively in the care of sick children. 'Partnership' evolves when outreach nurses work closely with primary healthcare professionals, retaining much nursing care themselves, but forming close links with the professionals, particularly during the early days of a child's illness. 'Disempowerment' arises when outreach nurses maintain more limited contact with primary healthcare professionals, informing them but rarely sharing skills or seeking their active participation in a child's care.

Whether outreach nurses 'empower' primary healthcare professionals, work in 'partnership' with them or 'disempower' them, depends on the degree to which hands-on care is provided by outreach nurses. 'Empowerment' is associated with outreach nurses who provide 'hands off' care to children in their own homes, 'partnership' arises when both 'hands on' and 'hands off' care is provided, and 'disempowerment' may be a result of 'hands on' care being retained by outreach nurses.

Whilst it might be appealing to outreach nurses to build very close relationships with sick children and their families, and to provide all nursing care themselves, the 'disempowerment' relationship described in this study indicates that there are problems for primary healthcare professionals with this approach. Adopting either 'empowerment' or 'partnership' relationships with primary healthcare professionals allows outreach nurses' knowledge and experience to cascade down to greater numbers of healthcare professionals, potentially benefiting more sick children and their families. Such approaches to healthcare provision have also underpinned government policy during the 1990s and have been equated with 'good practice' (e.g. Department of Health 1993, 1994, 1996, 1998, Dorrell 1996, National Health Service Management Executive 1996).

FURTHER READING

Breton M 1994 On the meaning of empowerment and empowerment-oriented social work practice. Social Work with Groups 17(3):23–37

This paper addresses two main questions: (1) What does it mean for people who are disempowered or unempowered to become empowered? and (2) What does it mean for practitioners to work within an empowerment-oriented approach? Five components are deemed essential for the disempowered to become empowered: (1) social action, (2) political awareness, (3) the right to say and 'have a say', (4) recognising oneself and being recognised as competent, and (5) the use of power. Collegiality is viewed as one of the principles of achieving empowerment-oriented practice within social work.

Casey A 1995 Partnership nursing: influences on involvement of informal carers. Journal of Advanced Nursing 22:1058–1062

Drawing on work that was conducted as part of a Master's degree, Casey views the partnership model, described in her earlier work, as rhetorical rather than a reality. Drawing on communication and nursing style, a framework to describe parental involvement is developed. This comprises: (1) communicating/nurse-centred: permission, (2) non-communicating/nurse-centred: exclusion, (3) non-communicating/person-centred: assumption and (4) communicating/person-centred: negotiation.

Darbyshire P 1994 Living with a sick child in hospital: the experiences of parents and nurses. Chapman & Hall, London

Darbyshire's doctoral study explores how parents adapt to living in hospital with a sick child and nurses' reactions to this 'living in' process. In his conclusions he challenges components of Foucauldian power discrepancy theories between healthcare professionals and patients, and suggests that valued caring practices of nurses are empowering for parents.

Gibson C H 1995 The process of empowerment in mothers of chronically ill children. Journal of Advanced Nursing 21:1201–1210

This paper draws on an empirical study which set out to describe the process of empowerment as it pertains to mothers of chronically sick children. Four components to the process emerged: (1) discovering reality, (2) critical reflection, (3) taking charge and (4) holding on. Empowerment was therefore viewed largely as a personal experience, although it is perceived as intertwining with interpersonal processes.

REFERENCES

Bacon C J 1989 Shared care in paediatrics. Archives of Disease in Childhood 64(14):8–9

Bignold S, Cribb A & Ball S J 1995 Creating a 'seamless web of care – the work of paediatric oncology outreach nurse specialists. In: Richardson A & Wilson-Barnett J (eds) Nursing research in cancer care. Scutari, London, p 67

Curnick S 1990 Domiciliary nursing care. Cited In: Baum J D, Dominica F & Woodward R N (eds) Listen, my child has a lot of living to do. Oxford University Press, Oxford, p 28

Department of Health 1993 Changing childbirth. HMSO, London

Department of Health 1994 Working in partnership: the report of the mental health nursing review. HMSO, London

Department of Health 1996 Child health in the community: a guide to good practice. The Stationery Office, London

Department of Health 1998 Working together: securing a quality workforce for the NHS. The Stationery Office, London

Dorrell S 1996 Primary care: the future. NHS Executive, London

Faulkner A, Peace G & O'Keeffe 1994 When a child has cancer. Chapman & Hall, London

Gibson F & Williams J 1997 Network of care for children and teenagers with cancer: an overview for adult cancer nurses. Journal of Cancer Nursing 1(4):200–207

Goldman A 1990 Domiciliary symptom control. In: Baum J D, Dominica F & Woodward R N (eds) Listen, my child has a lot of living to do. Oxford University Press, Oxford, p 38

Greener T 1998 Children's and families' perceptions of paediatric oncology shared care. BSc dissertation, University of Surrey

Hooker L & Williams J 1996 Parent-held shared care records: bridging the communication gaps. British Journal of Nursing 5(12):738–741

Hulley M & Hyne J 1993 Using parent-held records in an oncology unit. Paediatric Nursing 5(8):15–16

Hunt J 1991 Partnership in care for children at home: the development of the peripatetic nurse specialist. Nursing Standard (Special Supplement) 5(45):18–19

Hunt J 1994a Nursing uniform: what nurses in mufti wear. Paediatric Nursing 6(6):16–18

Hunt J A 1994b Paediatric oncology community nurse specialists – towards a model of good practice. Interim report to the United Kingdom Children's Cancer Study Group, Royal College of Nursing, Society of Paediatric Nursing, Paediatric Oncology Community Nurses Special Interest Group and the Paediatric Oncology Nurses Forum, London

Hunt J A 1995 The paediatric oncology community nurse specialist: the influence of employment location and funders on models of practice. Journal of Advanced Nursing 22:126–133

Hunt J A 1996 Paediatric oncology outreach nurse specialists: the impact of funding arrangements on their professional relationships. A report to the Paediatric Oncology Nurses Forum and the Paediatric Oncology Outreach Nurses Special Interest Group, Royal College of Nursing and the UK Children's Cancer Study Group.

Hunt J A 1998a Mixed funding within the British health care system: an examination of the effects on professional relationships between paediatric oncology outreach nurse specialists and other health care professionals. PhD thesis, University of Surrey

Hunt J A 1998b Empowering health care professionals: a relationship between primary health care teams and paediatric oncology outreach nurse specialists. European Journal of Oncology Nursing 2(1):27–33

National Health Service Management Executive 1996 Patient partnership: building a collaborative strategy. NHSME, Leeds

Patel N, Sepion B & Williams J 1997 Development of a shared care programme for children with cancer. Journal of Cancer Nursing 1(3):147–150

Peace G, O'Keeffe C & Faulkner A 1994 Whose role is it anyway? Child Health 1(6):239–243

12 Philosophy and ethics of home care

Imelda Charles-Edwards

KEY ISSUES

- Parental consent and partnership with families
- Consent to treatment
- Children's rights
- Advocacy
- Acting in a child's best interests

INTRODUCTION

This chapter explores ethical problems faced by all children's nurses but set within the context of community nursing. The starting point of this discussion is the case history of Freddy Shepherd, a 10-year-old boy with severe cerebral palsy. Freddy was cared for by his parents, the community children's nurses (CCNs) and also his local hospital children's unit. The impact of his location on the outcome of decisions made about Freddy exemplifies the value of considering ethical dilemmas in community as opposed to hospital practice.

Underpinning this discussion of some of the ethical dilemmas that face CCNs are foundations of moral philosophy. These are implicit rather than being made explicit, and the interested reader is given references for further reading.

The chapter will conclude with a brief discussion of the difficulty the law experiences in making decisions about children in areas such as child protection and juvenile crime. These issues are relevant for all children's nurses but are particularly so for community nurses working within primary healthcare and for a child's normal environment.

CASE STUDY *Freddy Shepherd's story*

The beginning

Freddy is 10 years old. He has cerebral palsy with profound mental and physical disabilities. His parents normally care for him at home with the help of the community children's nursing team, but because of repeated chest infections he has been admitted to the local hospital. Initially, and with the agreement of all, Freddy was given oxygen but not antibiotics and a 'do not resuscitate' decision was made. At this point the aims of Freddy's care were palliative; however, his paediatrician requested investigations to determine whether Freddy's chest infections were caused by a poor swallowing mechanism. It was shown that this was indeed the case. Mary and Tim, Freddy's parents, described this as 'death by drowning'.

Questions:

1. *Is it more difficult to continue palliative care rather than active treatment in hospital than it is in a child's home? If Freddy had not been admitted to hospital, investigations, with the potential that the results would prompt active treatment, would not have been performed.*
2. *Did Mr and Mrs Shepherd understand the significance of the investigation – that the result could lead to active medical intervention? Should they have been more fully informed?*
3. *What is the effect of partnership with parents on the process of giving consent?*

The next phase

Mary and Tim, his parents, described Freddy's aspiration on swallowing as 'killing him by drowning' and they supported the institution of enteral feeding. Initially a nasogastric tube was used for feeding but then the advantages of a gastrostomy were accepted by Mary and Tim, and Freddy was admitted for this procedure. The possibility of performing a Nissen procedure to minimise gastric reflux and aspiration was mooted. After some months at home Mary and Tim expressed ambivalence to the CCNs about the prolonging of Freddy's life.

Questions:

1. *Should Freddy's key worker, such as the CCN, have been asked to contribute to the implicit decision to change the aims of Freddy's care and act as an advocate and uphold his rights?*
2. *If Freddy had physical disabilities only and was able to participate in the decisions about his future, how should the options have been discussed with him and what value should be placed on his point of view?*

The last phase

Freddy started to put on weight. His activity was minimal but enteral feeding allowed his nutritional intake to be increased to a level approximating his expected weight. Mary and Tim experienced increasing difficulty in moving Tim. While the CCNs were trying to arrange a hoist for the family, Freddy went into heart failure. His parents refused to allow him to be admitted to the children's ward as they were concerned that no purpose would be gained by treating his heart failure actively and, with the agreement of all, Freddy was cared for at home by his parents and the community children's nursing team, supported by their GP and paediatrician until his death.

Question:

1. *What might be the moral rationale for maintaining Freddy's life through enteral feeding and then for withdrawing active treatment?*

THE BEGINNING OF FREDDY'S CASE HISTORY: PARENTAL CONSENT AND PARTNERSHIP

The first phase of Freddy's case history raises questions about the way decisions are made about a non-autonomous child's treatment in the face of a life-limiting condition. This is not to suggest that the care of such children will necessarily comprise a major part of a CCN's workload, but that children with life-threatening or limiting conditions may pose a critical range of dilemmas. A discussion of a difficult case, therefore, should encapsulate the key issues embedded in parental consent.

The ethical concept of autonomy is central to healthcare ethics in Western societies, which espouse the notion of individual rights. The right of individual autonomous patients to give or refuse consent to treatment or to being research subjects has been seen as the main safeguard against unjustified professional paternalism and, in extreme cases, treating people as if they had no human rights, as occurred in World War II concentration camps. The ethical concept of autonomy and the legal concepts of competence and capacity to make decisions are closely related.

The problem with children is, of course, that autonomy develops gradually during childhood. Freddy, however, is non-autonomous: he will never attain the competence to make decisions about himself. The Shepherds' situation exemplifies the heartache experienced by parents faced with making a proxy decision – always more difficult than making a decision for oneself.

Some decisions about healthcare are relatively straightforward, particularly where the predicted risks are low and the benefits high. Few parents would hesitate over giving consent for a 3-year-old child to have treatment for diabetes. Where risks increase and the benefits become less certain, the decision becomes more fraught and the risk–benefit equation becomes more difficult to calculate. Cases such as Freddy's exemplify real uncertainty over assessing likely benefits and risks. Mary and Tim Shepherd will be attempting to make an evaluation of the possible effects of treatment on the quality and quantity of Freddy's life, making judgements about what might do good and hoping to avoid harm. Applying beneficence, the ethical principle of doing good, versus non-maleficence, the principle of avoiding harm, can, in such circumstances, seem like two sides of the same coin with little certainty about which way the coin will fall when flipped. This illustrates the difficulty of resolving moral dilemmas when there are at least two possible courses of action and neither is clearly preferable.

Information about the child's future aspirations and values is not available to parents of young children and they can only attempt to judge what might be in the child's best interests. As has been suggested, making a calculation of potential risks and benefits may not be easy. By the same token, determining what might be in a child's best interests may not be straightforward; the 'best interests test', the legal criterion for such a judgement, is not a neat formula leading automatically to an objectively valid answer.

The best interests test also puts all the emphasis on the child, giving little space for the needs of the family. An often-quoted American court judgement (Prince v Massachusetts 1944) stated that parents are not entitled to make martyrs of their children. But, particularly in the context of the care for a child at home, one may be tempted to ask whether the parents are required to make martyrs of themselves and other family members. A child with complex health needs will have a permanent effect on the family; while many parents feel that overall the experience is positive, negative consequences, often arising out of insufficient support from the local health and social services and a lack of community children's nursing teams, may be evident.

In deciding what might be in their child's interests, parents will seek expert professional advice to inform them about possible actions and their likely outcomes. As all experienced children's nurses know, there is a subtle balance between the decision-making duties of the parents and those of the professionals with their own duty of care for the child. Adherence to the philosophy of partnership, with its emphasis on respect for parental views, does not absolve nurses and their colleagues from this duty (Charles-Edwards 1997). Mutual understanding and family empowerment should be supported by the fact that in community practice the partnership relationship between the family and professionals takes place in the home, the parent's 'place', and that the relationship is often sustained over a long period of time. In Freddy's case, the decision to investigate the cause of his chest infection further without explicit consent disempowered his family.

Whatever the complexity or simplicity of the decision about care or treatment, there are three ingredients that must be present for consent to be valid. Invalid consent can lead to an action for negligence. First, the patient/parent must have the competence or capacity to understand and, second, information to make the decision and, third, consent must be freely given without coercion. In the case of Mary and Tim Shepherd, the critical issue was whether they were given sufficient information to agree to the investigation of Freddy's swallowing mechanism. In practice, parents are rarely explicitly asked for consent to investigations; their consent is taken as implied by their compliance. Perhaps we should question how often, whether in hospital or community practice, consent over significant issues is sought or simply taken as implied, and whether this is justified. In Freddy's case the investigations signalled a real change in the aims of Freddy's care and led to a cascade of consequent actions. Also, if Freddy had not been admitted to hospital but had stayed at home while his chest infection was treated, would the option of investigating his pathology have arisen at all?

McHaffie and Fowlie (1996) discuss the technological imperative that can drive the continuation of treatment on beyond what is in a child's interests. It is easy to think that, because an intervention is possible, it is required. This is not the case. A child's best interests and the avoidance of harm may on occasion be better served by not treating. It is possible to argue that this technological imperative is easier to resist when a child is being cared for at home.

SECOND PHASE OF FREDDY'S CASE HISTORY: ADVOCACY, RIGHTS AND CONSENT AND THE CHILD

Listening to conversations amongst children's nurses, the terms advocacy and children's rights are often heard. A straw poll would probably support the assertion that both concepts are important to the philosophy and practice of CCNs, and yet we rarely analyse their complexities or reflect on the way they are implemented. In reality, both the practice of advocacy and the support of rights are problematic, particularly in relation to children.

Brykczynska (1993) describes different ways of understanding the concept of rights which illustrate why children have difficulty in having their rights recognised. Legal rights are awarded to a person through law or rules, and such rights can be removed by those in power in the same way as they are given. Moral rights are claimed by or for an individual in recognition of their moral status as a human person. Some moral philosophers deny that babies are fully human with the same moral rights as older children and adults, with philosophical discussion about the characteristics required for 'personhood'. Positive rights require another to do something for you, imposing an obligation on others which they may be reluctant to recognise, and negative rights are the right to be free to follow your own decision and course of action. Negative rights are rarely accorded to children; the reluctance to recognise children's right to refuse treatment is an example of this. Rights can also be understood as existing to protect the position of the strong or to protect the vulnerable and weak. Children in our society are weak, dependent on adults to recognise their needs and to take action to secure their rights. Children do not have the power to claim their own moral rights.

The description of rights as positive or negative reflects an understanding of liberty as positive and negative (Berlin 1969), which has relevance for the practice of advocacy. Negative liberty, classically described by Mills (1974), is freedom 'from' unwarranted interference, permitting an autonomous individual to be allowed to follow their own course of action. Others have a duty to ensure that the individual knows the risks but are not morally required to prevent the person from taking a foolish course. Berlin (1969) suggested, on the other hand, that positive liberty is more interventionist and answers the question: 'What or who is the source of control or interference that can determine someone to do, or be, this rather than that?' (p 122).

We should proceed to consider whether advocacy is more closely related to positive or negative liberty, and differentiate between advocacy and acting in a child's best interests. It is postulated here that clarity would be best served if we related advocacy to negative liberty in order to remind ourselves that acting as an advocate means ensuring that the family and the child have their own views represented, and to limit our role to ensuring that they understand the risks and benefits of treatment and care. The family's view may indeed not be in accord with our own. To substitute one's own opinion for the family's is paternalism rather than advocacy. The essential quality of an advocate is to be able to hear and represent another. However, our duty of care requires us to safeguard the interests of patients and to contribute to decisions, but this is not the same activity as advocacy. Using our professional expertise to safeguard the interests of patients is closely related to ideas about positive liberty.

Literature about advocacy (Gates 1995) emphasises further difficulties that professionals experience when attempting to act as an advocate. For example, our position as paid employees and as colleagues of other powerful team members may make the neutrality demanded of an advocate impossible to achieve. It is for these reasons that independent advocates are used within some organisations. However, few CCNs would debate that children and their parents, such as the Shepherds, at times need to have someone who can speak up for them. The challenge in fulfilling this role is to be a neutral non-judgemental advocate.

If Freddy had physical handicaps alone, he would be able to express his own view about his treatment plans. As children develop, they become more able to participate in decisions and then, eventually, become the main decider (Alderson and Montgomery 1996). One of the snags in the law of consent and children is that the right to participate remains in the gift of adults: parents and doctors. Note the relationship here to children's difficulty in claiming rights. Although the judgement in the Gillick case (Gillick v West Norfolk and Wisbech Area Health Authority 1985) led to the assumption that, as children matured, the power to give or refuse consent transferred to them from their parents, recent cases (Re: R 1991, Re: W 1992, Re: E 1993) have undermined this position. In an appraisal of the current law, Alderson and Montgomery (1996 p 38) point out that 'under current case law, treatment decisions for everyone under the age of 18 may be negotiated between doctors and parents without any reference to the child's view.' English law conceives competence to consent as either present or not, giving no place to a child's right to participation. Article 12 of the United Nations Convention on the Rights of the Child, however, supports the right of the children to express their views and, despite the paternalistic view of the law, best practice suggests that, as children become able, they should have the their views sought and taken seriously. Alderson and Montgomery (1996) describe a code of practice that would formalise this right.

To return to the 'what if' scenario: if Freddy were able to have a viewpoint about his treatment, the law might not uphold his right to be heard, but best practice, founded on the ethical principle of respect for his developing autonomy, would respect his participation and maturation towards becoming the main decider.

This discussion of children and consent is built on the premise that children are told the truth. One of the most difficult dilemmas faced by children's nurses is when a child appears to want information but the parents demand that the truth be withheld. In this situation it is impossible to respect the autonomy of both the child and the parents, and the trust of the child and the parents in the nurses is threatened. A resolution that satisfies all can be found in helping the parents to come to terms with their child's need to know and their own feelings about this.

WITHDRAWAL OF TREATMENT: THE LAST PHASE OF FREDDY'S STORY

During the first part of Freddy's history, a decision was made to withdraw active treatment; this position was returned to in the final phase of his illness. The Royal College of Paediatrics and Child Health (RCPCH 1997) has published guidance on withholding or withdrawing treatment, based on ethical principles and the philosophy of partnership with parents, in which five situations are outlined in which curative treatment may no longer be appropriate: the brain-dead child; the child in a permanent vegetative state; the 'no chance' situation; the 'no purpose' situation; and the 'unbearable' situation. It is suggested that Freddy falls into the no purpose situation. His mental disabilities prevent him from interacting with others and, superimposed upon this, is now a severe medical condition. Withdrawal of treatment raises complex moral issues around the difference between acts and omissions related to the practice of euthanasia. These pivot around the debate over intention. In both an act and an omission, the intention may be the same, leading to questions about whether there is any moral difference between the two. The RCPCH guidance (1997 p 12–13) addresses this concern by pointing out that redirecting the aims of care to palliation does not represent a withdrawal of care, and that in palliative care death occurs as a result of the disease process rather than as a result of an intended action. This is associated with the 'doctrine of double effect', used widely by doctors to support increasing the dosage of analgesia with the intention of alleviating pain rather than the possible secondary consequence of hastening death.

The guidelines provide a framework within which such decisions may be ethical and legal. They offer suggestions about the process leading to withdrawal or withholding of treatment based on the experience of the authors and working from ethical principles including respect for children's rights, respect for the parents' and older child's views, and the professional's duty of care to do good and avoid harm.

FURTHER THOUGHTS ABOUT DECISIONS CONCERNING CHILDREN

There is ambiguity in the way the law and the legislature treat children. Two problems persist: (1) finding the proper balance between the responsibilities of the state, acting through its agencies, and the responsibilities of the family for making decisions about child care, and (2) the relationship between young people and their parents. This second point is illustrated by the earlier discussion of children and consent. The first point, achieving a balance between the role of the state and the family, is an active contemporary issue as politicians debate the value of state guidance over good parenting. The history of child protection is replete with examples of swings between increased state intervention, via social and health services, and the contrary belief that intervention causes more problems than it solves.

King and Piper (1995) explore a similar ambiguity around the way in which the law deals with children who offend, and swings between, on one hand, the priority of justice as a punishment and a deterrent and, on the other hand, the belief that children who commit crimes are in need of remedial help to promote their welfare rather than punishment. The purpose of the criminal law is to determine guilt or innocence and it is not designed to cope easily with uncertain and complex areas of family relationships and developmental maturity. The same problems confront the law in the context of consent to treatment and child protection. The children's nurse who seeks a clear legal background against which to make ethical decisions, therefore, will be disappointed.

In community children's nursing the philosophy of empowerment emphasises the importance of respect for the autonomy of the family and the developing maturity of the child. This brings into even greater relief the complexity of all ethical decisions concerning children: that of the interplay between the child, parent and professional, and the uncertainty as to what extent the child's interests are necessarily the same as those of the parents and family (Alderson and Montgomery 1996, Charles-Edwards 1997). It is in raising these dilemmas that the philosophy of partnership with families challenges community children's nurses.

FURTHER READING

Alderson P 1990 Choosing for children. Oxford University Press, Oxford
In this book Alderson explains the outcome of research, performed in the 1980s, on how parents make difficult decisions about treatment for their children. The research was based on two cardiac surgery centres. It makes important points about parental proxy consent.

Alderson P 1993 Children's consent to surgery. Open University Press, Buckingham

This is a full discussion of the research Alderson carried out on the involvement of children in giving consent and some of the examples from the Alderson and Montgomery book given in the reference list comes from this source.

Dunnett A 1999 Euthanasia. Hodder and Stoughton, London

This is a valuable introduction to the euthanasia debate. The book comprises interviews with well-known protagonists on both sides of the debate; this format makes it easy to read and understand while introducing the important moral problems that need to be understood. The discussion does not address children in particular but can easily be related to children's nursing practice.

Freeman M 1983 The rights and wrongs of children. Frances Pinter, London

Although published some time ago, this book includes helpful discussion about the tension between family privacy and state intervention in bringing up children.

REFERENCES

Alderson P & Montgomery J 1996 Health care choices: making decisions with children. Institute for Public Policy Research, London

Berlin I 1969 Four essays on liberty. Oxford University Press, Oxford

Brykczynska G 1993 Ethical issues in paediatric nursing. In: Glasper A & Tucker A (eds) Advances in child health nursing. Scutari Press, London, ch 14, p 155

Charles-Edwards I 1997 Personal reflection on a paediatric nurse's duty of care. Journal of Cancer Nursing 1(4):197–199

Gates B 1995 Whose best interest? Nursing Times 94(4):31–32

King M & Piper C 1995 How the law thinks about children. Arena, London

McHaffie H & Fowlie P 1996 Life, death and decisions: doctors and nurses reflect on neonatal practice. Hochland and Hochland, Cheshire

Mills J S 1974 On liberty. Penguin Classics, London

Royal College of Paediatrics and Child Health 1997 Withholding or withdrawing life saving treatment in children. RCPCH, London

LEGAL CASES

Gillick v West Norfolk and Wisbech Area Health Authority 1985 3 All ER 402, 421 Prince v Massachusetts 1944 321 US 158 at 170

Re: R 1991 4 All ER 177, 185

Re: W 1992 4 All ER 627, 633

Re: E 1993 1 FLR 386

13 Home care for ventilated children: an analysis of the application of ethical reasoning

Julia Muir & Kim Gordon

KEY ISSUES

- Application of the evidence to children with high dependency needs in the community
- The increasing number of ventilator-dependent children being cared for at home in the UK
- Conflicting evidence on the positive and negative effects on the child and family
- The application of ethical reasoning to the issue is necessary in order to guide policy planning
- Ethical theories have difficulty in providing definitive answers
- There is a need for a systematic approach to discharge planning, taking ethical reasoning into account alongside fiscal matters and healthcare policy

INTRODUCTION

Community children's nurses (CCNs) increasingly support children with high dependency needs and their families in the community. More recently, children requiring ventilatory support are among this group. The number of children requiring long-term ventilatory support has risen considerably in the UK in the last decade (Jardine et al 1999). A logical consequence has been the increase of home care. This chapter will analyse the ethics of home care for such children from a number of philosophical perspectives. These principles may be applied to other children with high dependency needs.

Ethical consideration has been of interest to philosophers throughout history and has been noted as being crucial to civilisation (Seedhouse 1994). Healthcare commentators acknowledge the influential position of practitioners and suggest that an ethical decision-making process should permeate practice to ensure decisions are made from a structured, systematic foundation rather than on opinion or intuition (Brykczynska 1992, Gibson 1993, Seedhouse 1994). Whilst the application of different theories to the same issue may provide different resolutions, such a process is useful, if not essential, to clarify values and advocate for patients. Grundstein-Amado (1993) notes that the process may be influenced by the development of new technology, scientific progress, economic constraints and increasing consumer expectations. Each of these issues is reflected in the emergence of home care for highly dependent and ventilated children.

Whilst home care for ventilated children is a relatively new phenomenon in the UK, it has grown considerably in America for two reasons. First, in 1981, President Reagan waived eligibility rules for federal payment to enable a ventilator-dependent child to return home (Lantos & Kohrman 1992). This move facilitated a more universal, systematic approach to discharge planning and subsequent home care. Second, in response to this initiative, American home-care agencies developed specialist nursing provision in order to provide the necessary home support (Anderson 1990). These two strategies have provided the foundation for a growing body of evidence outlining the benefits and limitations of home care for such children. Whilst the transferability of these findings must be handled with caution, given the vastly different healthcare systems and cultures, the results offer some guidance and insight into the development of home care for ventilated children in this country.

REVIEW OF THE LITERATURE

The decision to initiate or undertake mechanical ventilation is rarely planned, but rather reactive to a preceding crisis. The uncertain nature of events compels parents and professionals to continue treatment. This situation has been described as 'the evolution of entrapment' (Orlowski 1993). At some stage, options for long-term care need to be identified. Existing alternatives to home care include paediatric or adult intensive care units, adapted rooms on children's wards and, in the USA, community-oriented units (Davies 1996, Goldberg et al 1984, Jardine et al 1999, Ward 1996). A more recent option has been home care, which has developed considerably since the 1980s (Jardine et al 1999). This initiative has been influenced by the scarcity of paediatric intensive care unit beds, the escalating numbers of people requiring ventilation, and increasing hospital costs.

A recent survey in the UK revealed the number of children requiring long-term ventilatory support as 141; of these, 93 were being cared for at home (Jardine et al 1999). In America it is estimated that between 2000 and 3000 ventilated children are cared for at home annually (Smith 1996).

The benefits of home care to the ventilated child are well documented, the most notable being the maximisation of the child's potential as social, emotional and developmental needs can be met (Jardine et al 1999). Home care promotes normalisation of family life and therefore long-term family well-being (Ward 1996), all of which appear to be in the best interest of the child. Fiscal matters also prevail, with home-care packages having been calculated at half the cost of paediatric intensive care units (Ward 1996). However, some argue that home care is only cost-effective if parents undertake the nursing care in the place of professional practitioners (Coffman 1995, Kirk 1998).

Alternative studies offer conflicting evidence and note the adverse effects of home care for ventilated children and their families, which could equally be applied to those with high dependency needs. Many consistent themes arise

BOX 13.1 ***Adverse effects of home care***

- Increased responsibility for the family
- Sleep deprivation
- Burnout
- Social isolation
- Lack of family normality
- Financial burden

within the literature, as identified in Box 13.1 (Coffman 1995, Kirk 1998, Smith 1996).

The financial burden on the family inevitably varies according to socio-economic status. Evidence suggests that there is often a deterioration of the family structure (Kirk 1998), and in some cases this results in the need for psychiatric intervention (Leonard et al 1993). Consequently, there is a need for competent, skilled carers to support families in order to overcome the possible detrimental effects of home care (Coffman 1995, Goldberg et al 1984). However, the cost of providing qualified skilled nurses for these children may compare with or even exceed the cost of hospital care (Harvey 1996).

This brief review demonstrates the complex issues involved in home care for ventilated children. The ethical underpinnings of such practice are particularly challenging and, as the evidence suggests, need to embrace the best interests of both child and family. Three prominent ethical theories have been identified within the literature to reflect a diverse view of the nature of ethical thought relevant to the area under study. These are: deontology, teleology and moral justice.

DEONTOLOGY

Deontology is concerned with the study of duty and derives from the work of Immanuel Kant (Seedhouse 1994). Kant stated that his theory was a natural consequence of the rational nature of human beings (Gillon 1986). His 'Supreme Moral Law' consists of three major concepts: duty as a motive, universal law, and the treatment of people as ends in themselves, not merely a means to an end (Gillon 1986).

Duty as a motive

First, deontology requires an individual always to perform a pre-ordained duty. Kant considered the fulfilment of duty to be the most superior motive when considering the moral value of an action (Seedhouse 1994). This demands placing the principle of duty above cognitive reasoning and projection of the potential consequences of an action. A truly moral action is one that aims to obey the purest motive of fulfilling this moral duty. An action can therefore be moral only if a person, group or organisation acts within boundaries set by duty. This implies that the motive of self-interest is not acceptable to deontologists. Will-power and conscious effort are considered to be acceptable in the effort to fulfil the expectations and demands of duty.

Can home care for ventilated children be considered to be practising within boundaries set purely by duty and without any prior consideration for self-gain or the potential consequences? This raises the dilemma of conflicting loyalties and is a problem that causes ethical writers to criticise Kant's theory heavily (Gillon 1986, Seedhouse 1994). It is often unclear where and to whom the duties lie.

The United Nations 'Convention on the rights of the child' (1992) acknowledges the vulnerability of children. It sets out principles that should be taken into consideration in the development of all child-related legislation, policy and practice. Many of these principles are reflected in the Children Act (Department of Health 1989). In both documents, the overarching duty for healthcare professionals is always to act in the best interest of the child.

The evidence clearly indicates that home care is in the best interest of the ventilated child through meeting their global needs. Home care can result in significant developmental progress and academic and spiritual growth, all of which may be affected adversely by long-term hospitalisation. Therefore, according to Kantian theory, healthcare professionals should pursue home care regardless of the potentially detrimental outcomes identified above. However, Lantos & Kohrman (1992), acknowledge that such practice would be immoral and that an approach considering the best interests of all concerned should be adopted.

The direction of duty is also unclear within Kant's theory. It can be argued that healthcare providers have a professional duty to meet Government targets, such as those identified in 'Our healthier nation' (Department of Health 1998). This document highlights mental health as a key target area and implies that healthcare professionals have a duty to examine the viability of home care carefully and consider its effects and consequences on all family members. This would contradict the deontological criteria necessary for the achievement of a truly moral act.

The poor definition and confusion over the boundaries and direction of duty within deontology have clearly caused problems and discrepancies within this attempt to apply deontological theory to the complex issues surrounding home care for ventilated children.

Universal law

The second major concept within deontology involves a consideration of whether the individual would desire the intended action to become universal law (Seedhouse 1994). The concept of universal law is designed to cause deliberation and action before implementation. In the UK, healthcare practitioners could not be accused of rash decision making, with one case taking 14 months before the first multidisciplinary discharge planning conference took place regarding a hospitalised ventilated child (Davies 1996). However, it is impossible and inappropriate to speculate here whether a healthcare professional would find home care acceptable for their own ventilated child, if they themselves were in such a position. This concept within deontology appears to have limited practical application within this context.

People as ends in themselves, and not merely as a means to an end

Lastly, Kant considers that all human beings should be treated as ends in themselves and not merely as a means to reach a set target. To abuse a position of power, freedom or possession in order to promote personal gain or self-interest would be condemned as immoral.

The development of home care for ventilated children has been influenced by the scarcity of paediatric intensive care unit beds and escalating hospital costs (British Paediatric Association 1993, Ward 1996). Alongside this, there have been two key political objectives: first, to develop a primary care-led National Health Service (NHS) and, second, to build a mixed economy of care (Department of Health 1994). As a result, primary care has experienced an increasingly dependent caseload with woefully inadequate resources to support the transformation. Consequently, the use of healthcare assistants and voluntary services to support technology-dependent children, including those requiring ventilation, is growing (National Health Service Executive 1998; Townsley & Robinson 1999) but the use of non-specialist carers can induce further anxiety in parents (Jennings 1990). It could be argued that, in this context, home care for ventilated children is seen as a means to an end. Advocating such care without skilled professional support could be seen as unethical practice, despite its clear benefits.

Deontology has been criticised for its inflexibility. Some critics believe it to have been developed on an intellectual rather than a pragmatic level (Gibson 1993, Seedhouse 1994). The lack of definition, the dilemma posed by conflicting loyalties, and the complicated motives involved in most actions and decisions seem to render the theory largely incapable of application to such complex and contemporary issues as home care for ventilated children. It would appear that this development is not driven purely by a sense and interpretation of duty, but by a combination of many influencing factors.

TELEOLOGY

This school was derived from the moral reasoning of Jeremy Bentham (1948, cited in Harrison 1948) and later developed by John S Mill (1962, cited in Trusted 1987). It is more commonly known as utilitarianism. The aims of individuals and society are to achieve the greatest good, or happiness, for the greatest number (Seedhouse 1994), with happiness and pleasure being the ultimate goals. The theory of utilitarianism seeks to maximise 'good' and to minimise 'evil' (Gillon 1986). In contrast to Kantism, it requires the actor to consider the consequences of their actions and, regardless of whether or not self interest or duty is involved, a morally right action is concerned with the amount of well-being it produces. Whilst utilitarianism considers that all individuals are of equal value, it simultaneously acknowledges that in order for the majority to benefit, a minority may suffer as a consequence (Seedhouse 1994, Trusted 1987).

Critics of this ethical school question the validity of pleasure as a uniform or measurable goal and note that definitions of 'good' and 'evil' are open to individual interpretation (Seedhouse 1994). Furthermore, these concepts must be measurable in order that a cost–benefit calculation can be made.

The greatest good for the greatest number

Aspects of home care for ventilated children can be considered to fit within the theory of teleology. Supporters of such practice note the financial benefit to the health service, proposing that the cost of home care may be less than half that of hospital care, particularly when parents substitute professional nursing care (Kirk 1998, Ward 1996). This releases valuable resources in paediatric intensive care units, whilst home care is deemed beneficial to the child.

Government policy also appears to reinforce this philosophy with the implementation of, for example, the continuing care policy (Department of Health 1995). This policy requires local authorities to produce eligibility criteria outlining and distinguishing health needs from social care. The main objectives are to develop more consistent arrangements for continuing healthcare and to ensure greater equal access. However, this notion has been challenged, with critics believing that the development of responsibility to local level leaves the prospect of developing equitable provision to chance (Henwood 1996, South 1997), penalising some individuals in the process. This is included and catered for within the boundaries set by teleology since utilitarians admit it is inevitable but acceptable that a minority will suffer.

Anti-utility: the counter-argument

There is a corresponding counter-argument which may be considered equally convincing in condemning aspects of home care for ventilated children as unethical within teleology.

First, teleology has been condemned for concluding in harsh calculations of 'cost versus benefit' within the healthcare arena (Seedhouse 1994). Davies (1996) proposes that home care for the ventilated child is 'not susceptible to financial analysis or even one using quality adjusted life years'. It is expensive, labour intensive and a burden on the family and health service. Often the calculations ignore the financial cost to parents and do not take account of the value of parents' time in the care-giving process (Lantos & Kohrman 1992). The financial burden on families, which may lead to notable hardship, can result in rehospitalisation and be a significant source of anxiety for parents (Kirk 1998).

The second relevant point in this counter-argument is that the acceptance of home care for ventilated children as ethical within the utilitarianism school is dependent on the predicted favourable health outcomes. Such assured success is disputed and challenged by those authors noting the detrimental consequences outlined above. Furthermore, studies have been criticised for using carefully selected samples, which do not necessarily reflect the social stratum (Lantos & Kohrman 1992). As a result, the detrimental effects and potential consequences could be underestimated and may not necessarily correlate with the amount of support actually provided (Coffman 1995).

Finally, this community-oriented theory conflicts with traditional healthcare ethics that focus on individualised care. An individualised approach is essential in the planning and delivery of such care in order for it to be beneficial. Issues such as family structure, family stability, parental motivation, community support and economic resources should all be taken into account (Lantos & Kohrman 1992).

The justification of home care for ventilated children within utilitarian theory is debatable. Whilst legislation is committed to the notion of community care, research demonstrates the potential unfavourable outcomes where there is a lack of financial support or specialist nursing provision.

MORAL JUSTICE

The concept of justice is founded on the principles of fairness. This school of ethical thought is commonly associated with Rawls (1973, cited in Gillon 1986), who assumes everyone to be egocentric, but, in order to maintain social stability, human survival demands sacrifices and restrictions. He theorises that ethical justice is contrived within a society through a theory of justice accomplished through a 'veil of ignorance'. This involves individuals hypothetically being oblivious of the role they are to have within society, leading them ultimately to choose a system of justice that promotes maximum liberty and equity for all (Gillon 1986). Rawlsian egalitarianism has difficulty assimilating the existence of inequity of power and possession with moral justice, unless this is beneficial to all, including the worst off in society (Gillon 1986). The law is concerned with retributive justice, but within philosophical reasoning there are three main forms of moral justice (Seedhouse 1994):

- Each according to their need: by equity
- Each according to their rights: by contract
- Each according to what they deserve: by meritocracy

This concluding part of the chapter will consider the first of these.

Equity

In both the USA and the UK, authors have commented on the inequitable allocation of support for families caring for a ventilated child at home. Some studies note that the type of support provided can vary significantly, from specialist professional nursing care to the employment of untrained care assistants (Jardine et al 1999, Leonard et al 1993). The amount of nursing care can vary from 24 hr cover to no assistance at all. In the USA, whilst this disparity relates to the reimbursement package from insurance companies, it has been shown to correlate directly with levels of depressive symptoms in parents (Leonard et al 1993).

It could be argued that these discrepancies exist in the UK, for a number of other reasons. First, just 50% of the country have access to community children's nursing services, of which only 10% offer a 24-hr service (Royal College of Nursing 1995). Clearly, then, the number of nurses with specialist experience will be limited. The national shortage of appropriately qualified nurses available for paediatric intensive care units is aggravated further by these community requirements. This deficit also relates to the inequitable geographical distribution of paediatric intensive care units (Department of Health 1997). Whilst core guidelines exist (Jardine & Wallis 1998), as yet there is no policy guidance advocating a unified standard for the delivery of nursing care for ventilated

BOX 13.2 ***Ethical issues that have not yet been addressed***

- The rights of parents when they wish to take their highly dependent child home and return to full-time employment
- The level of home health care that these families are entitled to
- The level of responsibility of parents within the home setting, to change ventilation levels for example, when receiving little or no nursing support
- The level of responsibility the nurse can assume when providing care to the highly dependent child alone in the home

children in the community. Together, these inequities form the basis for the development of this neophyte service.

Equity within healthcare is universally valued and commended, but is rarely reflected within practice. Rawls's theory of social justice through the 'veil of ignorance' does not seem applicable here. A system of justice that promotes maximum liberty and equity for all is indisputably desirable. However, it is easy to project hypothetical situations within theoretical debate, but the problems facing some families are a harsh reality. Once again, ethical reasoning appears to have been inapplicable and remote when related to complex and practical experience.

CONCLUSIONS

Just three ethical theories have been included in this chapter. Each theory has facilitated the consideration and discussion of many diverse issues. However, weaknesses, inconsistencies and confused definitions have often prevented a clear, simple application of theory to practice. Although selected for their common use and diversity, they can by no means be considered to include all aspects of ethical thought. Indeed, as high-dependency care gains momentum within the realms of community children's nursing practice, further ethical issues will arise that have not yet been addressed by current research. These are concerned with the principles of autonomy and rights in relation to the points outlined in Box 13.2.

From this analysis, it would appear that aspects of home care for ventilated children are unethical in the light of the available evidence. Competing external factors, such as fiscal matters and healthcare policy, influence the decision-making process but fail to be considered within some schools of thought. Teleology, perhaps, offers the most feasible and realistic theory to be applied to healthcare practice owing to its pragmatic recognition that some must inevitably suffer to benefit the majority. However, ultimately the theories appear to be somewhat idealistic and naive. They are unable to satisfy the demands of complex ethical problems contained within the constraints of a financially challenged healthcare system. It must be concluded that the ethical reasoning of philosophers does not always provide a viable, systematic or workable framework for application to current and practical issues. Rationalised, logical theory becomes easily clouded and contaminated with the complications and demands of the real, subjective and often emotional social world.

FURTHER READING

Jardine E & Wallis C 1998 Core guidelines for the discharge home of the child on long term assisted ventilation in the United Kingdom. Thorax 53:762–767

This article provides much needed core guidelines which were developed by a working party of people from a wide range of professional disciplines. The paper draws on three case scenarios to illustrate the valuable points made.

National Health Service Executive 1998 Evaluation of the pilot project programme for children with life threatening illnesses. The Stationery Office, London

The results of the pilot projects are drawn together in this document and provide insightful practical advice into the experiences of families and professional teams. One of the appendices offers a very user-friendly example of a 'home ventilation training programme'.

REFERENCES

Anderson J 1990 Home care management in chronic illness and the self-care movement: an analysis of ideologies and economic processes influencing policy decisions. Advances in Nursing Science 12(2):71–83

British Paediatric Association 1993 The care of critically ill children: report of a multidisciplinary working party on intensive care. British Paediatric Association, London

Brykczynska G M 1992 Ethics in paediatric nursing. Chapman & Hall, London

Coffman S 1995 Crossing lines: parents' experiences with pediatric nurses in the home. Rehabilitation Nursing Research 4(4):136–143

Davies R H 1996 Home ventilation of a child with motor and sensory neuropathy. British Medical Journal 313:153–154

Department of Health 1989 The Children Act. A new framework for the care and upbringing of children. HMSO, London

Department of Health 1994 Working in partnership: a collaborative approach to care. HMSO, London

Department of Health 1995 NHS responsibilities for meeting continuing health care needs. HSG(95)8 LAC(95)5. HMSO, London

Department of Health 1997 Government response to the reports of the health committee on health services for children and young people. The Stationery Office, London

Department of Health 1998 Our healthier nation. The Stationery Office, London

Gibson C H 1993 Underpinnings of ethical reasoning in nursing. Journal of Advanced Nursing 18:2003–2007

Gillon R 1986 Philosophical medical ethics. John Wiley, Chichester, UK

Goldberg A I, Faure E A M, Vaughn C J, Snarski R & Seleny F L 1984 Home care for life-supported persons: an approach to program development. Journal of Pediatrics 104(5):785–795

Grundstein-Amado R 1993 Ethical decision-making processes used by health care providers. Journal of Advanced Nursing 18:1701–1709

Harrison W (ed) 1948 Jeremy Bentham's fragment on government and introduction to the principles of morals and legislation. Blackwells, Oxford

Harvey I 1996 Commentary: reach beyond metaphor to assess value. British Medical Journal 313:154

Henwood M 1996 Silent progress. Health Service Journal 21 November: 24–25

Jardine E & Wallis C 1998 Core guidelines for the discharge home of the child on long term assisted ventilation in the United Kingdom. Thorax 53:762–767

Jardine E, O'Toole M & Wallis C 1999 Current status of long term ventilation of children in the United Kingdom: questionnaire survey. British Medical Journal 318:295–299

Jennings P 1990 Caring for a child with a tracheostomy. Nursing Standard 4(30):24–26 & 4(32):38–40

Kirk S 1998 Families' experiences of caring at home for a technology-dependent child: a review of the literature. Child: Care, Health and Development 24(2):101–114

Lantos J D & Kohrman A F 1992 Ethical aspects of pediatric home care. Pediatrics 89(5):920–924

Leonard B J, Dwyer Brust J & Nelson R P 1993 Parental distress: caring for medically fragile children at home. Journal of Pediatric Nursing 8(1):22–30

National Health Service Executive 1998 Evaluation of the pilot project programme for children with life threatening illnesses. The Stationery Office, London

Orlowski J P 1993 Ethical and quality-of-life issues in ventilator-dependent children. Clinical Pediatrics December:714–717

Royal College of Nursing 1995 Challenging the present, improving the future. Royal College of Nursing, London

Seedhouse D 1994 Ethics: the heart of health care. John Wiley, Chichester, UK

Smith C E 1996 Quality of life and caregiving in technological home care. Annual Review of Nursing Research 14:95–118

South J 1997 Themes and variations. Health Service Journal 26 June: 32–33

Townsley R & Robinson C 1999 What rights for disabled children? Home enteral tube feeding in the community. Children and Society 13:48–60

Trusted J 1987 Moral principles and social values. Routledge & Kegan Paul, London

United Nations 1992 The convention on the rights of the child. HMSO, London

Ward T A 1996 Commentary: need for a nationally consistent approach. British Medical Journal 313:155

14 Legal aspects of the community care of the sick child

Bridgit Dimond

KEY ISSUES

- Accountability
- Decision making and consent within the family
- Rights and responsibilities
- Changing structures in the delivery of care

INTRODUCTION

This chapter provides the reader with the framework for the law that relates to the care of the sick child in the community (Dimond 1996). Further reading is offered for those who wish to study the law in more depth. The topics to be covered are:

- The law and guidance
- Accountability
- Accountability for negligent advice and instruction
- Parental sharing in the care
- Decision making and disputes with parents
- Consent by the child: 16 and 17 years; under 16 years
- Confidentiality
- Children Act 1989; child protection issues
- Parental rights and responsibilities
- Education
- Palliative and terminal care:
- Changing National Health Service (NHS) structure: primary care groups and community care; clinical governance, National Institute of Clinical Excellence (NICE), Commission for Health Improvement (CHIMP)
- Role of the voluntary sector

THE LAW AND GUIDANCE

The law relating to the care of sick children derives mainly from statutes (i.e. Acts of Parliament) (see Box 14.1) and case law (otherwise known as common law or judge-made law). Increasingly, however, there are international

BOX 14.1 ***Statutes relating to the care of sick children***

Children Act 1989
Education Act 1993
Education Act 1996
Family Law Reform Act 1969, section 8(1) and 8(2)
Health Services Bill 1999, clause 13(4)

charters that set out the rights of the child. The United Nations (UN) Convention on the Rights of the Child was adopted on 20 November 1989. It is not directly enforceable in the courts of England and Wales. The European Convention of Human Rights, to which this country was a signatory in 1950, has in the past been enforceable by application to the Court in Strasbourg. However, with the enactment of the Human Rights Act 1998, the articles of the convention will be directly enforceable in the courts of England and Wales from 2000. For example, article 3 states that 'no person should be subjected to torture or to inhuman or degrading treatment or punishment'.

It may be that some of the conditions in which sick children in the community are being kept are in breach of this article. The child would have a right to take action in the courts of this country against any public organisation or organisation that performs public functions. Other charitable organisations have drawn up charters promoting standards in the care of children, but these, like the Patient's Charter (Department of Health 1992), are not directly enforceable in the courts of England and Wales. The Audit Commission (1993), whose functions may be taken over by CHIMP (see below), published a report on community child health and social services. It gave detailed guidance for managers and practitioners, including an agenda for providers of community child health services. The Department of Health (National Health Service Executive 1996) has issued a guide to good practice in caring for children in the community. It emphasises the importance of 'better co-ordination, adoption of good practice, better targeted support, and more effective collaboration' and recommends that purchasers should take account of the UN Convention on the Rights of the Child in planning contracts for child health services.

ACCOUNTABILITY

All professionals caring for sick children in the community are personally and professionally accountable for any harm which they cause or for any failure to follow an approved standard of care. Any person at fault could face criminal proceedings, civil proceedings, disciplinary proceedings brought by the employer, and professional conduct proceedings by the registration body: United Kingdom Central Council for Nursing, Midwifery and Health Visiting (UKCC), the General Medical Council (GMC) or the Council for Professions Supplementary to Medicine (CPSM).

Criminal proceedings

An unexpected death would be followed by an investigation by the coroner, who can order an autopsy to be performed and decide whether an inquest should be held. At any stage in the proceedings the coroner can adjourn the inquest for criminal proceedings to take place. Gross negligence or recklessness which led to the death of the child could be subject to criminal proceedings, and a health professional could be liable for the death if his or her gross recklessness caused the death (R v Adomako 1994).

Civil proceedings

Health professionals owe a duty of care to the patient. Failure to provide a reasonable standard of care, which results in reasonably foreseeable harm, could lead to a civil action for compensation. The child's parents could sue on behalf of the child, but, if they fail to do so, the child has 3 years from attaining the age of majority (i.e. 18 years) to sue on his or her own behalf for harm caused while a child. The action would be brought against the employer of the health professional, since the employer is vicariously liable for the negligence of an employee whilst acting in the course of employment. For example, a child might suffer from pressure sores as a result of failure to protect tissue viability. It may be that the community children's nurse (CCN) has failed to ensure that parents have been provided with a pressure-relieving mattress for their child or the CCN has failed to provide instruction on how to care for the child appropriately.

The determination of whether there is a breach of the duty of care is based on what has become known as the Bolam Test, that is, what is the reasonable standard of care?

> '[A doctor] is not guilty of negligence if he has acted in accordance with a practice accepted as proper by a responsible body of medical men skilled in that particular art ... Putting it the other way round, a man is not negligent, if he acts in accordance with such a practice, merely because there is a body of opinion who would take a contrary view.' (Bolam v Friern Hospital Management Committee 1957)

The House of Lords has emphasised that experts who give their opinion on what would be competent practice must ensure that such expert opinion flows logically, and reasonably, from the specific circumstances:

> 'The use of the adjectives "responsible, reasonable and respectable" (in the Bolam case) all showed that the court had to be satisfied that the exponents of the body of opinion relied upon could demonstrate that such opinion had a logical basis.' (Bolitho v City & Hackney Health Authority 1997)

Accountability for negligent advice and instruction

If a health professional were to give negligent advice to a patient or to the carers and, in reliance on that advice, harm was caused, then, if the advice was given knowing that it would be relied upon, the health professional or the employer could be held accountable and required to pay compensation. A physiotherapist might instruct parents on how to carry out percussion physiotherapy; if these instructions were negligent and the child suffered harm, the parents could sue the employer of the physiotherapist.

Disciplinary proceedings

Under the contract of employment, there are implied terms that require the employee to act with reasonable care and skill and to obey the reasonable instructions of the employer. Failure to comply with these implied terms could lead to disciplinary proceedings with the ultimate sanction of the employee being dismissed. The employee could bring an application for unfair dismissal to the industrial tribunal, claiming compensation and reinstatement.

Professional conduct proceedings

A registered employee is subject to professional conduct proceedings by his or her own registration body. At present the UKCC, GMC and CPSM all have different definitions of the nature of misconduct that could lead to a striking off the register. UKCC-registered practitioners are liable to professional conduct proceedings if they are guilty of misconduct, defined as 'conduct unworthy of a nurse, health visitor or midwife', but this definition is now likely to be changed following the review conducted by J M Consulting Ltd on the Nurses, Midwives and Health Visitors Acts of 1979 and 1992.

PARENTAL SHARING IN THE CARE; DECISION MAKING AND DISPUTES WITH PARENTS

Community care of the sick child is a partnership between the multiagency, multiprofessional team and the family. Health professionals have a considerable responsibility to ensure that the family and other carers have the necessary instructions to enable the child to be safely cared for. For example, the role of a domiciliary physiotherapist in the treatment of children with cystic fibrosis was reviewed by Rogers and Goodchild (1996). They show that the provision of a domiciliary physiotherapy service for cystic fibrosis has been a major development, allowing patients and their families increased access to physiotherapy both in the clinic and at home. Compliance with physiotherapy has been improved by discussion and demonstration in the home. They conclude that there is room for improvement in the service, but more detailed feedback is required from patients and their families.

Sometimes parents are asked to sign an exemption form when they undertake treatments at home. Such notices would be invalid if they were relied upon to exempt the health professional from liability for negligence. For example, parents might agree that they will undertake intravenous administration of drugs at home for their child. They may be asked to sign a form which states that they have had reasonable instruction and will not hold the Trust or its employees liable for any harm that occurs. If the nurse instructing the parents on how to carry out the intravenous injections fails to tell them about warning signs such as a rash or sudden change in temperature, for example, and the child were to suffer harm, the notice the parents signed would not prevent the Trust being held vicariously liable for the negligence of its staff. The Unfair Contract Terms Act 1977 prevents a person from relying on a notice or contract term to exempt them from negligence if personal injury or death is caused. A notice can be relied upon for exemption for negligence that leads to damage or loss of property, if such reliance is considered reasonable.

Good communication with parents would be considered to be part of the duty of care owed to the child, and health professionals should ensure that parents have easy contact with health professionals for advice and support.

CONSENT BY THE CHILD: 16 AND 17 YEARS; UNDER 16 YEARS

A child of 16 or 17 years has a statutory right to give consent to medical, surgical and dental treatment, and this includes diagnostic procedures and other ancillary procedures including anaesthetics (Family Law Reform Act 1969). At 18 years the child becomes an adult and no person can then give consent on their behalf, including the parents. In the case of mental incapacity of an adult, others can act in the best interests of that person on the basis of the common law power to act out of necessity recognised by the House of Lords in the case of F v West Berkshire Health Authority (1989).

The parent can also give consent on behalf of a child up to the age of 18 years. Where a child of 16 or 17 years is refusing treatment which is in her or his best interests, the refusal of the child can, in exceptional circumstances, be overruled. This was the principle established by the Court of Appeal in the case of Re: W (1992), when it upheld the decision of the High Court judge to order a child of 16 years who was suffering from anorexia nervosa to undergo medical treatment against her will.

Jehovah's Witness parents of a boy aged $15\frac{3}{4}$ years, who was suffering from leukaemia, pleaded with the court that his refusal to have a blood transfusion should be upheld, but they were overruled on the grounds that the boy needed the transfusion as part of his treatment (Re: E, Family Division 1993).

A child below the age of 16 years does not have a statutory right to give consent to treatment, but the House of Lords has held that if the child is competent to understand the nature of the proposed treatment and its effects then he or she can give a valid consent to treatment (Gillick v West Norfolk and Wisbech Area Health Authority 1986). As a result of this case (which was brought by Mrs Gillick, who claimed that a Department of Health memorandum permitting doctors to give family planning advice to girls under 16 years without parental involvement was invalid), we now have the expression 'Gillick competent'.

CONFIDENTIALITY

General

There is a duty of care, originating in professional codes of conduct, to respect the confidentiality of information about the child and family. However, this is subject to many exceptions, which are shown in Box 14.2.

Information provided by the child

Where the child gives information to the health professional in the expectation that this will be kept secret, including from the parents, the health professional

BOX 14.2 ***Exceptions to the duty of confidentiality***

1. Consent of the parents (and of child if 'Gillick competent')
2. In the best interests of the patient
3. Order of court
4. Statutory exceptions (e.g. notification of infectious diseases)
5. Public interest

BOX 14.3 ***Principles of the Children Act 1989***

1. The welfare of the child is the paramount consideration in court proceedings.
2. Wherever possible, children should be brought up and cared for in their own families.
3. Courts should ensure that delay is avoided, and may make an order only if to do so is better than making no order at all.
4. Children should be kept informed about what happens to them, and should participate when decisions are made about their future.
5. Parents continue to have parental responsibility for their children, even when their children are no longer living with them. They should be kept informed about their children and participate when decisions are made about their children's future.
6. Parents with children in need should be helped to bring up their children themselves.
7. This help should be provided as a service to the child and the family, and should:
   a. be provided in partnership with parents
   b. meet each child's identified needs
   c. be appropriate to the child's race, culture, religion and language
   d. be open to effective independent representations and complaints procedures
   e. draw upon effective partnership between the local authority and other agencies, including voluntary agencies

should warn the child that an absolute assurance of confidentiality cannot be given. Clearly, the younger the child, the less likely it will be that information will be kept from the parents. If the child is reporting abuse of any kind, the health professional would have a duty to initiate appropriate steps in accordance with the procedures for the Area Child Protection Committee.

CHILDREN ACT 1989; CHILD PROTECTION ISSUES

The Children Act 1989 provides a clear framework for the lawful intervention in the care of the child and for reconciling disputes between parents. The involvement of the child in the decision making is clearly emphasised. It sets out the principles that should underline the care of children, shown in Box 14.3. The overriding principle is that 'The child's welfare shall be the court's paramount consideration'.

PARENTAL RIGHTS AND RESPONSIBILITIES

Even after parents are divorced, both still retain responsibilities in relation to the child. If disputes arise between parents over the care and treatment of their children, an application can be made to court for a prohibited steps order. This will prevent certain action being taken in respect of a child, unless the court's agreement is obtained.

EDUCATION

Those caring for sick children should ensure that every effort is made to support their continuing tuition, so that they do not suffer educationally as a result of the illness. The education authority has a statutory duty to provide home tuition, but this is subject to different interpretations.

The Education Act 1993, section 298(1), which came into effect on 1 September 1994 (now consolidated in the Education Act 1996) placed a duty on local education authorities to provide suitable full-time or part-time education for children of compulsory school age who, by reason of illness, exclusion from school or otherwise, may not for any period receive suitable education unless such arrangements are made for them. Health professionals should liaise with the parents, school and education authority to ensure that this statutory duty is met.

PALLIATIVE AND TERMINAL CARE

Pressure may sometimes be brought upon health professionals to assist in the speedy death of a terminally ill child. It would be a criminal offence for the health professional or the parent/carer to undertake such an action. The law recognises no right to accelerate the process of dying. Such an action would constitute murder or manslaughter. This does not mean, however, that medication for pain relief cannot be given, if an unintended effect of that medication is that life is thereby shortened. This was the ruling in the case of Dr Bodkin Adams (Bedford 1961). The law also draws a distinction between killing and letting die. The former is a criminal offence; the latter may be part of the duty of care. The House of Lords recognised the distinction in the Tony Bland case, when it allowed artificial feeding of a patient in a persistent vegetative state to be discontinued (Airedale NHS Trust v Bland House of Lords 1993). Annie Lindsell, who suffered from motor neuron disease, brought an action in court for a declaration that her doctor would be allowed to let her die peacefully and with dignity, but withdrew her action after an assurance that that would be the doctor's duty of care to her, even though administration of pain relief may inadvertently shorten her life (Wilkins 1997).

The Association for Children with Life-Threatening or Terminal Conditions and their Families & the Royal College of Paediatrics and Child Health (1997) have developed a charter for the care of children. It emphasises the principle that every child shall be treated with dignity and respect and shall be afforded privacy, whatever the child's physical or intellectual ability. Guidance has also been published by a working party which included the British Paediatric

Association and the King's Fund on the care of dying children and their families (Thornes 1988).

THE CHANGING NHS STRUCTURE

The White Paper on the NHS (Department of Health 1997) envisaged major reorganisation and new organisations within the NHS. In April 1999 the internal market in healthcare and general practitioner fund-holding was abolished. Primary care groups (PCGs) in England (local health groups in Wales) were established to arrange provision of healthcare for patients in their catchment area, including the agreements with providers for secondary and tertiary services. Eventually some of these PCGs will receive Trust status. The effect will be that the emphasis in healthcare should be on primary care. This may, therefore, give an impetus to the provision of more day surgery and increasing community care of sick children. Community child health professionals should be part of the multiprofessional team employed by the PCG to provide care at home.

In addition, the establishment of the National Institute for Clinical Excellence (NICE) and the Commission for Health Improvement (CHIMP) should ensure that research findings on clinically effective care are disseminated and that research-based practice is implemented. CHIMP will have powers of inspection and audit. There will be a statutory duty upon primary care and NHS Trusts to put and keep in place arrangements for the purpose of monitoring and improving the quality of healthcare provided to individuals. Healthcare is defined as meaning 'services for or in connection with the prevention, diagnosis or treatment of illness' (Health Services Bill 1999). National standard frameworks will also be published across the specialities to ensure high standards of provision. A national standard for the community care of the sick child should assist professionals in pressing for the necessary resources to ensure high standards of care for children being cared for at home.

The legal effect of these statutory changes is that, in future, parents who claim that their child has suffered harm as a result of a failure to provide a reasonable standard of care will be able to point to published league tables and national evidence of research and standards which local providers have not implemented. In other words, the Bolam Test, when applied to a situation of alleged negligence, will be based on these national standards. Even where harm has not occurred (so an action for negligence is not possible), parents will still be able to use national evidence to draw attention to deficits in local standards as the basis for a complaint. This, potentially, could have a positive influence on the development of community children's nursing services. At the moment there are great inequalities; for example, 50% of the country has no access to such services (Health Committee 1997). National standards should ensure that such inequalities are highlighted and ended.

ROLE OF THE VOLUNTARY SECTOR

No analysis of the care provided in the community for sick children would be complete without a consideration of the role that is increasingly being played by the voluntary sector. All health professionals should be sure that they are aware of the local services provided for children by the many charities that care for children and provide specific advice on different disorders. The organisation, Action for Sick Children, has published a charter on the rights of the child (cited in Dimond 1996). Other charities provide hospice care and Macmillan nurses. Support from these voluntary groups can assist families in carrying the burden of a sick child and provide them with essential respite.

CONCLUSION

The pressure on those who care for sick children in the community will continue to increase: shorter lengths of stay, day surgery and the preferred option to avoid hospitalisation for sick children will lead to more children being cared for at home with increasingly complex technological equipment and treatment regimens. Community staff must ensure that they are competent to practise in new areas of professional development. In addition, they must be aware of the publications from the new NHS institutions on best practice and national standards, and ensure that their local services meet increasingly higher standards of care.

FURTHER READING

Dimond B 1996 The legal aspects of child health care. Mosby, London

This book gives an overview of the law relating to the healthcare of the child, covering all the issues raised in this chapter and specifically considering practical aspects of child care in the community in more depth.

White R, Carr P & Lowe N 1990 A guide to the Children Act 1989. Butterworths, London

This book gives a comprehensive analysis of the provisions of the Children Act 1989.

Dimond B 1996 The right to die, euthanasia and advanced directives. In: Greaves D & Upton H (eds) Philosophical problems in health care. Avebury, London

This chapter sets out the law relating to letting die and killing.

Dimond B 1997 Legal aspects of care in the community. Macmillan, London

All chapters in this book are relevant.

REFERENCES

Association for Children with Life-threatening or Terminal Conditions and their Families & Royal College of Paediatrics and Child Health 1997 A guide to the development of children's palliative care services. Association for Children with Life-threatening or Terminal Conditions and their Families, London

Audit Commission 1993 Seen but not heard: coordinating child health and social services for children in need. HMSO, London

Bedford S 1961 The best we can do. Penguin Books, London

Department of Health 1992 The patient's charter. HMSO, London

Department of Health 1997 The new NHS. Modern, dependable. The Stationery Office, London

Dimond B 1996 The legal aspects of child health care. Mosby, London

Health Committee 1997 House of Commons select committee. Health services for children

and young people in the community: home and school. Third report. The Stationery Office, London
National Health Service Executive 1996 Child health in the community: a guide to good practice. The Stationery Office, London
Rogers D & Goodchild M 1996 Role of a domiciliary physiotherapist in the treatment of children with cystic fibrosis. Physiotherapy 82(7):396–402
Thornes R 1988 The care of dying children and their families. National Association of Health Authorities, Birmingham
Wilkins E 1997 Dying woman granted wish for dignified death. The Times 29 October

LEGAL CASES

R v Adomako 1994 2 All ER 79
Bolam v Friern Hospital Management Committee 1957 2 All ER 118
Bolitho v City & Hackney Health Authority 1997 3 WLR 1151
F v West Berkshire Health Authority and another 1989 2 All ER 545
Re: W (a minor) (medical treatment) 1992 4 All ER 627
Re: E (a minor) (wardship: medical treatment) Family Division 1993 1 FLR 386
Gillick v West Norfolk and Wisbech Area Health Authority 1986 1 AC 112
Airedale NHS Trust v Bland House of Lords 1993 1 All ER 821

15 Health promotion in community children's nursing

Lisa Whiting & Sue Miller

KEY ISSUES

- Health
- Health education and health promotion
- Child health promotion
- Health promotion within community children's nursing

INTRODUCTION

The aim of this chapter is to explore the role of the community children's nurse (CCN) in relation to child health promotion. Tannahill's model (1996) will be used as a framework for the discussion and will include a consideration of primary, secondary and tertiary disease prevention.

In the first instance, it is important to clarify the concepts of 'health' and 'health promotion'. This will be followed by a brief overview of the value of community involvement in health promotion initiatives and the importance of promoting health to children and their families.

HEALTH

The critical examination of 'health' is fundamental to the practice of health promotion. Without an understanding of its many perspectives, there is a danger that professionals will 'continue to do what they have always done, because *they know* that they are right' (Seedhouse 1986 p 9).

A great many authors have debated the concept of health, offering a range of definitions (Downie et al 1990, King 1990, Nutbeam 1986, Seedhouse 1986, World Health Organization 1984). These vary from a rather simplistic biomedical view in which it is argued that health is the absence of, or mirror image of, disease, to those that provide much broader approaches. Perhaps one of the most well known and frequently quoted is that produced by the World Health Organization (WHO) (1946, cited by Dines and Cribb 1993 p 5) which states that health is:

> 'a complete state of physical, mental and emotional well-being and not merely the absence of disease or infirmity.'

This definition has been heavily criticised as being unrealistic, idealistic and static (Dines and Cribb 1993, Ewles and Simnett 1995, Maben and Macleod Clark 1995). In addition, it has been argued that no-one could claim to be healthy if this view is adhered to. It is, however, important to remember that this description was written more than 50 years ago; since then more modern definitions and explanations have been offered (Downie et al 1990, Nutbeam 1986, Seedhouse 1986). For example, Seedhouse (1986 p 61) describes health as 'the state of the set of conditions which fulfil or enable a person to work to fulfil his or her realistic chosen and biological potentials'.

The WHO has also given further consideration to its original work and in more recent publications has provided this updated version:

> 'Health is therefore seen as a resource for everyday life, not the objective of living; it is a positive concept emphasising social, personal resources, as well as physical activities.' (WHO 1984 p 5)

A number of authors have discussed the importance of enabling individuals to fulfil their potential so that quality and quantity of life can be enhanced (Ewles and Simnett 1995, Seedhouse 1986, Tones 1990). This is perhaps of particular relevance to the role of the CCN, who may have to acknowledge that return to complete health may not be feasible for every child (although the child and family could still be enabled to achieve their full potential).

Having briefly explored the concept of 'health', it is also essential to examine the term 'health promotion', before considering its relevance to the role of the CCN.

HEALTH PROMOTION

It is important to distinguish between the terms 'health education' and 'health promotion'. Although some authors, for example Dines and Cribb (1993), state that the two terms are frequently used synonymously, most theorists make quite clear distinctions in their definitions. Recently, there has been considerable debate about the role and purpose of both 'health education' and 'health promotion' (Catford and Nutbeam 1984, French 1985, Seymour 1984, Speller 1985, Tannahill 1985). Ewles and Simnett (1995) argue that this is because of the tremendous range of activities that are undertaken to facilitate optimum health. Health education has been defined as:

> 'any planned activity which promotes health or illness related learning, that is, some relatively permanent change in an individual's competence or disposition.' (Tones 1990 p 2).

This view is reinforced by Tannahill (1985 p 167), who says that it is concerned with 'enhancing well-being and preventing or diminishing ill-health'. According to Tones and Tilford (1994), health education may operate at a series of levels which range from one-to-one interactions, to addressing large sections of the general population and utilising a whole array of resources.

In summary, it could be said that health education is just one aspect of health promotion. The literature concerning 'health promotion' is not so clear and concise. The WHO (1984 p 4) suggests that:

BOX 15.1 *Key aspects of health promotion*

- A broad definition of health and its determinants which embraces social and economic contexts within which health – or, more precisely, non-health – is produced
- Movement beyond earlier emphasis on individual lifestyle strategies to broader social and political strategies
- Embracement of the concept of empowerment – individual and collective – as a key health-promoting strategy
- Advocating participation of communities in identifying health problems and in the development of strategies to address these perceived problems

> 'Health promotion is the process of enabling people to increase control over, and to improve, their health.'

Bunton and Macdonald (1992 p 7) provide a broad description by stating that health promotion: 'represents at the very simplest level ... a strategy for promoting, in some positive way, the health of whole populations.'

The view that individuals are not only able to make choices about their health needs but also able to take control of the decision-making process seems to have been widely accepted (Dines and Cribb 1993, Downie et al 1990, Saan 1986, Tones 1990, Whitehead 1989). It could be argued that the goals of health promotion are more challenging and include political, economic and social changes. Robertson and Minkler (1994 p 296) highlight key aspects of health promotion, as identified in Box 15.1.

Health promotion may be divided into three areas: primary (elimination of the health risk), secondary (striving to enhance the individual's quality of life) and tertiary (the instigation of social change aimed at promoting the health of everyone) (Wass 1994). Some authors suggest that nurses appear to have different understandings of the term and claim to be practising health promotion when, in fact, they are carrying out health education activities (French and Milner 1993, Maben and Macleod Clark 1995). In addition, different terms are used by professionals and this may lead to confusion (Caplan 1993). There is no doubt that health promotion is open to interpretation, but it is important for individual practitioners to clarify their role as a health promoter. There are no precise answers, but personal values should be reflected upon and examined.

A number of frameworks for the promotion of health have been offered (Beattie 1991, Tones & Tilford 1994). Perhaps one of the most popular and user-friendly tools is that produced by Tannahill (1996), which will be referred to later in the chapter and used to illustrate possible health promotion strategies.

COMMUNITY PARTICIPATION AND HEALTH PROMOTION

The value of community participation within health promotion initiatives has been acknowledged (Department of Health 1998a, Ewles and Simnett 1995) and the WHO (1986) emphasises the importance of empowering communities, thereby enabling them to develop 'ownership' and gain control of their futures.

In terms of community health promotion, it is necessary to define the 'community'. Baric and Baric (1991 p 204) state that it is 'a large number of people living together and sharing certain values and interests, as well as interacting for a certain purpose'. There appears to be consensus that the sharing of a goal is central to the ethos of a community. In terms of community children's nursing, this may be a group of parents who have children with special needs, campaigning for improved respite facilities. Alternatively, it may be a cystic fibrosis group who are concerned about levels of air pollution in local built-up areas. This may lead to schools, councillors, local press and health professionals all working together to influence local policy.

The Government suggests that a healthier nation will be achieved only if everyone works together (Department of Health 1998a). With this in mind, health action zones have been instigated in England to target inequalities in health by bringing together a partnership that includes local authorities, community groups, the voluntary sector, local businesses, as well as health professionals. One area identified in the publication which may be particularly applicable to community children's nursing is the Healthy Schools initiative. This initiative aims to increase the awareness of children, teachers and families about a whole range of health issues, including diet, exercise and environment, with the aim of improving the mental and physical health of children and young people. The high priority that the health of children and their families deserve is reiterated by the Department of Health (1998b). It is clear that health professionals have a central role in ensuring that health promotion is directed towards the younger population (Bagnall and Dilloway 1996, Hall 1996). CCNs are in an ideal position to facilitate child health promotion initiatives, but this must reflect a philosophy of family-centred care, and include working in collaboration with a range of other personnel.

CHILD HEALTH PROMOTION

In the past, a large proportion of child health promotion initiatives have either been directed towards the family and carers, rather than the children themselves, or, the problems have been identified by adults (Kalnins et al 1994). These initiatives were frequently linked with conditions that led to unnecessary mortality and morbidity (Kalnins et al 1994). Whilst the CCN should work in partnership with the parents promoting the health of the whole family, it is equally important to address the health of the child as an individual. Lee (1998) emphasises the importance of children having freedom to choose, and Campbell (1994) suggests that, if the locus of control is with the child, a lifestyle change is more likely to occur. Certainly, projects that have been initiated by children do appear to have some success. For example, Treseder (1997) describes a programme developed by youngsters who have complex and multiple disabilities at Chailey Heritage in the south of England. The aim was to solve problems and share points of view about a range of issues including relationship difficulties and experiences of disability. Support was provided by staff, and the commitment and attendance by the group members was evident throughout.

Kalnins et al (1994 p 195) state that 'children have to be seen as partners in health promotion rather than as a special group needing protection'. This view now appears to be widely accepted and has been reiterated by others (Lee 1998,

BOX 15.2 ***Key issues related to child health promotion***

- The local healthcare needs of the children should be identified, taking into account age, development, culture and sociopolitical factors.
- A range of innovative health promotion strategies should be employed.
- It is imperative that the views of the children are obtained.
- Appropriate health professionals are required to be available.
- Children should have the freedom to choose the 'way forward' and be given the locus of control, if this is feasible.
- A philosophy of partnership between the professional and child is important.
- Teamwork with a range of other personnel may be necessary, for example the community at large, other health professionals, schools and voluntary organisations.
- A strategy for evaluating the initiative should be considered.

Riley 1998, Seymour and Dean 1997). For example, Seymour and Dean (1997) conducted a study amongst 206 13–14-year-old children with the aims of determining the extent of teenage smoking and discovering methods that adolescents felt would be effective in preventing them from starting to smoke. The importance of pupil involvement in a 'stop smoking group' was highlighted by 66.6%. In addition, other ideas were suggested and included the production of stronger educational material (53.3%), inviting someone who had a smoking-related illness to speak to them (26%) and banning the tobacco sponsoring of sporting events (13%). One of the prime conclusions was that not only are health visitors and nurses in an ideal position to coordinate projects between the school, family and community, but in addition they have a knowledge of how to influence policies.

Although a range of child health promotion initiatives has been instigated throughout the UK, it is clearly not feasible to discuss them in detail here. However, it is evident that a number of issues should be considered when promoting the health of children, as summarised in Box 15.2.

Whilst current child health promotion projects are clearly valuable, there remain many opportunities for CCNs to explore additional areas. CCNs are in a key position to influence the future of child health promotion positively and to ensure that a range of innovative and purposeful programmes is implemented.

ROLE OF THE COMMUNITY CHILDREN'S NURSE IN RELATION TO HEALTH PROMOTION

Clearly the CCN does have a health promoting role, although the extent of that role has yet to be defined. It is also debatable as to how the role should extend in the future, given the current changes impacting on care delivery, including the formation of primary care groups in England.

The example of childhood constipation will be used to explore the role of the CCN in relation to health promotion. Care of these children constitutes a significant component of the workload of many CCNs (Health Committee 1997). Children may suffer with constipation for a variety of organic reasons; however, the majority have idiopathic constipation (Clayden 1992). These

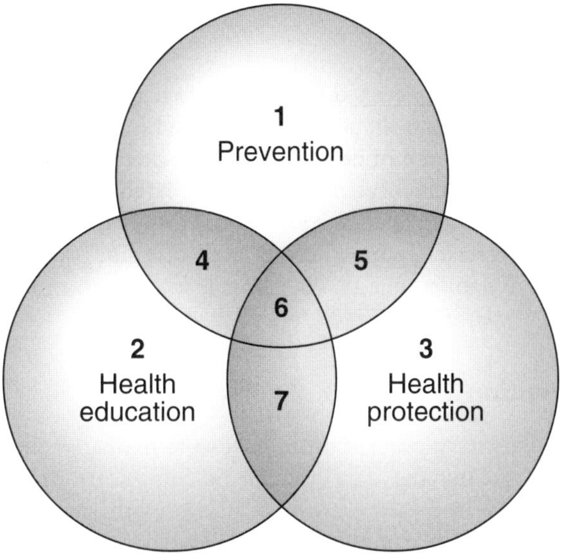

Figure 15.1 Tannahill's model (1996)

children may exhibit a wide range of related problems affecting their psychological, educational, physical, spiritual, emotional and social well-being (Chaney 1995, Kelly 1996, Lewis and Muir 1996) which could have detrimental effects on their overall development.

Tannahill's (1996) model (Fig. 15.1) will be used as a framework to consider how the CCN may promote the health of these children and their families in a number of ways. This model has been chosen as it was specifically designed as a tool to aid the implementation of health promotion strategies. It is composed of three overlapping circles – health education, prevention, and health protection. The spheres encompass seven domains, each of which will now be discussed.

1. Preventive activities

A number of authors (Downie et al 1990, Tones and Tilford 1994) have established a classification for disease prevention with three levels of intervention being commonly identified: primary, secondary and tertiary.

Primary prevention

This may include the provision of adequate toilet facilities which ensure privacy, comfort and cleanliness. For the school-age child, the CCN may be required to liaise with school personnel to ensure appropriate facilities are available. Alternatively the focus may be directed towards the family, providing opportunistic advice concerning an adequate diet and fluid intake to avoid constipation.

Secondary prevention

This is concerned with the early detection of a disease. It may include identifying those children already known to be at risk of constipation, for example the child who is immobile as a result of a fractured shaft of femur, the child who has profound cerebral palsy or those having enteral feeding. In these situations, the CCN will spend time with the family discussing the child's normal bowel habits, exercise regime and diet, and offering proactive advice. Insight into the family dynamics can also be gained, so that emotional as well as practical support can be offered.

Tertiary prevention

Tertiary prevention involves the management of existing constipation to avoid or limit the development of complications. The CCN may have an extensive role in these cases. First, liaison with and possible referral to other professionals, such as a paediatrician, psychotherapist, health visitor, teacher or play therapist, may be necessary. Second, it is important to gain insight into the family's understanding of the constipation, so that adherence to the programme of care can be enhanced. This, in turn, may avoid hospitalisation and maintain a holistic and continuous approach to care. Time will need to be spent ascertaining the most appropriate way of managing the child's individual problems so that solutions can be identified. For example, the teenager with constipation and overflow is likely to be concerned about the associated soiling and odour. Discussing realistic strategies to manage this may prevent social isolation. Adolescence is a time when body image, relationships with peers, and sexuality are important aspects of development. The teenager may therefore have many individual concerns which need to be identified and discussed in private.

2. Preventive health education

This includes strategies that may influence lifestyle in the interests of preventing ill health (Tannahill 1996). It might include discussing with parents the need to provide their children with adequate and suitable fluids and a diet that contains an appropriate amount of fibre. The CCN should be especially aware of the needs of children who are at greater risk of developing constipation as a result of immobility, poor appetite or certain medications, in order that appropriate contemporaneous advice can be given. Much of this support may be of an opportunistic nature.

3. Preventive health protection

This section relates to policy commitment to provide preventive measures (Tannahill 1996). Therefore, it would be important for the CCN to be aware of school policies in relation to toilet provision. It may not be possible to be familiar with all the protocols, but working in collaboration with other professionals such as the school nurse may help to achieve this. For example, the constipated child, who experiences pain on defaecation, may exhibit a range of emotional changes, perhaps becoming withdrawn, frightened or aggressive. Working with the multidisciplinary team and following the school policies may help to ensure that the child has the necessary privacy and understanding in relation to the health problem. This, in turn, may enhance school attendance and the child's self-esteem. In addition, the CCN should be aware of the resources available to support children and their families if they require additional psychological help. This may include professionals or organisations that may run 'self-help' groups. If these services are unavailable, or the waiting list is so long as to make the help untimely, the CCN may consider lobbying for increased resources.

4. Health education for preventive health protection

This does not occur spontaneously, so the education of policy makers is important (Tannahill 1996). This is perhaps an aspect of health promotion which some CCNs may be less familiar with. For example, liaising with head teachers may highlight the importance of the role that schools have in reducing the incidence of constipation amongst pupils, through provision of adequate drinking facilities and suitable toilets. Alternatively, it could include liaising with local councillors to improve public toilets to make them more child friendly.

5. Positive health education

This encompasses two categories: health education aimed at influencing behaviour on positive health grounds, and that which seeks to help individuals and groups to develop positive health attributes (Tannahill 1996). For instance, one of the factors that may contribute to the increasing numbers of young people suffering constipation is the speed with which many children leave for school in the morning. This may reduce the time required for elimination. Discussion with the young person and their parents may lead to an earlier rising and more time to visit the toilet. There is no doubt that the involvement of parents is central to community children's nursing (Procter et al 1998) and, by working in partnership, problems such as these may be resolved with relative ease.

6. Positive health protection

This aims to make healthy choices easier choices. The CCN may wish to identify policies regarding school meals and snacks available to pupils. It will be easier for school-age children to make healthy choices if meals and snacks offer healthy options that are high in fibre and low in fat; this is, of course, particularly important for the child who is prone to constipation. Perhaps one key issue here is the concept of empowerment, a central tenet of health promotion. Everyone needs to have the opportunity to feel in control of their lives, and young people are no exception. Therefore, consultation with young people about their dietary needs is crucial. The child with constipation is far more likely to adhere to a dietary programme if they have been involved in its development.

CCNs may also have a role in assisting families who have limited finances, which may make the purchase of fruit and vegetables difficult. The CCN may be able to help them identify foods that are high in fibre but relatively inexpensive. In addition, they may require advice on claiming the benefits to which they are entitled.

7. Health education aimed at positive health promotion

This includes raising awareness of and seeking policy commitment to positive health education (Tannahill 1996). Asserting the need for more CCNs could be viewed as protective health education. An increase in community children's nursing services may enable more young people who suffer from constipation to receive help sooner, thus minimising long-term difficulties. It may also enable children to receive care in their own homes rather than being admitted to hospital for treatment which may, in some cases, aggravate the child's development.

SUMMARY

From this exploration, it can be seen that many of the activities that the CCN undertakes could be considered to be health promoting. Indeed, it has been claimed that almost anything can be undertaken in a health-promoting way (Maben and Macleod Clark 1995).

Whilst this is just one practice example, it does demonstrate the potential scope of the health-promoting role of the CCN, which could be further extended. For example, the need for rigorous oral and dental hygiene for children who are totally dependent on enteral nutrition, is an area which would benefit from specific attention.

However, all health-promoting activities are time consuming and can present nurses with difficulties in justifying the time required when the outcomes are not always tangible or measurable (Robinson and Hill 1998). This is particularly pertinent since there are increasing pressures to provide evidence of success in order to justify utilisation of finite resources.

If the health-promoting role of the CCN is extended, other professionals may feel threatened. This could lead to conflict and defensiveness, particularly in the light of the Health Committee recommendations (1997). Procter et al (1998) state that the roles of CCNs, health visitors and school nurses have merged and that the need for a common knowledge base, which can be adapted for the professional caseload, is important. It could be argued that this will have the additional benefit of facilitating communication and enhancing campaign strategies in which professionals may be involved.

CONCLUSION

It is apparent that health promotion is an important aspect of community children's nursing. However, it is for individual practitioners to clarify the meaning of health promotion and be accountable for their decisions in relation to these responsibilities.

Many nurses have been prepared by educational programmes based on a sickness model, such that health promotion was perceived to be an 'added extra' provided only when there was sufficient time. Nurses need to accept that this is no longer the case: health promotion is an essential aspect of care and not a luxury we can ill afford.

Whilst CCNs should adopt a wider health-promoting role, the importance of evaluating any activity should not be underestimated, particularly within the remit of the clinical governance and evidence-based practice agendas. However, adequate education is required in order for CCNs to feel they have the skills, knowledge and competence to take on a wider health-promoting role. This will equip them with the confidence to participate in local and national campaigns in a more effective manner.

FURTHER READING

Downie R S, Fyfe C & Tannahill A 1990 Health promotion: models and values. Oxford University Press, Oxford

A comprehensive overview of the key concepts surrounding health promotion. There is also discussion of models in action.

Ewles L & Simnett I 1995 Promoting health. A practical guide, 3rd edn. Scutari Press, London

A generic, user-friendly, practical guide for professionals working as health promoters.

Lucy J 1999 The role of health promotion in childhood soiling. Journal of Community Nursing 13(4):24–28

This article discusses the role that health promotion can play when caring for children who have a soiling problem. Particular attention is paid to the importance of working in partnership with the whole family.

Procter S, Biott C, Campbell S, Edward S, Redpath N & Moran M 1998 Preparation for the developing role of the community children's nurse. English National Board, London

Research commissioned by the English National Board for Nursing, Midwifery and Health Visiting. The study explores the needs of families caring for sick children at home, considering the perspectives of children, carers, children's nurses, service managers and educationalists. It also examines aspects of disease prevention and health-promoting models of practice.

REFERENCES

Bagnall P & Dilloway M 1996 In a different light: school nurses and their role in meeting the needs of school-age children. Queens Nursing Institute and Department of Health, London

Baric L & Baric L F 1991 Health promotion and health education, 2nd edn. Barns Publications, Altrincham

Beattie A 1991 Knowledge and control in health promotion: a test case for social policy and social theory. In: Gabe J, Calnan M & Bury M 1991 (eds) The sociology of the health service. Routledge, London, pp 162–202

Bunton R & Macdonald G 1992 Health promotion: disciplines and diversity. Routledge, London

Campbell S 1994 The well and sick child. In: Webb P (ed) Health promotion and patient education. A professional's guide. Chapman and Hall, London, pp 80–97

Caplan R 1993 The importance of social theory for health promotion: from description to reflexivity. Health Promotion International 8(2):147–157

Catford J & Nutbeam D 1984 Towards a definition of health education and health promotion. Health Education Journal 43(2):38

Chaney C 1995 A collaborative protocol for encopresis management in school age children. Journal of School Health 65(9):360–364

Clayden G 1992 Management of chronic constipation. Archives of Diseases in Childhood 67:340–344

Department of Health 1998a Our healthier nation. A contract for health. The Stationery Office, London

Department of Health 1998b Independent inquiry into inequalities in health report. (Chairman Sir Donald Acheson). The Stationery Office, London

Dines A & Cribb A (eds) 1993 Health promotion: concepts and practice. Blackwell Scientific Publications, Oxford

Downie R S, Fyfe C & Tannahill A 1990 Health promotion: models and values. Oxford University Press, Oxford

Ewles L & Simnett I 1995 Promoting health. A practical guide, 3rd edn. Scutari Press, London

French J 1985 To educate or promote health? Health Education Journal 44(3):115–116

French J & Milner S 1993 Should we accept the status quo? Health Education Journal 52(2):98–101

Hall M B (ed) 1996 Health for all children, 3rd edn. Oxford University Press, Oxford

Health Committee 1997 House of Commons Third Report of Session 1996–7 Health services for children and young people in the community: home and school. HMSO, London

Kalnins I, McQueen D V, Backett K C, Curtice L & Currie C E 1994 Children, empowerment and health promotion: some new directions in research and practice. In: Gott M & Moloney B (eds) Child health: a reader. Radcliffe Medical Press, Oxford, pp 191–198

Kelly C 1996 Chronic constipation and soiling in children. A review of the psychological and family literature. Child Psychology and Psychiatry Review 1(2):59–66

King M 1990 Health is a sustainable state. Lancet 336:664–667

Lee P 1998 Childhood accidents: how a health promotion model may help. Journal of Child Health Care 2(3):128–131

Lewis C & Muir J 1996 A collaborative approach in the management of childhood constipation. Health Visitor 69(10):424–426

Maben J & Macleod Clark J 1995 Health promotion: a concept analysis. Journal of Advanced Nursing 22:1158–1165

Nutbeam D 1986 Health promotion glossary. Health Promotion 1(1):113–126

Procter S, Biott C, Campbell S, Edward S, Redpath N & Moran M 1998 Preparation for the developing role of the community children's nurse. English National Board, London

Riley R 1998 Foundations for a healthy future. Journal of Child Health Care 2(1):20–24

Robertson A & Minkler M 1994 New health promotion movement: a critical examination. Health Education Quarterly 21(3):295–312

Robinson S & Hill Y 1998 The health promoting nurse. Journal of Clinical Nursing 7:232–238

Saan H 1986 Health promotion and health education: living with a dominant concept. Health Promotion 1(3):253–255

Seedhouse D 1986 Health. The foundations for achievement. John Wiley, Chichester, UK

Seymour H 1984 Health education versus health promotion – a practitioner's view. Health Education Journal 43(2):37–38

Seymour L & Dean A 1997 Adolescent smoking trends: a local investigation. Health Visitor 70(5):185–187

Speller V 1985 Defining health promotion: service implications. Health Education Journal 44(2):96

Tannahill A 1985 What is health promotion? Health Education Journal 44(4):167–168

Tannahill A 1996 A model of health promotion. In: Downie R, Tannahill C & Tannahill A (eds) Health promotion: models and values. Oxford University Press, Oxford, pp 50–75

Tones K 1990 Why theorise? Ideology in health education. Health Education Journal 49(1):2–6

Tones K & Tilford S 1994 Health education: effectiveness, efficiency and equity. Chapman and Hall, London

Treseder P 1997 Empowering children and young people – training manual. Save the Children, London

Wass A 1994 Promoting health: the primary care approach. W B Saunders–Baillière Tindall, London

Whitehead M 1989 Swimming upstream: trends and prospects in education for health. King's Fund Institute, London

World Health Organization 1984 Health promotion. A discussion document on the concept and principles. World Health Organization, Copenhagen

World Health Organization 1986 Ottawa Charter for Health Promotion: an international conference on health promotion: the move towards a new public health. WHO, Copenhagen

16 Cultural issues in community children's nursing

Paula Kelly & Saleha Uddin

KEY ISSUES

- Impact of culture on the care for sick children at home
- Exploring definitions of culture
- Health and ethnic minorities in the UK
- Examination of practice examples highlighting the components of culture
- Recommendations for practice developments in community children's nursing to achieve culturally sensitive care

INTRODUCTION

This chapter will explore the impact of culture on the care of sick children in the home setting and the implications this has for the continued development of community children's nursing practice (Procter et al 1998). By exploring definitions of culture and how these relate to practice, issues of health for minority ethnic cultures in the UK will be considered. A number of practice examples will illustrate four key concepts:

1. How childhood is viewed
2. The home environment of care
3. Communication
4. Health beliefs

Anthropological studies indicate that these concepts are not necessarily held in the same way by all cultures (James & Prout 1997). Since there are limited primary data to inform and guide nursing practice (Gerrish et al 1996, Scott 1998), the intention of this chapter is to stimulate debate rather than to present solutions or 'cultural checklists' (Mares et al 1985). Through an ongoing examination of key issues community children's nurses (CCNs) can develop dynamic models of care that respond effectively to the needs of children and their carers.

DEFINITIONS OF CULTURE

There are many ways in which culture can be defined and therefore explored (Helman 1994). Simplistic definitions, although attractive at first, can limit understanding (Richardson 1998). Kuper (1994) suggests two key variants within the overall concept of culture. First, culture may be seen as a tradition, learnt from generation to generation, that teaches how to behave and act. Second, this teaching distinguishes different human populations from one another. This may relate to religion, marriage practices, language and many other identifying behaviours. This concept highlights two important facets of culture. All humans, all societies have culture, and participation within a culture often gives a sense of identity and belonging. However, at the same time, culture can be excluding, in that it is what often marks us out as different from one another. This does not imply that within a culture there is homogeneity, whether the 'culture' in question is Jewish, black, nursing or childhood. All 'cultures' will have explicit and implicit divisions within them (Prout 1996). In some situations this leads to the emergence of a subculture; thus paediatric nursing could be seen as a subculture within the wider culture of nursing (Armitage 1998). Neither should we assume that a cultural perspective is static or unchanging. Baumann (1996), in examining the experiences of identity in multiethnic London, suggests that, for young people in particular, the notion of minority ethnic groups as static homogeneous communities is inaccurate and simplistic.

In addition to exposing the lack of homogeneity, we must also consider the fact that culture does not exist within a political vacuum. Some groups within a society hold more power and their 'culture' may dominate; for example, within the healthcare profession, medical concerns may at times carry more weight than nursing concerns. For recipients of healthcare, cultural differences may have a negative effect when it comes to securing resources or communicating across cultures (Department of Health 1995, Gates 1995, Murphy & Macleod Clark 1993).

To comply with item 7 of the United Kingdom Central Council (UKCC) 'Code of professional conduct' (1992) nurses need to apply modes of care that will effectively meet the needs of all cultural groups. In an effort to improve nursing practice and avoid the negative effects of 'cultural imposition', Leininger (1995) developed the concept of transcultural nursing. She argues that an understanding of cultural diversity is essential to the provision of safe and effective care. It could be argued that CCNs, operating outside the constraints imposed by hospital culture, are in a unique position to provide transcultural nursing. Furthermore, in the home setting, the child and their carers may feel more able to assert their cultural needs.

HEALTH AND MINORITY CULTURES IN THE UK

In British healthcare literature the term culture, as discussed above, seems to be almost synonymous with ethnicity (Balarajan & Raleigh 1993). Although this is problematic, a focus on ethnicity has served to highlight some of the key issues in meeting the cultural needs of recipients of healthcare (Madood 1997). Data from the last census, which estimates minority ethnic groups as 5.9% of the UK population (Office of Population Censuses and Surveys 1991), and from ethnic monitoring within the NHS, have the potential to provide information on the healthcare outcomes for some groups of patients (Gilthorpe et al 1997). There is considerable evidence of inequalities of access to, and delivery of, healthcare for minority ethnic communities (Banatvala & Jayaratnam 1996, Cortis 1998, Fernando 1991, Heathley & Yip 1991, Murphy & Macleod Clark 1993, Rocheron et al 1989, Samanta et al 1987, Scott 1998, Slater 1993, Weatherall 1991). Just one study relates directly to the needs of sick children from minority ethnic communities within a hospital setting (Slater 1993).

Caring at home for children with complex chronic or acute conditions is a rapidly developing area in children's nursing (Tatman & Woodruffe 1993). Research in this field has focused on evaluating professional support services, particularly community children's nursing services (Bignold et al 1994, Tatman et al 1992, While 1991), and assessing the ability of parents to carry out technical skills to support the care of their child at home (Evans 1992, Wilson et al 1998). Furthermore, the literature on family experiences has focused either on a particular disease process, such as childhood cancer (Bluebond-Langer 1978), cystic fibrosis (Coyne 1997, Whyte 1992) and juvenile arthritis (Jerret 1994), or on parental participation in their child's care during hospital admissions (Alderson 1993, Darbyshire 1994). As yet, there are few published UK studies that focus on the impact of culture on care in the home setting. Whilst the above studies offer insight into the stress and burden of care faced by caregivers (usually mothers) and thus could be said to indicate the development of appropriate support services (Coyne 1997), they are problematic when considering the cultural needs of families since they regard the care both given and received as culturally neutral (Good 1994).

For CCNs to deliver culturally sensitive and therefore effective care, there is a need to recognise and reflect upon the implications of our personal and professional cultural backgrounds, in addition to increasing our knowledge of the cultural needs of individual children and families through assessment (Narayan 1997).

CULTURAL CONSTRUCTION OF CHILDHOOD

Conceptualisations of 'childhood' are not universal (Prout 1982). This is evident in the historical review of the change in attitude towards child abuse in Britain (Jenks 1996). Similar variations exist, between social class and ethnic groups, in child-rearing practices (Mayall 1991, Ochs & Schieffelin 1984, Swanwick 1996). Examining parental perceptions in immigrant Chinese families of children with chronic illness, Elfert et al (1991) demonstrated that the illness was frequently described as having a global effect on many aspects of the child's present and future life. This was compared with Euro-Canadian parents who described the illness or disability as affecting only particular aspects of the child's life. Hillier & Rahman's (1996) study of Bangladeshi families in east London argued that, in child psychiatry, clinical care could be improved by setting the concerns of the family in a cultural context, by exploring notions of child development held by parents. How a particular family conceptualises childhood will therefore affect their response to the illness and treatment, and how it is managed.

One way in which these responses can be seen as significant within the realms of community children's nursing is illustrated in the case study below. Here, the notion of childhood as a time of freedom from responsibility was challenged by a sibling's involvement in nursing care.

CASE STUDY

Samera was the fifth child of Bangladeshi parents. She was born at 28 weeks' gestation and required mechanical ventilation for several weeks. Although able to maintain adequate oxygen saturation levels within air, extubation proved difficult. A tracheostomy was performed and a diagnosis of subglottal stenosis was made. Before discharge her parents were taught all aspects of her nursing care including changing the tracheostomy tube. The teaching programme was facilitated by ward nurses and members of the local community children's nursing team. On a home visit, several weeks after discharge, the CCN was surprised to find Samera in the sole care of her 14-year-old sister. Her parents and the other children were visiting the general practitioner at the time.

Discussion

In this case, the teaching programme before discharge had failed to highlight that within this family it was expected that older daughters would have care responsibilities for younger children. This had potentially exposed both Samera and her older sibling to an unsafe situation. With help from the team's link worker, the expectations of care responsibilities for Samera were re-negotiated between the nursing team and the family. This process enabled the team to recognise that their own views on childhood were based within a particular legal, ethical and philosophical framework which was, in this case, challenged by a different conceptualisation of childhood.

ENVIRONMENT OF CARE

The home environment provides the physical structure within which care is managed in community nursing. The household is the area where families manage the majority of their responsibilities, into which the many aspects of care for the sick child need to be incorporated. The home provides the context where the care actually takes place. Helman (1984) indicates that, in healthcare, context has a considerable impact on the style and content of information giving by health professionals. Therefore CCNs need to consider how different areas of the house are managed, for example the use of reception rooms for visitors only or the separation and behaviour of ages and genders within household space. This physical environment can have tremendous implications for nursing practice, particularly for children with complex needs who may be dependent on technological advances.

CASE STUDY

A nurse specialist in nutrition at a regional cardiac centre referred John, aged 6 months, to his local community children's nursing service. Following interim surgery for a complex congenital cardiac malformation, John had failed to gain weight in the hospital or home setting. A trial of nasogastric feeding (before possible gastrostomy formation) was planned. John's family was living on a permanent site for travellers and expected to be there for the next few months. They spend half of the year travelling around sites in the south of England and the remainder of the year in Ireland. The site had a water supply from a standpipe. A portable generator supplied electricity to each caravan during the day.

Discussion

The management of equipment in this setting was an initial concern for the CCNs. Their own expectations of a 'home' did not extend to a caravan. Visiting the family revealed that the way in which the space was used by the family to organise their day-to-day needs could safely incorporate an enteral feeding system. The caravan, spacious during the day when John would have bolus feeds, was adapted at night to accommodate the sleeping needs of a large family in a confined but highly organised space. Together with the family the CCN decided to run the overnight feeding pump on batteries rather than rely on the generator. John already slept close to his parents, so problems during the night could be dealt with, causing minimal disruption for the rest of the family. The main difficulty arose with the delivery of feeding sets. The site was not recognised by the delivery service as an address, highlighting the practical issues faced by the family in receiving appointments and other information sent by post. This aspect was resolved by a local pharmacist agreeing to receive and store the supplies, which the family collected on a regular basis. In this example both physical and political aspects of the household in question needed to be considered to achieve safe and appropriate care.

COMMUNICATION

Communicating effectively with patients and caregivers is fundamental to nursing care (Burnard 1989). Child health nursing curricula devote considerable time for students to develop knowledge and communication skills with children of different developmental stages. As developmental age may be a barrier to communicating with children, so language may be a barrier for communicating with caregivers and children. Families for whom English is not the first language may receive a reduced quality of care because of communication difficulties (Slater 1993). It is acknowledged that the provision of skilled interpreters in the health service is inadequate (Audit Commission 1993, Cortis 1998). The cost of provision may seem prohibitive when the minority ethnic population is small or extremely diverse in terms of language needs. The use of relatives, especially children, or other health service staff is usually problematic since they lack the skills required by a trained interpreter in addition to the conflicts of confidentiality. Where interpreters or link workers are available, their effectiveness may be hampered by healthcare professionals' lack of experience in their use. The provision and use of skilled interpreters, by healthcare professionals, has received little attention in healthcare training (Heathley & Yip 1991). For CCNs visiting families in the home setting, other practical concerns arise concerning flexibility of visiting (if interpreting services have to be booked in advance) and maintaining continuity by visiting with the same interpreter (Twinn 1997).

CASE STUDY

At 6 years of age, Ifat was diagnosed with acute lymphoblastic leukaemia. His parents are Turkish speaking and he lives at home with them and his elder sister. During his hospital admission, interpreters had been used to convey details of Ifat's diagnosis and planned medical treatment. Following Ifat's extended hospital admission the CCNs worked with a community-based Turkish interpreter to establish rapport with the family in their own home. Re-establishing home routines was an initial priority, in particular adapting the style of giving oral medication to a manner more suited to the family's needs. The seriousness of the diagnosis had led to a rigid interpretation of administering the medicines. As confidence in the CCN team developed, the family became more involved in the management of Ifat's central venous access line. The role of the interpreter was crucial in this and it quickly became apparent that visiting without the interpreter meant halting the teaching programme, despite the fact that both parents had some understanding and expression of English.

Discussion

The facility of a skilled experienced interpreter was essential to ensure that Ifat and his family received appropriate care. Concerns about his long-term prognosis and reintegration into school were raised by the family in an environment where they were able to communicate their needs. The nurses were also able to give more detailed explanations because of the quality of the interpreting services. It was recognised that language was just one potential communication barrier. Styles of verbal and non-verbal communication also became a key aspect of care delivery. Written information on the care of the central venous line was not available in the family's own language. Consequently, the CCNs were able to have this information translated and supplemented by the team's own pictorial teaching tool (Sexton et al 1996, Smettem 1999). This not only helped to reinforce verbal information given but also gave access to information for other family members who were not always present on visits. This practice example also illustrates how a simplistic approach to culturally sensitive care could be problematic as both the gender and political views of the interpreter in this case were very important to the family, who were refugees. The use of specific dialect should also be considered in planning interpreting service needs.

HEALTH BELIEFS

The perceived neutrality of biomedical explanations of health and illness is problematic when considering the care needs of patients (Good 1994). Medical anthropologists suggest that, regardless of culture, most of us hold a range of explanations of health and illness (Helman 1994). Furthermore these explanations may be invoked to a greater or lesser extent depending on the context. Eade's (1997) review of beliefs and practices among Bangladeshis in Tower Hamlets indicates that, although 'experts' often demarcate the differences between medical, Islamic and folk models, 'ordinary people' operate with less rigid boundaries.

Much of the literature on the response to illness in children from specific ethnic groups is comparative (Chen 1986, Pachter et al 1995, Watson 1984). A comparative approach is problematic since it implies or explicitly sets the study group against a perceived standard of compliance or appropriate use by another population. This stance demonstrates the difficulties that Good (1994) outlined, in exposing the tendency for biomedical explanations to be regarded as facts and other models as beliefs. He suggests that medical anthropologists experience a tension between wishing to give weight to traditional explanations of ill health or misfortune and yet feeling an obligation to ensure access to 'biomedicine', therefore privileging that explanation. Nurses wishing to be culturally sensitive in their practice may experience the same tension. Weller (1994) advocates the use of an assessment framework, by nurses, to evaluate the impact of traditional health beliefs and practices on child and family health.

CASE STUDY

Blessing is 3 years old and has had eczema for the last year. Her mother is West Indian and has recently begun to supplement her daughter's prescribed treatment with herbal remedies in an effort to control her distressing symptoms.

Discussion

In discussion with Blessing's mother the CCN became aware that her expectations of the effects of biomedical treatment were rather unrealistic. She had anticipated that compliance with the skin care regimen would result in Blessing's skin returning permanently to 'normal'. Initially family and friends had encouraged her to use a range of other treatments, but she had felt that the 'prescribed' treatment would be the best. Her disappointment had reduced her confidence in all aspects of the healthcare system. Although the CCN considered it important to make her aware of the potential harmful effects of herbal treatments, she also wished to support the mother's own decision about her child's care. By continuing to visit, despite the use of 'unorthodox' treatments, the nurse was able to re-establish confidence in other aspects of the healthcare service. The experience gave an opportunity to explore in more detail this method of management and to recognise that at different times in the child's illness the preferred explanation or treatment could change. As Blessing's skin condition went into a more stable phase, her mother felt that she could revert to a more biomedical explanation and treatment. This example focused on 'complementary or alternative' treatments in its explorations of health beliefs. Other topics for consideration could have included the impact of dietary, religious or spiritual explanations and treatments.

CONCLUSION

This chapter has illustrated some of the issues that may impact on the care of sick children in a community setting from a cultural perspective. There are several implications for practice.

Education programmes at pre- and post-registration level need to increase the opportunities for learning about culture (Gerrish et al 1996), giving students the opportunity to explore issues such as differences in family structure and how these may impact on the planning and delivery of nursing care. The work of Martinson et al (1997), on expectations of support for Chinese families caring for children with chronic illness, demonstrates the need for awareness of changing family structures. CCNs need to be constantly mindful of the context for individual families and children. This may mean that a particular family will approach care through their previous experience, which may include immigration experiences, racism within or outside the health service, and a range of vulnerabilities and strengths.

The case studies used have focused predominantly on meeting the 'cultural' needs of carers. Ethnographers have demonstrated how children are active in constructing their own cultural identities (Briggs 1970, James 1993, Mayall et al 1996, Toren 1990). Hall's (1995) study illustrated how fluid this cultural identity could be where British Sikh teenagers graded their behaviour more or less towards traditional expectations depending on the context. Practice models will need to balance potential conflicting and changing interpretations of culture to meet the needs of children and carers.

Assessments and evaluations of care need to incorporate an opportunity for cultural needs to be explored and the extent to which care given meets these needs (Chevannes 1997, Narayan 1997). Whyte's (1996) work on family nursing represents one potential framework that could be used in this way.

There continues to be a need to develop research in this area that can inform and guide practice. Any investigation into the care needs of children and families in a community setting should address cultural needs. In addition, focused research on assessment and evaluation would be a valuable starting point in developing culturally sensitive care. Finally, as suggested above, how children construct their own cultural identities in sickness and health could provide a fruitful and fascinating area for collaborative research projects between health and social sciences.

FURTHER READING

Dwivedi K N & Varma V P 1996 Meeting the needs of ethnic minority children. Jessica Kingsley, London

Addresses the social and health care of children from minority ethnic families in the UK, with a particular focus on meeting the psychological and emotional needs of children.

Helman C G 1994 Culture, health and illness, 3rd edn. Butterworth–Heinemann, London

Medical anthropology text, well organised into chapters that enable the reader to dip into an area of interest. Little direct information on children but useful for the insights it provides into the culture of medical care.

Prout A 1996 Families, cultural bias and health promotion implications of an ethnographic study. Health Education Authority, London

Ethnographic study examining the impact of culture on health promotion in the family. Detailed case studies give the reader an insight into the complexities of how families make decisions about health. Particularly useful for the attention that it draws to children's own contribution, which may have resonance when considering the decisions made by children with chronic illness.

Slater M 1993 Health for all our children: achieving appropriate health care for black and ethnic minority children and their family. Action for Sick Children, London

Report of a study reviewing the experiences of minority ethnic families within the health service. Provides examples of good practice and an associate training package which could be adapted as a foundation for developing standards of care in the community setting.

Wyke S & Hewison J 1991 Child health matters: caring for children in the community. Open University Press, Milton Keynes

Collection of writings, mainly from a sociological perspective. Takes the stance that, as parents are the main providers of healthcare for children, professions need to understand their perspective. Sections 2 and 3 on perspectives on health and use of health services are particularly useful for community children's nurses planning care to meet the cultural needs of children and families.

REFERENCES

Alderson P 1993 Children's consent to surgery. Open University Press, Buckingham

Armitage G 1998 Analysing childhood: a nursing perspective. Journal of Child Health Care 2(2):66–70

Audit Commission 1993 What seems to be the matter? Communication between hospitals and patients. HMSO, London

Balarajan R & Raleigh V S 1993 Ethnicity and health: a guide for the NHS. Department of Health, London

Banatvala N & Jayaratnam P 1996 The experiences of East London's minority ethnic community. Health in the East End: Annual Public Health Report 1995/6. Department of Public Health,

East London and City Health Authority, London
Baumann G 1996 Contesting culture: discourses of identity in multi-ethnic London. Cambridge University Press, Cambridge.
Bignold S, Ball S & Cribb A 1994 Nursing families of children with cancer: the work of the paediatric oncology outreach nurse specialists. Cancer Relief Macmillan Fund/Department of Health, King's College London.
Bluebond-Langer M 1978 The private world of dying children. Princeton Press, Newhaven, New Jersey
Briggs J 1970 Never in anger. Harvard University Press, Cambridge, Massachusetts
Burnard P 1989 Teaching interpersonal skills: a handbook of experiential learning for health professionals. Chapman & Hall, London
Chen L C 1986 Primary health care in developing countries: overcoming operational, technical and social barriers. Lancet 29 November:1260–1265
Chevannes M 1997 Nurses caring for families – issues in a multi racial society. Journal of Clinical Nursing 6(2):161–167
Cortis J D 1998 The experiences of nursing care received by Pakistani (Urdu speaking) patients in later life in Dewsbury, UK. Clinical Effectiveness in Nursing 2:131–138
Coyne I T 1997 Chronic illness: the importance of support for families caring for a child with cystic fibrosis. Journal of Clinical Nursing 6(2):121–129
Darbyshire P 1994 Living with a sick child in hospital. The experiences of parents and nurses. Chapman & Hall, London
Department of Health 1995 Variations in health. What can the Department of Health and the NHS do? HMSO, London
Eade J 1997 The power of the experts: the plurality of beliefs and practices concerning health and illness among Bangladeshis in contemporary Tower Hamlets, London. In: Marks L & Worboys M (eds) Migrants, minorities and health. Routledge, London, pp 250–271
Elfert H, Anderson J M & Lai M 1991 Parents' perceptions of children with chronic illness: a study of immigrant Chinese families. Journal of Pediatric Nursing 6(2):114–120
Evans M 1992 An investigation into the feasibility of parental participation in the nursing care of their children. Journal of Advanced Nursing 29:477–482
Fernando S 1991 Mental health: race and culture. Macmillan Press, Basingstoke
Gates E 1995 Culture clash – the nursing care of dying children from cultural backgrounds that are different from the nurses. Nursing Times 91(7):42–43
Gerrish K, Husband C & Mackenzie J 1996 Nursing for a multi-ethnic society. Open University Press, Buckingham
Gilthorpe M S, Lay Yee T, Wilson R C, Walters S, Gryfiths R K & Bedi R 1998 Variations in hospitalisation rates for asthma among black and ethnic minority communities. Respiratory Medicine 92(4):642–648
Good B J 1994 Medicine rationality and experience an anthropological perspective. Cambridge University Press, Cambridge
Hall K 1995 There's a time to act English and a time to act Indian: the politics of identity amongst British Sikh teenagers. In: Stephens S (ed) Children and the politics of culture. Princeton University Press, Princeton
Heathley P T & Yip R Y W 1991 Analysis of general practice consultation rates among Asian patients. British Journal of General Practice 41:476
Helman C 1984 The role of context in primary care. Journal of the Royal College of General Practitioners 34:547–550
Helman C G 1994 Culture, health and illness, 3rd edn. Butterworth–Heinemann, Oxford
Hillier S & Rahman S 1996 Childhood development and behavioural and emotional problems as perceived by Bangladeshi parents in East London. In: Kewllerher D & Hillier S (eds) Researching cultural differences in health. Routledge, London, pp 38–68
James A 1993 Childhood identities: self and social relationships in the experience of the child. Edinburgh University Press, Edinburgh
James A & Prout A 1997 Constructing and reconstructing childhood: contemporary issues in the sociological study of childhood. Falmer Press, London
Jenks C 1996 Childhood. Routledge, London
Jerrett M D 1994 Parents' experiences of coming to know the care of a chronically ill child. Journal of Advanced Nursing 19:1050–1056
Kuper A 1994 Anthropological futures. In: Borofsky R (ed) Assessing cultural anthropology. McGraw Hill, New York, pp 113–118
Leininger M 1995 Transcultural nursing: concepts theories and practices. John Wiley, New York
Madood T 1997 Ethnic minorities in Britain, diversity and disadvantage. PSI Press, London
Mares P, Henley A & Baxter C 1985 Health care in multi racial Britain. Health Education Council National Extension College
Martinson I M, Armstrong V & Qiao J 1997 The experience of the family of children with chronic illness at home in China. Pediatric Nursing 23(4):371–375
Mayall B 1991 Ideologies of childcare: mothers and health visitors. In: Wyke S & Hewison J (eds) Child health matters: caring for children

in the community. Open University Press, Milton Keynes
Mayall B, Bendelow G, Barker S, Feltman M & Storey P 1996 Children's health in primary schools. Falmer Press, London
Murphy K & Macleod Clark J 1993 Nurses' experiences of caring for ethnic minority clients. Journal of Advanced Nursing 18:442–450
Narayan M C 1997 Cultural assessment in home health care. Home Health Care Nurse 15(10):663–670
Ochs E & Schieffelin B 1984 Language acquisition and socialisation: three developmental stories and their implications. In: Shweder R A & Le Vine R A (eds) Culture theory: essays on mind, self and emotion. Cambridge University Press, Cambridge, Massachusetts
Office of Population Censuses and Surveys 1991 Census reports. HMSO, London
Pachter L M, Cloutier M M & Bernstein B A 1995 Ethnomedical (folk) remedies for childhood asthma in a mainland Puerto Rican community. Archives of Paediatric Adolescent Medicine 149(9):982–988
Procter S, Biott C, Campbell S, Edward S, Redpath N & Moran M 1998 Preparation for the developing role of the community children's nurse. English National Board for Nursing, Midwifery and Health Visiting, London
Prout A 1982 Children and childhood in the sociology of medicine. COMAC, Workshop on Medicine and Childhood
Prout A 1996 Families, cultural bias and health promotion, implications of an ethnographic study. Health Education Authority, London
Richardson J 1998 Culture and the child health ambulatory setting. In: Glasper E A & Lowson S (eds) Innovations in paediatric ambulatory care: a nursing perspective. Macmillan, London
Rocheron Y, Dickinson R & Khan S 1989 Evaluation of the mother and baby campaign. University of Leicester, Leicester
Samanta A, Campbell J, Spalding D, Panja K, Neogi S & Briden A 1987 Dietary habits of Asian diabetics in a general practice clinic. Human Nutrition, Applied Nutrition 41a:160–163
Scott P 1998 Lay beliefs and the management of disease amongst West Indians with diabetes. Health and Social Care in the Community 6(6):407–419
Sexton E, Paul L & Holden C 1996 A pictorial assisted teaching tool for families. Paediatric Nursing 8(5):24–26
Slater M 1993 Health for all our children: achieving appropriate health care for black and minority children and their families. Action for Sick Children, London
Smettem S 1999 Welcome/Assalaam-u-alaikam: improving communications with ethnic minority families. Paediatric Nursing 11(2):33–35
Swanwick M 1996 Child rearing across cultures. Paediatric Nursing 8(7):13–17
Tatman M A & Woodruffe C 1993 Paediatric home care in the UK. Archives of Disease in Childhood 69:677–680
Tatman M A, Woodruffe C, Kelly P J & Harris R J 1992 Paediatric home care in Tower Hamlets: a working partnership with parents. Quality in Health Care 1:98–103
Toren C 1990 Making sense of hierarchy: cognition as social process in Fiji. Athlone Press, London
Twinn S 1997 An exploratory study examining the influence of translation on the validity and reliability of qualitative data in nursing research. Journal of Advanced Nursing 26:418–423
UK Central Council for Nursing, Midwifery and Health Visiting 1992 Code of professional conduct. UKCC, London
Watson E 1984 Health of infants and use of health services by mothers of different ethnic groups in East London. Community Medicine 6:127–135
Weatherall D 1991 Bookshelf the sickle cell patient. Lancet 337:1590
Weller B 1994 Cultural aspects of children's health and illness. In: Lindsay B (ed) The child and family: contemporary nursing issues in child health and care. Baillière Tindall, London, pp 96–107
While A E 1991 An evaluation of a paediatric home care scheme. Journal of Advanced Nursing 16:1413–1421
Whyte D 1992 Family nursing approach to the care of a child with a chronic illness. Journal of Advanced Nursing 17:317–327
Whyte D 1996 Explorations in family nursing. Routledge, London
Wilson S, Morse J M & Penrod J 1998 Absolute involvement: the experience of mothers of ventilator dependent children. Health and Social Care in the Community 6(4):224–233

SECTION

3 DIMENSIONS OF COMMUNITY CHILDREN'S NURSING PRACTICE

The ability of community children's nursing to be responsive and proactive is influenced by many factors which require consideration. The aim of this section is not to provide a comprehensive review of clinical practice, but to offer the reader the opportunity to explore some of its diverse aspects. These include team composition alongside organisational issues and information management. An examination of dependency measurement provides a necessary foundation to the increasing range of dependency encountered in practice. The fact that children and young people often act as carers is recognised and the broader implications of this for practitioners are rightfully explored.

SECTION CONTENTS

17 Issues for the composition of community children's nursing teams

Maybelle Tatman & Suzanne Jones

KEY ISSUES

- The necessity for team leadership within community children's nursing services
- Generalist and specialist practice
- Adjusting skill mix to meet the needs of children and their families

INTRODUCTION

This chapter outlines the inter-related issues when planning or reviewing the structure of a new or developing community children's nursing team. These are identified as team composition, team competencies and specialism, skill mix, and the roles of the other disciplines and of parents.

TEAM COMPOSITION

Community children's nursing has developed diversely in Britain, with patchy coverage by often small services, some generalist and some specialist, based either in acute units or in the community (Tatman & Woodroffe 1993). These services have often consisted of one or two whole-time equivalent nurses, working autonomously, at a high level of competence and often under considerable stress (Miller 1992). Currently community children's nursing teams are increasing in both number and size, raising the possibility of a wider skill mix, including junior team members who can work under supervision. This is also required to meet the needs of community children's nurses (CCNs) in training for supervised placements.

In the future, community children's nursing services may be integrated, which will mean that all nurses who work with children, whether CCN, health visitor or school nurse, will be qualified as children's nurses and able to give hands-on care as well as carrying out child health surveillance and health promotion (Health Committee 1997). This cannot happen without clear definition of the roles that generic nurses fulfil within a community children's nursing service or clinical supervision of individual nurses. It is essential, therefore, that teams include a clinical leader with the management skills to develop the service in response to identified unmet needs (Parkin 1998).

BOX 17.1 *Skills and abilities required by CCNs*

- To work with a high level of independence in a child's home, without immediate recourse to other clinicians
- To assess complex needs of children requiring nursing in the community, and of their families
- To formulate individual care plans
- To teach and support families in carrying out their child's nursing care
- To monitor the child's progress, solve problems, and adapt the care plan accordingly
- To manage their time and workload to provide a reliable and responsive service
- To liaise with and teach other professionals and coordinate their input
- To establish and audit service standards, policies and procedures
- To teach and support other team members

BOX 17.2 *The seven broad areas in which CCNs work (Whiting 1998)*

1. Neonatal and post-neonatal care, including care of babies with congenital disorders and those with sequelae of prematurity
2. Caring for children with acute nursing needs to reduce the length of hospital admission
3. Supporting children undergoing planned surgery
4. Supporting the families of children with long-term nursing needs
5. Follow-up care of children requiring emergency treatment to enable early discharge from hospital
6. Supporting children with a disability
7. Supporting children's palliative care

Leadership may be summarised as (Colquhoun & Dougan 1997, Malone 1996).

- Vision – acting as a change agent to set strategic direction
- Risk taking – having the confidence to implement innovative practice
- Boundary management – reviewing professional roles
- Empowerment – enabling team members to assume a leadership role and share vision
- Mentoring – training and clinical leadership to demonstrate reflective and evidence-based practice

In formulating a strategy to meet identified needs, the required competencies of the team must be considered and the team leader must be able to determine the level of training and supervision required by individual team members.

TEAM COMPETENCIES

The competencies required by CCNs, either autonomously or with supervision, are shown in Box 17.1 and the seven broad areas in which CCNs work are outlined in Box 17.2.

These areas include a number of subspecialities such as oncology and cystic fibrosis care, and no individual CCN could reasonably be expected to provide the same high level of competency in each. Some diagnosis-based specialisation is inevitable within teams if competencies are to be maintained across a wide range of diagnoses. This may conflict with the need for the team members: (1) to retain insight into one another's work, (2) to cross-cover for one another, including out-of-hours cover where this is an aim of the team, (3) to work with a geographical patch with the aim of improving liaison with primary care, and (4) to avoid practising in isolation. In developing a team, the identification and assessment of unmet needs is essential to determine service priorities and the competencies and level of specialisation required in each clinical area.

SPECIALISATION IN THE CONTEXT OF COMMUNITY CHILDREN'S NURSING

There are two separate dimensions to specialisation:

- Concentration of practice in a disorder-specific subspeciality
- Increased level of expertise, in the sense of advanced practice

Benner's work (1984) has been widely embraced because she encapsulated much of the early theory on advanced practice by explaining competencies in terms of five levels of practice from novice through to expert. The distinctions between these levels continue to be debated as nurses have examined the boundaries of advanced clinical practice.

In 1994 the United Kingdom Central Council (UKCC) for Nursing, Midwifery and Health Visiting recognised the concepts of specialist and advanced practice in the UK for the first time. It described specialist practitioners as demonstrating 'higher levels of clinical decision making and being able to monitor and improve standards of care through supervision of practice, clinical nursing audit, developing and leading practice, contributing to research, teaching and supporting colleagues.' The clinical nurse specialist has been described as a clinical expert, resource/consultant, educator, change agent, researcher, advocate and mentor (Miller 1995). Hamric (1996) identified eight core competencies to define the advanced nurse practitioner role as expert clinical practice, expert guidance and coaching, consultation, research skills, clinical and professional leadership, collaboration, change agent skills and ethical decision making. Advanced practitioners are defined as 'Specially prepared nurses who are working in roles which demand a lot of nursing experience, education at master's degree level, and nursing skills that contribute to meeting the complex needs of vulnerable people and the need to be continuously questioning the fundamentals and boundaries of nursing' (Castledine 1996).

These definitions overlap, and a survey of specialist and advanced nursing practice in England (McGee et al 1996) found that there was still a need for clarification of the interface between the two roles and that of doctors. Maclaine (1998) suggested that the nurse practitioner had a more generalist range of practice than a nurse specialist and also used diagnostic skills including physical examination, but that many aspects of their roles were the same.

The concept of a 'higher level practitioner' has been introduced to include both specialist and advanced practice (UKCC 1998, Waller 1998).

The generalist CCN practises with a high degree of skill and autonomy and takes responsibilities corresponding to those of a specialist (Fradd 1992). Procter et al (1998) described the relationship between generalist and specialist roles. Of the community children's nursing teams identified in a postal survey carried out in England, they classified those with more than two whole-time equivalent nurses as 'large'. They divided these teams into community-based teams with and without clinical nurse specialists, and acute-based teams with and without members with community qualifications. Their subsequent fieldwork found that teams classified as community-based generalists in fact worked alongside specialists who were not located within the team and also that some specialist nurses functioned in a more generalist role. Services based on subspecialities could be left with gaps, creating the need for generalists with wider skills or for specialists to broaden their expertise. They argued that the multi-skilled generalists were advanced practitioners in community children's nursing: '"Generalist" may be used in the sense of "not yet having acquired specialist expertise in a particular area" or in the sense of "having moved beyond narrow specialisation into an expert role, capable of coping with a range of specialisms". In the latter may lie the true meaning of advanced practice' (Procter et al 1998).

As CCNs achieve recognition and status as higher level practitioners, the opportunity arises for the introduction and training of junior members of the team, leading to the consideration of the issue of skill mix.

NURSING SKILL MIX

McKenna (1995) reviewed the conflicting evidence on skill mix and quality of care. Some studies suggested that a highly qualified skill mix was expensive and unproductive, and others found the reverse. Skill mix should be appropriate to the nature of work required, and be reviewed and adjusted as the needs of the caseload change.

Many community children's nursing services comprise one or two highly skilled nurses (Tatman & Woodroffe 1993) and have been too small to introduce skill mix. In contrast, Peter & Torr (1996) described the successful first year of a Hospital at Home scheme providing 24-hour care with nine whole-time equivalents, including seven staff nurses, working on a rotation system through the wards. The children treated had mainly acute conditions such as bronchiolitis, febrile illnesses and gastroenteritis. Evaluation of a similar, longer established, service (Jennings 1994) revealed that a high standard of care was received by children but that community liaison and clarification of medical responsibilities needed addressing. As a result, one nurse became team leader and adopted a key worker role, coordinating the long-term follow-up of children with chronic conditions. A paediatric registrar post was linked to the service. The team became smaller and more highly qualified, and home visiting was separated from ward work. These changes may be interpreted as an increase in specialisation and skill levels in response to the needs of children with complex and chronic conditions, and illustrate the need to review provision as the caseload changes.

ROLE OF OTHER DISCIPLINES

There is a further dimension to skill mix beyond that of nursing competence, which is to consider the needs of patients in a holistic way and how these can be met by other disciplines. This means valuing the complementary skills of others. An example is the role of play specialists in home visiting. Wilson (1992) described how play therapy helped children to cope with renal transplantation and needle phobia.

Thornes (cited in National Health Service Executive 1998) described multidisciplinary teams that had been set up within a pilot project programme for children with life-threatening illnesses. CCNs provided coordination, and the range of needs necessitated a wide mix of skills and disciplines within the teams which included social workers, clinical psychologists, community paediatricians, bereavement carers, and volunteers providing domestic help. Domiciliary respite care was provided in some teams by CCNs and in others by healthcare assistants. Healthcare assistants, trained by CCNs, provided a good standard of care with the overall responsibility being retained by the nurse.

WORKING WITH PARENTS

Coyne (1995), in a review of the literature, identified an expectation that parents will be extensively involved in the care of their sick child, in hospital and at home. There was a lack of clarity among both nurses and parents about the boundaries of parental participation. Surveys of home-care schemes (Procter et al 1998, Tatman et al 1992, While 1991) have identified a high level of nursing tasks undertaken by families while key elements of the CCN's role were teaching and supporting the parental care of the child. A higher level of competency is required for the CCN to focus on the supportive role rather than on direct physical care (Procter et al 1998).

CASE STUDY

Edward had a rare syndrome requiring artificial ventilation during sleep. By 2 months of age, his ventilation was stable. At this time he was resident on the regional paediatric intensive care unit using equipment that would be suitable for home use. Discharge planning began, including multidisciplinary meetings and, in the absence of national guidelines, consultation with providers of home ventilation services elsewhere. A package of care was negotiated with funding authorities to include 24-hour care from a nursing team and alterations to the family home. At 7 months of age, Edward was transferred to his local hospital, with ward nurses having been seconded to learn his care.

Recognising that recruitment and retention of nurses for this work would be difficult, the home ventilation team was planned to include a coordinator and to be sufficiently staffed to enable nurses to undertake further education and rotate through the existing generalist community children's nursing team. Despite this, only four of seven posts could be filled, and as a result the coordinator's post was over-committed to hands-on nursing and the staff could not rotate as planned.

The team was able to take Edward, now aged 18 months, home during the day, returning to the ward at night. As the home alterations were incomplete, Edward was nursed in an upstairs bedroom. Uncertainties over the alterations and team recruitment were stressful for the parents and nurses and, despite prior preparation, tension arose between them because professional boundaries became blurred. The parents expected the nurses to 'become part of the family' and contribute to parental roles. The nurses preferred to maintain their professional role but at times required parents to adopt some nursing roles.

As Edward's sleep pattern became predictable, a reduction in daytime nursing was negotiated with the aim of introducing nursery nurses and concentrating nursing input at night. The home alterations were completed and Edward was discharged from hospital aged 27 months. Nursery nurses were recruited and trained in the ventilation techniques. They also contributed to Edward's waking needs for play and stimulation, and accompanied him to nursery school, acting as class helpers. The parents' need for respite was acknowledged and this was provided in such a way that they could have a break away from the home.

Despite the rarity of the child's diagnosis, this case study illustrates some pitfalls in developing a new service:

- There was a need to release the coordinator from hands-on care to lead the team effectively and pursue managerial issues.
- The skill mix should have incorporated nursery nurses earlier.
- The skills of parents must be recognised but managed with care: they too can burn out.

CONCLUSIONS

Leadership is necessary for the development of a team in which there is appropriate skill mix, with support and mentorship for junior members, and close cooperation between senior members. 'Generalist' community children's nursing is a recognised specialisation in itself, necessitating a high level of competency and autonomy within the nursing team. Once implemented, a team should maintain a service development plan based on ongoing review of caseload needs and adjustment of skill mix and team size accordingly. Cognisance should be taken of the contribution of other disciplines.

FURTHER READING

Procter S, Biott C, Campbell S, Edward S, Redpath N & Moran M 1998 Preparation for the developing role of the community children's nurse. English National Board for Nursing, Midwifery and Health Visiting, London

This research was carried out to inform the development of a training programme for community children's nursing, based on the needs of families caring for sick children at home. It provides a valuable snapshot of different models of care and considers in detail the issues explored in this chapter.

National Health Service Executive 1998 Evaluation of the pilot project programme for children with life threatening illnesses. The Stationery Office, London

Provides an overview of the diverse multidisciplinary services set up for children with life-threatening illnesses, with many examples of good practice.

Colquhoun M & Dougan H 1997 Ensuring that the specialist nurse is special. Palliative Medicine 11:381–387

This analysis of primary, specialist and advanced roles within the context of adult palliative care nursing provides a table of performance standards for each level of practice.

Hamric A B, Spross J A & Hanson C M (eds) 1996 Advanced nursing practice: an integrative approach. W B Saunders, Philadelphia

A key text for advanced practice.

REFERENCES

Benner P 1984 From novice to expert: excellence and power in clinical nursing practice. Addison-Wesley, Menlo Park, California

Castledine G 1996 The role and criteria of an advanced nurse practitioner. British Journal of Nursing 5:288–289

Colquhoun M & Dougan H 1997 Ensuring that the specialist nurse is special. Palliative Medicine 11:381–387

Coyne I T 1995 Parental participation in care: a critical review of the literature. Journal of Advanced Nursing 21:716–722

Fradd E 1992 Working with the specialists. Community Outlook June:29–30

Hamric A B 1996 A definition of advanced nursing. In: Hamric A B, Spross J A & Hanson C M (eds) Advanced nursing practice: an integrative approach. W B Saunders, Philadelphia, pp 42–56

Health Committee 1997 House of Commons Health Select Committee. Health services for children and young people in the community: home and school. Third report. The Stationery Office, London

Jennings P 1994 Learning through experience: an evaluation of 'Hospital at Home'. Journal of Advanced Nursing 19:905–911

McGee P, Castledine G & Brown R 1996 A survey of specialist and advanced nursing practice in England. British Journal of Nursing 5(11):682–686

McKenna H 1995 Nursing skill mix substitutions and quality of care: an exploration of assumptions from the research literature. Journal of Advanced Nursing 21:452–459

Maclaine K 1998 Clarifying higher level roles in nursing practice. Professional Nurse 14(3):159–163

Malone B 1996 Clinical and professional leadership. In: Hamric A B, Spross J A & Hanson C M (eds) Advanced nursing practice: an integrative approach. W B Saunders, Philadelphia, pp 213–228

Miller S 1992 The cost of caring. Paediatric Nursing 4(9):15–16

Miller S 1995 The clinical nurse specialist: a way forward? Journal of Advanced Nursing 22:494–501

National Health Service Executive 1998 Evaluation of the pilot project programme for children with life threatening illnesses. The Stationery Office, London

Parkin P 1998 An approach to management for community health professionals. British Journal of Community Nursing 3(8):374–381

Peter S & Torr G 1996 Paediatric hospital at home; the first year. Paediatric Nursing 8(5):20–23

Procter S, Biott C, Campbell S, Edward S, Redpath N & Moran M 1998 Preparation for the developing role of the community children's nurse. English National Board for Nursing, Midwifery and Health Visiting, London

Tatman M & Woodroffe C 1993 Paediatric home care in the UK. Archives of Disease in Childhood 69:677–680

Tatman M A, Woodroffe C, Kelly P J & Harris R J 1992 Paediatric home care in Tower Hamlets: a working partnership with parents. Quality in Health Care 1:98–103

UK Central Council for Nursing, Midwifery and Health Visiting 1994 The future of professional practice: policy statement. UKCC, London

UK Central Council for Nursing, Midwifery and Health Visiting 1998 A higher level of practice: consultation document. UKCC, London

Waller S 1998 Clarifying the UKCC's position in relation to higher level practice. British Journal of Nursing 7(16):961–964

While A 1991 An evaluation of a paediatric home care scheme. Journal of Advanced Nursing 16:1413–1421

Whiting M 1998 Expanding community children's nursing services. British Journal of Community Nursing 3(4):183–190

Wilson L 1992 The home visiting programme. Paediatric Nursing 7:10–11

18 Needs analysis and profiling in community children's nursing

Julie Hughes

KEY ISSUES

- Needs assessment – defining and identifying needs
- Profiling – defining the community in the context of community children's nursing
- Needs analysis – how to assess and analyse need
- Determining a need for a community children's nursing service
- Production of a business plan to support service development

INTRODUCTION

The principles of undertaking needs analysis and profiling of a defined population are essential skills for all community healthcare nurses. Comprehensive and effective needs analysis of individual client groups is essential in order to maximise use of finite resources. The community children's nurse (CCN) must possess these necessary skills to provide accurate evidence of the needs of the client group and to sustain and develop the service.

With the developments in primary care and the commissioning process (Department of Health 1998) the CCN needs to be aware of how to assess, plan, implement and evaluate a service. The assessment and planning stages of service development require needs assessment and profiling from which a business plan should be produced in the evaluative stage. This chapter will endeavour to examine the skills required for each of these stages in the context of community children's nursing.

NEEDS ASSESSMENT

The principles of needs assessment are historically rooted within the health visiting profession (Tinson 1995) but can and should be applied to all specialist areas of community nursing. To facilitate this process, the specialist practitioner should consider first the definition of need and, second, the meaning of the word community in the context of their specialist practice.

What is need?

The concept of need takes on different meanings for different people. Consequently, definitions remain nebulous as sociologists and health professionals define need from their own perspective. Two of the most functional theoretical frameworks have been developed by Bradshaw (1972) and Orr (1985).

Bradshaw (1972) identifies need as:

- **Normative** – need based on the professional perspective
- **Felt** – need identified by members of the community
- **Expressed** – felt need that has progressed to a demand for a service
- **Comparative** – need identified by comparison with another area

As a contrast, Orr (1985) refers to need as:

- **Social** – need according to standards of communal life
- **Relative** – meaning of need will vary across people and society
- **Evaluative** – need is based on value judgements

When defining the needs of the child and their family the CCN should explore the relative needs from a range of perspectives including social, cultural and educational. In addition, the ideas of the professional and voluntary services involved in the child's care should be considered in order to identify a unified normative need. The recognition and incorporation of these broad and potentially conflicting associated meanings is challenging and demands, amongst other things, an awareness of the community in which they are located.

What is the community?

The concept of a community is complex and diverse. Definitions of a community vary according to the context in which it is defined. Quite simply, Collins Dictionary defines a community as 'a body of people with something in common e.g. district of residence'. For community children's nursing teams a much wider perspective of the community is required. The catchment area of the team will be determined by the organisational model within which they work. The most common models are identified as (Eaton & Thomas 1998, Sidey 1995, Winter & Teare 1997):

- Hospital outreach: generalist
- Hospital outreach: specialist
- Community-based team
- Hospital at home

Given the range of organisational models, boundaries may be set by either primary healthcare teams or the acute hospital service. Often the geographical area will be vast and is likely to include urban and rural localities, neighbourhoods of wealth and deprivation, and ethnic and cultural diversity. The client group will be children and young people (usually aged 0–18 years) with a health need and their families. To determine the size of the potential client group, the CCN can obtain information on the numbers of children residing in their geographical area from the Office of Population Censuses and Surveys (OPCS) (1991).

BOX 18.1 *Sources of information with respect to geographical area*

- Community health council
- Health authority
- Public health department
- Public library
- Social services unitary authority
- Housing department
- Local education unitary authority

BOX 18.2 *Sources of information on the client group*

- OPCS (to identify client group)
- Hospital statistics, including patterns of admissions, length of stay, children regularly attending clinics and wards, etc.
- Community paediatricians
- Caseload profiles of similar community children's nursing teams

Having identified and defined the community, the next stage is to compile the data in the format of a profile.

COMPILING A PROFILE

The NHS and Community Care Act (Department of Health 1990) advocates the compilation of profiles for all community healthcare workers as a tool to identify healthcare need. Within community nursing, profiling is seen as a vital and specific skill which can empower nurses in service development and be used to influence policy (Royal College of Nursing 1993, Tinson 1995). A profile should be a comprehensive picture of the population targeted by the service (Billings & Cowley 1995). For the CCN this will include information on the community as a geographical area and on the children with a healthcare need residing in this area.

A profile can be compiled using epidemiological and demographic data from the population census (OPCS 1991) and from specific information applicable to the community available from other sources (Box 18.1).

Information gained from these sources will provide the foundation to the profile specifically in relation to the geographical area. The community children's nursing service profile must also include data relating to the actual or potential client group. Sources of information for this element are shown in Box 18.2.

Once data have been collected, they should be assessed and analysed concurrently to provide a meaningful source of evidence. Many would argue that some of the data are inherently flawed. Census data are available only on a 10-year basis, and many of the community data may be subjective (Billings & Cowley 1995, Thomas 1997). Despite these obvious limitations, profiles are an essential component to service development.

BOX 18.3 *PEST analysis*

Political	Having compiled a profile it is important for the CCN to consider political influences that may affect the service both locally and nationally. For example, the CCN may incorporate recommendations from the Health Committee report (1997) in order to provide arguments to support local service developments.
Environmental	Consideration should be given to the positive and adverse effects of the local environment on children's health. For example, the incidence of asthma may be exacerbated in an urban area with heavy traffic congestion (Hall 1996).
Sociological	Sociological analysis is a well-researched component of community nursing. It is recognised that improvements in the overall health of a community have always come from changes in the social environment (Brown 1993, Department of Health 1998). Consideration should be given to areas such as undesirable living conditions, stress and poverty (Hall 1996).
Technological	The number of technology-dependent children requiring support in the community has increased significantly over the last decade (Jardine et al 1999). Local hospital statistics may demonstrate that these children occupy a significant number of bed-days. Combining this type of evidence with an economic evaluation may provide a sound argument for developing or expanding a community children's nursing service.

ASSESSING AND ANALYSING THE DATA

Clearly only a small component of the child population will require the services of a CCN and it may be useful to consider epidemiological factors within the identified community. This will provide information on the frequency, distribution and determinants of health and illness, and the tracing of disease occurrence within the defined population (McMurray 1993). Tinson (1995) suggests that the knowledge level of the nurse will influence the quality of a needs analysis exercise. She recommends a literature search to ensure appropriate evidence is assimilated into the process. This evidence may be supported by political, environmental, sociological and technological data to provide a more comprehensive account of the findings (Buchan & Grey 1990) (Box 18.3).

Buchan & Grey (1990) argue that the analysis of need involves value judgements on the part of healthcare professionals and should therefore be balanced by the acquisition of qualitative data from children with a health need and their families. Similarly, it is also necessary to elicit views of other stakeholders.

An accurate and comprehensive needs analysis can raise awareness and identify the need for resources. It promotes a collaborative approach to care delivery as promoted by the Government (Blackie 1998).

BOX 18.4 ***Example of a SWOT analysis***

Strengths

- A well-established community children's nursing team to assess and plan nursing care
- A child development centre with children's therapy services on site
- Knowledge of the community from social, environmental, political, economic and cultural perspectives
- Links with social, education and voluntary sectors
- Children and families are key to the strategic planning of the health authority

Weaknesses

- Provision of a fragmented package of health and social care
- Limited resources within the community children's nursing team to introduce a key worker role
- Limited resources for providing complete and comprehensive care packages to meet the needs of families (e.g. respite care, sibling support, psychological support)
- Social services under enormous pressure owing to their own statutory obligations

Opportunities

- Provision of a key worker for all children and families with life-threatening or life-limiting illnesses
- Provision of a coordinated, collaborative package of care from health, social, education and voluntary sectors
- Development of a supportive culture for staff from a variety of professional backgrounds
- Improved networking and communication across health, social and educational boundaries

Threats

- Difficulties convincing commissioners of the need to invest in new services
- Moral and ethical implications of developing a service with short-term investment
- Emotional fatigue of team members
- Acknowledgement of service development in a climate of change

DETERMINING THE NEED TO DEVELOP THE COMMUNITY CHILDREN'S NURSING SERVICE

Having considered the components of profiling and needs analysis, the next stage is to demonstrate the need for developing a community children's nursing service. Demonstrating the need for a service development to potential commissioners requires data that are current, reliable and measurable. Analysing the statistics gathered from the hospital and community services, and considering previous patterns of care for these children, would be one way of demonstrating a service gap (Royal College of Nursing 1994). Ward attenders and hospital inpatient stays are measurable and could be costed against the provision of a CCN service.

A SWOT (strengths, weaknesses, opportunities and threats) analysis could be used to present the data. This is a strategic analysis of every aspect of an operation which enables objectives to be assessed and developed (Young 1986). An example of a SWOT analysis is illustrated in Box 18.4.

A SWOT analysis is a useful tool, whether initiating or developing a service, as it focuses on the issues that will be of importance to the commissioners.

Whether the service is in its initial stages of development or well established, it is likely that annual business planning will be required. As advocates for the community children's nursing profession, and ultimately for children and their families, business planning skills are an essential prerequisite for community children's nursing team leaders.

COMPILING A BUSINESS PLAN

The business plan should include retrospective achievements and a projection of service developments. There is a dearth of literature relating to business planning for nurses, which reflects its relatively recent assimilation into the profession, although it is interesting to note that the concept of 'planning' in nursing has been well researched for many years. Hyett (1988) indicates that planning will be undertaken on macro, meso and micro levels:

- The Trust plan
- The department plan
- The team plan

It is important to consider the broader perspective when producing a business plan and to ensure that the service plan integrates with that of the Trust and health authority. A proposed structure is offered in Box 18.5.

CONCLUSIONS

This chapter has outlined the complexities associated with profiling, needs assessment and analysis, and the production of business plans. Acquiring these skills can enhance the autonomy of the nursing profession and nurses' ability to negotiate resources for service development (Royal College of Nursing 1998). The need for CCNs to embrace these concepts is essential to ensure that a 'bottom-up' assessment of services informs developments rather than a 'top-down' approach (Tinson 1995). Experienced CCNs may be familiar with these processes. Networking and sharing the relevant knowledge and skills between teams may contribute to the ultimate aim of establishing an equitable service nationwide.

BOX 18.5 ***Proposed structure for a business plan***

- Mission statement
- Service aims
- Existing service provision (e.g. location, facilities, human resources)
- Analysis of activity
- Analysis of the community (e.g. PEST)
- Analysis of service (e.g. SWOT)
- Statement of need
- Proposal for meeting the need
- Action plan

FURTHER READING

Blackie C 1998 Community health care nursing. Churchill Livingstone, London

This text explores many of the dimensions of the common core of knowledge for all branches of community healthcare nursing. It explains the organisation of community care against the background of healthcare reforms and provides a clear account of the attitudes and skills that are common to all community healthcare nurses.

Cain P, Hyde V & Howkins E 1995 Community nursing: dimensions and dilemmas. Arnold, London

While some sections of this book are out of date, there are some useful sections covering client relations.

REFERENCES

Billings J & Cowley S 1995 Approaches to community needs assessment: a literature review. Journal of Advanced Nursing 22:721–730

Blackie C 1998 Community health care nursing. Churchill Livingstone, London

Bradshaw J 1972 The concept of social need. New Society 30:640–643

Brown V 1993 Health care policies, health policies or policies for health. In: Gardner H (ed) Health policy development, implementation and evaluation. Churchill Livingstone, Melbourne

Buchan H & Grey J A 1990 Needs assessment made simple. Health Service Journal 100:240–241

Department of Health 1990 NHS and Community Care Act. HMSO, London

Department of Health 1998 The new NHS. Modern, dependable. The Stationery Office, London

Eaton N & Thomas P 1998 Community children's nursing: an evaluative framework. Journal of Child Health Care 2(4):170–173

Hall D M B (ed) 1996 Health for all children, 3rd edn. Oxford University Press, Oxford

Health Committee 1997 Third report. Health services for children and young people in the community: home and school. House of Commons Session 1996–97. The Stationery Office, London

Hyett K 1988 Nursing management handbook. Churchill Livingstone, London

Jardine E, O'Toole M & Wallis C 1999 Current status of long term ventilation of children in the United Kingdom: questionnaire survey. British Medical Journal 318:295–299

McMurray J W 1993 Community health nursing, 2nd edn. Churchill Livingstone, London

Office of Population Censuses and Surveys 1991 General household survey. HMSO, London

Orr J 1985 Individual and family needs. In: Luker K & Orr J (eds) Health visiting. Blackwell Scientific, Oxford, pp 67–120

Royal College of Nursing 1993 The GP practice population profile. Royal College of Nursing, London

Royal College of Nursing 1994 Wise decisions. Developing paediatric home care teams. Royal College of Nursing, London

Royal College of Nursing 1998 Marketing community and specialist nursing. Royal College of Nursing, London

Sidey A 1995 Community nursing perspectives. In: Carter B & Dearmun A (eds) Child health care nursing. Concepts, theory and practice. Blackwell Science, London, pp 33–41

Thomas E 1997 Community nursing profiles: their role in needs assessment. Nursing Standard 11:37,39–42

Tinson S 1995 Health needs assessment. In: Cain P, Hyde V & Howkins E (eds) Community nursing: dimensions and dilemmas. Arnold, London, pp 144–166

Winter A & Teare J 1997 Construction and application of paediatric community nursing services. Journal of Child Health 1(1):24–29

Young A 1986 The manager's handbook. The practical guide to successful management. Sphere, London

19 Dependency scoring in community children's nursing

Sue Facey

KEY ISSUES

- What is dependency scoring and why is it needed?
- Example of a dependency scoring tool
- Elements of a community children's nurse's workload
- Benefits of dependency scoring

INTRODUCTION

Much has changed in the way sick children are nursed, from the custodial style wards of years ago, where parents were permitted only occasional visits, to – in many cases – the care of the sick child by parents, often in their own home. This shift has been accompanied by escalating productivity in the National Health Service (NHS) (Royal College of Nursing 1994). In June 1994 Virginia Bottomley, the Secretary of State for Health, reported that the output of NHS employees had risen by almost 30% between 1982 and 1991 (Royal College of Nursing 1994). The volume of work and the dependency of the patients have increased as the 'new' NHS strives, like all public sector organisations, to be more efficient and effective. Increased demands upon staff to be more productive require specific strategies to allocate work within teams as well as to ensure that resources match the work to be done. This will help to ensure high-quality care within a framework of good economic management, which should meet the requirements of clinical governance (Department of Health 1998).

DEPENDENCY SCORING

Dependency scoring is essential to avoid imbalances, which could have a detrimental effect on staff and patients, and provides 'an assessment of a patient's ability to care for themselves, for instance with regard to feeding, personal hygiene, mobility' (Audit Commission 1992). The measurement of nurse dependency should embrace the patient's total needs for nursing care including education, rehabilitation and psychological care (Audit Commission 1992). This identification of the patient's needs allows for appropriate allocation of nursing resources to either a ward of patients, a community nurse's caseload, or for individual patients.

Patient dependency and nursing workload are closely associated concepts and, without a dependency score, the allocation of resources is highly problematic. This may lead to arbitrary and possibly mismatched staff utilisation and time management. The time required to provide care, the nursing skill-mix, the quality of care and patient needs must all be considered if the equation of resources is to be in any way balanced (Mersey Regional Health Authority 1991).

Healthcare resources are not available on a demand basis and, to ameliorate inequities in delivery, staff should be required to offer evidence for resources and have tools to ensure their best use. Dependency scoring is one such tool. However, from the outset, it must be recognised that the dependency of patients is often measured by nursing activity, which assumes that nurses are actually in touch with, and able to accurately identify, the patient's needs. Within community children's nursing this requirement is made more difficult, given that care is focused upon the needs of the whole family rather than the individual child, and where the child may be unable to articulate their own needs. This is further complicated by the significant change in the whole approach to the care of children from an almost custodial one to the more child-centred approaches now used, and the impact this has on staffing.

Most of the work relating to dependency scoring has been based on acute-care settings, and in particular in critical care (Royal College of Nursing 1995). Little about dependency scoring in the community, or in the area of community children's nursing, is available. Nursing colleagues in health visiting, mental health and learning disability have made some inroads into non-acute-care dependency assessment (Frame and O'Donnell 1996).

Dependency scoring systems and tools are also described as caseload management tools, which indicates their value, but within this chapter the term dependency scoring is used throughout.

WHEN TO BEGIN TO MEASURE DEPENDENCY

There is no right or wrong time to begin dependency scoring, but the sooner the better. In a newly established team, where funding may be for a fixed period, dependency assessment may provide valuable evidence for repeat funding. In more established teams, it will assist in ensuring efficiency and effectiveness, the latter being a key feature of the clinical governance agenda.

WHAT IS BEING MEASURED?

As a team, it is essential to consider what needs to be measured, for example:

- To itemise each single nursing activity and the time it takes
- To aggregate the time spent with/for each patient regardless of the activity

The former is clearly more accurate, but time consuming to collect, liable to collector error, and needs complex and expensive information technology to analyse and interpret. The latter, whilst more of a guestimate of time per trained nurse per patient, is easier to use and more likely to be adopted by staff. An example of the latter approach is provided in Box 19.1.

BOX 19.1 ***Dependency scoring tool***

Direct patient contact	Indirect patient-related activity	Non-patient-related activity
Calculated per week as follows: Visit frequency × length of visit	For example: Travel, record keeping, liaison, etc.	For example: Clinical supervision, professional development, team meetings, etc.
	Method of scoring	
Frequency is scored: × 2 per day = 14 points × 1 per day = 7 points × 2 per week = 2 points × 1 per week = 1 point × 2 per month = 0.5 points Monthly or less = 0.25 points	Length of visit is calculated per 15 min: 15 min = 1 point 30 min = 2 points 45 min = 3 points 60 min = 4 points > 60 min = 5 points	Record the amount of activity spent over several weeks in order to identify an average per week in hours. Transfer to a point scale by multiplying by 4 to match the direct patient contact score (i.e. per 15 min)

Example 1: A family requiring fortnightly visits, of 1 hour's duration, scores 2 points (0.5 × 4).
Example 2: A family requiring three visits per week, of 40 min each, scores 9 points (3 × 3).

Example of a dependency scoring tool

Frame and O'Donnell (1996), working in adult community nursing, devised a method of scoring dependency based upon aggregation of time. The system has three main components: (1) direct patient contact, (2) indirect patient-related activity and (3) non-patient-related activity, compared with staff availability. It is calculated on a weekly basis (see Box 19.1).

Using the scores

1. Each team member is allocated a ceiling score based on the total number of hours worked per week, multiplied by 4 (to break the time into 15-minute units). For example, a full-time community children's nurse (CCN), working 37.5 hours per week, would have 150 points available; a part-time CCN, working 22.5 hours per week, would have 90 points available.
2. Deduct the score for non-patient-related activity. This will vary for each team member, depending on grade, study commitments, etc. For example, the team leader will have less time available for patient-related activity than other team members. The remaining score will indicate the points available for indirect and direct care for each team member.

Pt. ID no.	Direct			Indirect			Non-patient-related activity		
	Frequency x duration score			Duration (15 minutes =1 point)			(15 minutes =1 point)		
	Visit frequency	(x by) Duration	= no. of points	Activity	Time	Points	Activity	Time	Points
		Total points			Total points			Total points	
			Points available					Total points recorded this sheet/week	

Figure 19.1 Example of a chart for recording dependency scores.

3. Score direct and indirect activity and allocate work accordingly. For example, 22.5 hours of direct patient activity scores 90 points (22.5 × 4) and 10 hours of indirect patient-related activity scores 40 points, giving a total of 130 points. As new children are admitted to the caseload, their dependency score is calculated. If the team does not have the capacity to take on new referrals, the child should remain in hospital where care can be provided and/or be placed on the team's waiting list.
4. It is possible to use this tool both retrospectively and prospectively. Comparison of the availability figures with the activity that the nurse is actually undertaking gives a clear indication as to the capacity for additional work or the need for assistance (see Figure 19.1).

ELEMENTS OF THE COMMUNITY CHILDREN'S NURSE'S WORKLOAD

In calculating the direct and non-direct time it is important to recognise the scope of the CCN's role. Box 19.2 is by no means exhaustive or in order of priority, but provides some indication of the complexity and example components of a CCN's workload. These components must be incorporated into a tool in order to represent the workload accurately. An element that is difficult to incorporate is the skill of the CCN undertaking the visit.

HOW WILL DEPENDENCY SCORING HELP?

Dependency scoring may help nurses and nursing in a number of ways, as shown in Box 19.3. The application of this dependency scoring system demonstrates demand placed on the team and its members, and allows for better distribution of work amongst the team members. However, it is evident that the information can be used for a number of additional purposes.

BOX 19.2 ***Components of the CCN's workload***

- **Meetings** (team, management, case conferences, discharge planning, etc.)
- **Associated clinical visits** (nursery, schools, outpatients, etc.)
- **Professional resource**
- **Supervision**
- **Documentation**
- **Advice and support** (carers, colleagues, students, etc.)
- **Liaison** (primary healthcare teams, voluntary and independent sectors, hospital staff)
- **Management** (time, team, caseload, etc.)
- **Telephone triage**
- **Professional development**
- **Administration**
- **Equipment and supplies** (organisation, ordering, maintenance)
- **Teaching** (students, families, colleagues)
- **Direct care requirements**
- **Health promotion**
- **Emergencies**
- **Risk analysis**
- **Travel time** (to take account of weather, geography, etc.)

BOX 19.3 ***Areas in which dependency scoring can help***

- Workload planning
- Staff planning
- Staff development
- Report writing
- Business planning
- Cost-effectiveness and efficiency
- Comparisons and benchmarking
- Value
- To ensure parity of workload within and between teams
- To provide an upper limit to caseload size

Workload planning

An appropriate dependency tool will aid all team members to plan workload on a day-to-day basis. For example, this can help ensure that appointments are kept on time and families are not inconvenienced by having to wait in for the CCN to call. A recent study noted that, whilst families highly value the CCN, waiting when the nurse arrives late increases the stress in the family (Procter et al 1998). The scores will also indicate, to an extent, the urgency of each visit and how best to manage individual workloads.

Report writing and business planning

Most teams and individuals are required to submit annual reports as part of the clinical governance agenda, whereby Trusts demonstrate they have effective staff, organisations and practices. It is possible that Trusts may pass this responsibility on to individual teams, requiring them to submit annual reports and audits of care. The inclusion of information that quantifies the workload of the team in a meaningful way will assist the team as well as the Trust.

Cost-effectiveness and efficiency

A significant number of CCNs work in isolation, and the lone worker or new team may be required to submit reports and evidence to demonstrate that they are providing a 'value for money' service. It is unlikely that the executive members of their Trust will have a good understanding of the role of the CCN. Therefore, a tool that gives some indication, and even a comparison, of the work will help to gain recognition along with continued if not extended funding.

Comparisons and benchmarking

It would be ideal if a nationwide tool could be developed that would suit all community children's nursing services. This would truly enable benchmarking with other teams and perhaps go some way to ensure that children in the whole country received a similar service.

Value

It is essential that teams recognise the contribution made by individual nurses within the team and that individuals gain job satisfaction. A tool that encourages team members to reflect on the work undertaken will enhance an individual's sense of purpose and motivation.

Ensure fair workload within and between teams

It must be emphasised that caseload figures alone give no indication of the volume of work. Frame and O'Donnell (1996) described a district nursing team who were concerned that they were working under increased pressure. There was no change in the admission or discharge rate, or variance in the number of face-to-face contacts, but the increased pressure was due to the increased complexity of care needed by patients. This can be identified only if the dependency of patients is measured over a sustained time period.

Upper limit to caseload size

An audit tool to measure patient dependency will also ensure safe patient care, by identifying critical ceiling levels for each nurse. When the local children's ward is full, no more children are admitted to ensure that staffing levels are appropriate to meet the needs of those in their care. This is not the case in the community, where the caseload of the CCN can grow to unmanageable proportions unless evidence can be offered to indicate a capacity has been reached. To be able to state that the current staffing offers a specified amount of care delivery time, and the current workload already demands more than that, will enable decisions to be made regarding the safety of taking on new patients. It also gives tangible evidence to managers that work has outgrown the team and funding is required for team expansion.

KEYS TO SUCCESS

- Involvement of all team members at the outset. As with any change in management, success is more likely with the cooperation of all those involved (Ottaway 1976). It is unreasonable to expect team members to complete long and complicated forms on a daily basis if they have no understanding of the need for gathering such data and what it will be used for.
- Information needs to be accurate and complete. It is therefore essential that each team member interprets and uses the tool in the same way.
- The information gained must be analysed from the outset and used to inform activity and planning to ensure the exercise has meaning to the team.
- Reductionist approaches to dependency analysis, which itemise all aspects of care, are time consuming to collect and collate, and require extensive information technology support.

CONCLUSION

Only one example of a patient dependency tool has been offered here, chosen in part for its simplicity. Others are available, although not published in detail, which have taken teams many years to develop and which are expensive to buy and far more complicated to use. The time has come for all teams to calculate dependency scores of patients to ensure appropriate resource use. It is also essential, with the increasing trend towards community care, to ensure that the needs of the child and family can be safely met. Every children's nurse is aware that the best place to care for a sick child is in the child's own home, but only if the support required by the family is available. If it is not available, the child and family may actually be better placed in hospital. Currently children may be discharged into the community without careful consideration of whether or not the community children's nursing team can accommodate the family on to the caseload, perhaps with an assumption that where a team exists, so does the nursing time. In reality, this may not be the case. Many teams who do not use a patient dependency tool may be placing the families on the caseload in an unsafe position, by accepting them into a community children's nursing 'ward', which is already full. This will put pressure on community nursing staff, and may in turn lead to increased sickness levels as well as a potentially unsafe environment for the child and family. This important aspect of caseload management demands much more consideration.

FURTHER READING

Eaton N 1998 Community children's nursing: an evaluative framework. Journal of Child Health Care 2(4):170–173

This article provides suitable criteria for evaluating a community children's nursing team, including efficiency, effectiveness and accountability – three areas in which dependency scoring can provide evidence of service.

Goldstone L & Ball J 1984 Manpower planning 4. The quality of nursing services. Nursing Times 80(35):56–58

Goldstone L & Ball J 1984 Manpower planning 5. Criteria for care. Nursing Times 80(36):55–58

These two articles describe Monitor and the North West Staffing Formula, and their application in acute medical and surgical wards. The North West Staffing Formula is a similar tool to that described above, but a few years earlier.

Roberts W & Ross R 1996 Make it so: leadership lessons from Star Trek: The Next Generation. Pocket Books, New York

Star Trek, the Next Generation is an excellent source of illustrations of good leadership qualities. This book highlights the importance of keeping logs and records. For example, Chapter 2 is entitled 'Urgency' and notes: 'Apathy, laziness, distraction, and interference can all lead to a self inflicted workplace crisis created by the failure to do what needs to be done within acceptable time limits, or according to established standards.'

Royal College of Nursing 1998 Guidance for nurses on clinical governance. Royal College of Nursing, London

A short booklet that provides definition, basic principles and key elements of clinical governance for nurses.

REFERENCES

Audit Commission 1992 Caring systems: a handbook for managers and nursing project managers. HMSO, London

Department of Health 1998 The new NHS. Modern, dependable. Department of Health, London

Frame G & O'Donnell P 1996 Weight-lifters. Health Service Journal 10 October:30–31

Mersey Regional Health Authority 1991 Using information in managing the nursing resource: workload. Greenhalgh

Ottaway R N 1976 A change strategy to implement new norms, new styles and new environment in the work organisation. Personnel Review 5(1):13–18

Procter S, Biott C, Campbell S, Edward S, Redpath N & Moran M 1998 Preparation for the developing role of community children's nurse. English National Board for Nursing, Midwifery and Health Visiting, London

Royal College of Nursing 1994 Nurses and NHS productivity. Royal College of Nursing, London

Royal College of Nursing 1995 Dependency scoring systems: guidelines for nurses. Royal College of Nursing, London

20 Information management

Anne Casey

KEY ISSUES

- Information is the most important resource in healthcare.
- Effective management of information improves care of children and families.
- The NHS Information Strategy provides guidance for the local development of standards, education and systems.
- The community children's nursing team requires a range of tools and methods to manage information effectively.

INTRODUCTION

Information management is about ensuring that relevant information is in the hands of those who need it, at the time they need it, and in a format that they can understand and use. In healthcare, information is needed by patients and carers, clinical staff, managers and administrators so they can:

- make sense of the situation
- make decisions about what to do

The right format for the information may be a laboratory report, a set of statistics, a video, a referral letter, or any of the range of methods available for presenting facts, opinions and concepts. Making the information relevant to the person receiving it and providing it at the right time can be more challenging, particularly in stressful situations.

Information management can be viewed as a number of processes in which information from different sources is collected, used, communicated and sometimes recorded. Within these processes, information itself can be regarded as a resource: information about an individual patient (e.g. name, address and medical diagnosis) is the single most important resource in healthcare. Unfortunately, the skills required for effective use of this critical resource are not well integrated into the training of health professionals, despite government and statutory body recommendations (English National Board 1997, National Health Service Executive 1998), and despite the fact that every year the main criticisms made by the health ombudsman relate to inadequate communication and poor record keeping.

This chapter begins with a brief overview of some principles of information management. It then addresses three aspects of information management for community children's nurses:

1. Meeting the information needs of children and families
2. Information management for care delivery
3. Management of aggregated information for purposes such as auditing and improving care, and for costing and planning services

In today's National Health Service (NHS), this last item is assuming greater importance for nurses and other clinical professionals as they take responsibility for the development of evidence-based care and contribute to clinical governance (Department of Health 1997a). The aims of this chapter are to emphasise the importance of information as a resource and to demonstrate that effective information management can improve care and make life easier for the community children's nurse (CCN).

PRINCIPLES OF INFORMATION MANAGEMENT

The first step towards effective information management is to identify information requirements. This exercise should always begin with the people who are to receive and use the information. CCNs often receive standard referral letters from other professionals, but how many of these letters were designed by the CCNs themselves to include the information that is important to them? Those giving the information usually decide what they think the other party needs to know, rather than asking what information they would like.

Within the information literature there is a range of methods for identifying information requirements systematically (Eaton 1994, Gassert 1990, Goossen 1996). These include modelling working practices, looking at information flows in the workplace or identifying problems that would be solved by information solutions. One of the problems that might face a community children's nursing team is obtaining up-to-date information on the full range of drugs they may come across in their work. Could the children's hospital provide a monthly bulletin on new drugs? Should every parent keep full drug information with the parent-held record? Can the nurse rely on being able to contact a pharmacist by phone if there is a problem? There will be a number of possible solutions which can then be evaluated to see whether they will meet the identified needs but also to assess whether they are appropriate for the nurses' working environment.

Consideration of the working context is the most important, and most neglected, principle of information management in healthcare. Nurses do not work at desks, yet many information solutions in the health service rely on desk-top computers (Cowley 1994). The context of care also includes prevailing philosophies and practices. Some information solutions do not fit with the view that the parents and child should have full access to the clinical record and use it to record their own care. If the context of information use is considered, meeting information requirements can be simple and effective, and may often involve continued use of pen and paper.

One way of ensuring sensible, practical solutions is to focus on another key information principle: 'fitness for purpose'. Do the information tools you use, including your nursing records, do the job that you require of them? If the answer is no or not very well, then you should seek advice from an NHS information specialist who can provide unbiased expertise. As the new NHS information strategy (NHS Executive 1998) gets underway, there will be an increasing number of such posts and improved educational input focusing on 'the long term development of an information culture, and not – as in the past – on short term training designed simply to get people using (computer) systems' (p 96).

INFORMATION FOR CHILDREN AND FAMILIES

In many situations the child and family will not know what information will be of use to them. However, they will usually have questions that indicate what they believe are their information needs. These questions are the starting point for the provision of meaningful information which can then be expanded to include what the nurse believes will be helpful to them in making sense of the situation and in deciding what to do. As with any other aspect of individualised care, no assumptions can be made about what the child already knows, what they should or should not be told, and what they are capable of understanding. In much the same way that a child's physical condition is regularly assessed so too should information requirements be identified: What does the child know? Has anything changed? What is likely to happen that the child needs to know about? And – with the goal of promoting independence – how can children be helped to access appropriate information themselves?

Everything from the telephone helpline through to the computer game and the Internet can be drawn upon to provide information tailored for the individual's needs and preferences. These advances can be looked at in two ways: as a threat to the authority and control of the health professional, or as an opportunity for patients and public to be better informed and participate more in their healthcare (Cross 1998).

Health information on the Internet is 'changing the balance of power between healthcare organisations and individual patients' (Cross 1998). But the quality of the information available from such sources is questionable as, at present, there may be no way of knowing whether what you are reading is the latest evidence-based clinical guideline or sales material from a drug company. The NHS information strategy (NHS Executive 1998) includes provisions for accrediting information from reliable sources and suggestions for delivering that information into the hands of people who may not have access to the expensive technology required. Public access to electronic health information is being tried in some areas in libraries, shopping centres, hospital foyers and clinics (Jones 1998).

Word processing and publishing software can be used to produce professional looking and easily updatable information, with cartoons and pictures added to bring the information alive for the child. Guidance on producing good-quality patient information is available from many sources (see Resources). There are software packages available to check your information material for jargon, giving it a 'plain English' rating. Many organisations now employ information officers and involve children and families in the production of information materials, ensuring that content is at an appropriate level for different age groups. Hopefully the badly photocopied sheet of paper listing instructions in nursing and medical language is a thing of the past.

Although the provision of information must be individualised, there is a place for standardised material and, as the Audit Commission (1997) suggested, this could be produced more efficiently if there were more coordination. It is wasteful for each community children's nursing team to produce and update its own material on managing febrile convulsions, when to call the doctor, storing drugs in the home, etc. With the UK-wide network provided by the Royal College of Nursing Community Children's Nursing Forum, it should be possible to share and re-use well-developed material to save others the time and expense of development.

The growth of information technology to support clinical practice brings with it the requirement for a new set of skills for nurses. Not least of these will be the skills of working with highly informed individuals who may question your advice or clinical judgement. How comfortable will you be negotiating with an 8-year-old child who questions their medical treatment by referring to details obtained from other patients on the Internet?

INFORMATION MANAGEMENT FOR CLINICAL PRACTICE

To care for the child and family effectively, the community team manages two distinct types of information. First, clinical and contextual information about each child and his or her family is obtained, used, recorded and communicated – managing information about the patient. Second, general information from professional literature, local policies, guidelines, drug manuals and so on is used to inform decisions about the most effective approaches to the child's care – decision-support.

Managing information about the patient

The child's clinical record is the main tool for managing this information. The information principle of 'fitness for purpose' can be used to assist development of new records or to evaluate the structure, content and location of existing records, whether on paper or computer. In deciding what information to record, in what format and where the information should be held, there is one key question to answer: what is the purpose of the record? Every professional who comes in contact with the patient needs to be able to make timely decisions about what care is needed and how best to deliver that care. If it is to be an effective information tool, the record should support this process of clinical decision making. A key purpose of records is communication between disciplines, which suggests that moves towards a single record, used by all professionals and possibly held by the child or parent, will help to achieve 'fitness for purpose'.

A recent review of information management in Community Trusts identified a number of problems around the collection and recording of individual patient data, particularly the inefficient duplication of records by different professionals and the lack of standards for what information should be recorded (Audit Commission 1997). In the Audit Commission study, over 25% of the district nurses who were surveyed reported problems in obtaining details of the patient's care to date. The report concluded that 'critical decisions on patient care can be based on incomplete or unchecked data' (Audit Commission 1997 p 17).

Although the United Kingdom Central Council (UKCC) publishes guidance on record keeping, the advice is at a very general level, stating only that the record should 'identify problems that have arisen and action taken to rectify them' and 'provide clear evidence of the care planned, the decisions made, the care delivered and the information shared' (UKCC 1998 pp 8–9). The decision about what to record and the amount of detail remains a question of professional judgement, but the simple 'fit for purpose' test can be done, perhaps as part of clinical supervision, by asking a colleague whether they could (a) find the patient record and (b) care for the child based on information in that record.

Decision-support

As the evidence base for practice grows, so will the need to provide easily accessible and up-to-date knowledge to the practitioner at the bedside or in the patient's home. Technology certainly has a role here, provided it is suited to the working environment of the nurse. Many nurses already use decision-support, particularly in primary care systems, which provide warnings on drug incompatibilities, remind the nurse to check the patient's blood pressure or weight, or prompt particular assessment questions depending on information already held about the patient. In one hospital system the nurse can click on a diagnosis, for example of 'RSV' (respiratory syncytial virus) bronchiolitis and choose from a list of help topics such as 'RSV investigations', 'RSV precautions' and 'RSV parent information'.

Future developments

To manage the information required to support the care of child and family, the nurse can draw on all the information tools available: spoken and written words, electronic equipment, computers, telephone, etc. Each has its place but the electronic and computer tools will become more useful once the NHS networks and systems are better developed. Clinical systems for community nurses (as distinct from administrative systems) are in their infancy, and more complex developments, like the electronic health record described in the NHS information strategy, will take some time to develop. As the strategy indicates, there are major issues to be addressed, such as enforcing confidentiality standards and integrating health centre, community and hospital systems. However, the biggest challenge continues to be to ensure that future systems meet information needs in ways that are appropriate to the community setting and that do not compromise fundamental principles such as child and family involvement (Cowley 1994).

The most useful contribution that individual nurses and teams can make is to be very sure about what information they need to do their jobs effectively. Each team could have someone who leads on information and records, so that, if any new systems are being planned in the Trust, there will be someone who can contribute the community children's nursing team's perspective. A significant lesson to date from the use of computers by community nurses is that using a system designed for management purposes does not benefit clinical practice (Audit Commission 1997, Cowley 1994).

MANAGEMENT OF AGGREGATED INFORMATION

Aggregations of small subsets of patient information that has been anonymised can be used for audit, costing and planning, and research. The community children's nursing team needs such information to demonstrate or improve the effectiveness and efficiency of its service. Three main issues need to be considered in the management of aggregated information:

1. Confidentiality and security of patient data
2. Ownership and control of the information
3. Uses and purpose of the aggregated information

The NHS strategy draws on the Data Protection Act (Data Protection Registrar 1998) and the Caldicott review (Department of Health 1997b) of the use of patient-identifiable information to address the first of these issues. But, as the UKCC code of conduct states, the nurse alone is personally accountable for her or his practice and it is the nurse who must protect the patient's confidential information (UKCC 1996). So, if you believe that patient information which you have obtained may be used by others in a way that could potentially identify the child and family, you are responsible for preventing that use.

There are several other reasons why the nurses themselves should manage the data about their patients and control how information is used and by whom. First, because nurses collect the data, they know how accurately it reflects the real situation. A statement that the child is 'much improved' can have a huge range of meanings. It may mean that the child is terminally ill but that pain relief is more effective. How would a distant administrator interpret the same statement? Second, the results from analysing aggregated patient data are most useful in the hands of those providing patient care. You cannot improve care or plan your service more efficiently if you do not have data to show you how you are doing. If you know what your own management goals are, you will be able to identify the information requirements for achieving those goals. One of your quality goals might be to ensure that all day cases are contacted within 24 hours of discharge. You could set up a method of collecting a list of day cases from the day ward and comparing it with the calls logged by the team over the same period.

A management goal might be to persuade the Trust Board to fund another full-time post. The information requirement to support this goal might include the data you collect routinely on the activity of the team, your data on parent satisfaction with the service, and some form of economic evaluation study presented graphically alongside reminders of NHS policy. With paper or computer systems in place to collect management data quickly and simply as part of nurses' routine work, you would have this information available when and where you needed it. This is the goal of effective information management.

CONCLUSION

Information management in healthcare is moving away from an emphasis on computerisation to a broader understanding of the total information picture. Effective solutions for meeting the information needs of patients and carers, clinical staff, managers and administrators will be those that:

- Identify the requirements of the users of the information
- Consider the working environment and context
- Focus on 'fitness for purpose' of tools and methods

Many of these solutions will not include computers, but where computers are a practical and sensible option they can bring significant benefits for patients and staff. One of the main benefits will be in the use of aggregated data about clinical practice to obtain visible evidence about what works and what could be improved. If CCNs across the UK could agree on some common assessment formats, outcome measures and intervention categories, it would be possible to undertake comparative studies of the effectiveness of interventions and of different services. But the collection, analysis and interpretation of UK-wide data and the dissemination of results need to be owned by the nurses and used by them to manage and develop their local service. Information is a powerful and important resource for CCNs. Its proper management is central to safe, effective practice and to the future of community children's nursing services as they spread throughout the UK.

FURTHER READING

Clinical Systems Group 1998 Improving clinical communications. Information Management Group of the Nattional Health Service Executive, Leeds

This report of three research studies demonstrates the complexity of clinical communications and makes recommendations for improving local and national action to improve records, communications, training and teamwork. One of the research case studies is of a child with special needs.

Information Management Group of the National Health Service Executive 1995 Strategic guidance on the effective use of information to support the management and delivery of nursing and midwifery care. The Stationery Office, London

Summarises the issues, actions and responsibilities for effective information management for nursing professionals, managers and Trust executives. A good place to start in developing a local information strategy.

Manworren R & Woodring B 1998 Evaluating children's literature as a source for patient education. Pediatric Nursing 24(6):548–553

Uses 'Curious George goes to hospital' to illustrate seven steps for evaluating books for children at different development stages. Of 23 books in the study, only four were suitable for use.

REFERENCES

Audit Commission 1997 Comparing notes: a study of information management in community trusts. Audit Commission, London

Cowley S 1994 Counting practice: the impact of information systems on community nursing. Journal of Nursing Management 1(6):273–278

Cross M 1998 All tangled on the web. Health Service Journal 19:22–23

Data Protection Registrar 1998 The Data Protection Act 1998: an introduction. Office of the Data Protection Registrar, Wilmslow, Cheshire

Department of Health 1997a The new NHS. Modern, dependable. The Stationery Office, London

Department of Health 1997b The Caldicott Committee report on the review of patient-identifiable information. The Stationery Office, London

Eaton N 1994 Information requirements analysis and evaluation. In: Wainwright P (ed) Nursing informatics. Churchill Livingstone, Edinburgh, ch 6, p 87

English National Board for Nursing, Midwifery and Health Visiting 1997 Information for caring: integrating informatics into learning programmes for nurses, midwives and health visitors. English National Board, London

Gassert C A 1990 Structured analysis: methodology for developing a model for defining nursing information system requirements. Advances in Nursing Science 13(2):53–62

Goossen W T F 1996 Nursing information management and processing: a framework and definition for systems analysis, design and evaluation. International Journal of Bio-medical Computing 40:187–195

Jones R 1998 Current research in consumer health informatics. Information Technology in Nursing 10(4):11–15

National Health Service Executive 1998 Information for health: an information strategy for the modern NHS 1998–2005. The Stationery Office, London

UK Central Council 1996 Guidelines for Professional Practice. UKCC, London

UK Central Council 1998 Guidelines for records and record keeping. UKCC, London

RESOURCES

Shanahan P 1996 Using and managing information for better health care. Churchill Livingstone, Edinburgh, 1996, ISBN 0 443 05331 6

Produced by Professional Development for Quality (PDQ) Care and accredited by Anglia Polytechnic University, this open learning pack contains exercises, reading material and case studies to help develop skills in information management.

Royal College of Paediatrics and Child Health 1997 A guide to child health information sources. Royal College of Paediatrics and Child Health, London, ISBN 1 900954 11 7

This book lists contact information for organisations and charities that can provide information from national statistics through to child-friendly literature.

Centre for Health Information Quality, Highcroft, Romsey Road, Winchester, SO22 5DH. Tel: 01962 863511 Ext 200. Fax: 01962 849079. e-mail: enquiries@centreforhiq.demon.co.uk

Set up in 1997 to help NHS staff and organisations improve the quality of information to patients and the public, the centre provides advice on all aspects of the development of consumer information.

21 Caring for the acutely ill child at home

Sarah Neill

KEY ISSUES

- The majority of childhood illness takes place at home with no recourse to professional care and support.
- Parents' ability to manage acute childhood illness at home appears to be directly related to personal control, itself related to the perceived degree of threat to the child's health.
- When parents seek help, children with acute childhood illness at home are often cared for by healthcare professionals with no specific qualification in child healthcare.
- Parents are reported to be often dissatisfied with care provided by general practitioners, wanting more reassurance and information.
- Rising demand means that alternatives to general practitioner care are needed to support children and their families during acute childhood illness at home.
- Future development of community services needs to provide this client group with services from appropriately qualified professionals, such as the community children's nurse, accessible to families from within the primary healthcare team.

INTRODUCTION

The majority of childhood illness is of short duration and takes place in the child's own home. However, research regarding community healthcare of children has, to date, focused primarily around the care of the chronically ill or highly dependent child. 'Theoretical developments regarding family process during acute illness have been limited' (Rennick 1995) to the experience of the hospitalised child. This chapter focuses on the acutely ill child at home. The literature is critically reviewed to identify what is known about the experiences of children and families, and the involvement of health services in their care at these times. From this analysis the chapter considers the implications of this knowledge for both contemporary and future models of care. Examples of contemporary practice are included. Throughout the chapter, where parents are referred to, the following definition will be applied: 'the child's birth parents, his/her legal guardians or permanent parent substitute (those who usually care for him/her)' (Neill 1996).

WHAT IS MEANT BY 'ACUTE CHILDHOOD ILLNESS' FROM A COMMUNITY PERSPECTIVE?

The Oxford Concise Medical Dictionary defines acute as 'a disease of rapid onset, severe symptoms, and brief duration'. Using this definition, acute childhood illness becomes 'childhood illness with rapid onset, severe symptoms, and brief duration'. At present, services to provide care for acutely sick children at home (i.e. those who develop severe symptoms) are not well developed in most areas (Meates 1997). This chapter is, therefore, concerned primarily with acute illness in children whose illness is not of sufficient severity to warrant hospitalisation. The term 'common childhood illness' is also often used to refer to acute childhood illness in the community. Such illness includes:

- coughs and colds
- upper respiratory tract infections
- childhood infectious diseases (mumps, measles, chickenpox)
- gastroenteritis
- acute exacerbations of chronic conditions such as asthma
- otitis media
- other febrile illness

The terms 'acute illness', 'minor illness' and 'minor ailments' will be used interchangeably, as these terms all appear in the literature reviewed.

HEALTHCARE SERVICE USE DURING ACUTE CHILDHOOD ILLNESS AT HOME: THE STATISTICS

Children aged under 16 years comprise 20% of the UK population (Central Statistical Office 1994). Some 9% of these are from minority ethnic groups. One-third of the ethnic minority population consists of children, in contrast to 20% of the total population of the UK. In some areas with large minority ethnic populations, the childhood population is continuing to expand (Leicester City Council 1997).

Morbidity statistics from general practice show that across the UK children make up 19% of consultations with doctors in general practice and 15% of consultations with practice nurses (McCormick et al 1995). The 0–4 years age group has the second highest consultation rate of all ages (Balarajan et al 1992). Acute childhood illness constitutes a high proportion of child consultations, with the most common reason for consultation being diseases of the respiratory system: 27.6% of consultations at both 0–4 and 5–15 years (Health Committee 1997).

Whilst no statistics are centrally available concerning the involvement of other community nursing services in the care of the acutely ill child at home, health visitors, school nurses and district nurses are variously involved in providing care to children in the community with minor ailments.

By chance, occasionally community children's nurses (CCNs) may also be involved.

IMPACT ON THE WORK OF HEALTHCARE PROFESSIONALS IN THE COMMUNITY

The statistics show that children with acute childhood illness at home constitute a significant proportion of the workload of general practitioners (GPs)and practice nurses, roughly parallel to the proportion of children in the population.

In areas with a higher proportion of children in the population, such as areas with large minority ethnic communities, this workload can be expected to be higher. For example, in the City East region of Leicester 39% of the population belongs to minority ethnic groups (Leicester City Council 1997), in contrast to the national figure of 5.5%. These figures are even more relevant when considered in the light of evidence that minority ethnic groups also have an increased incidence of socioeconomic deprivation (Webb 1996). This potentially leads to higher rates of health service use per head of the population due to the associated increased morbidity. These suggestions are supported by the findings of Clarke and Hewison (1991), who found higher consultation rates in 'Asian' groups with increased scores for severity of illness, and Watson (1991) who found that Bengali children were reported to suffer more severe symptoms, coughs and colds than children from the indigenous group.

A further factor affecting the uptake of health services for the acutely ill child in the community is poverty. Parents from lower socioeconomic groups are more likely to present to the doctor with their child (Gillam et al 1989). This statistic is not surprising as virtually all aspects of health are worse in children living in poverty than those living in affluent families (Reading 1997). These children are likely to represent a considerable proportion of healthcare professionals' workload, as approximately one-third of children are living in conditions of poverty in Britain (Graham 1994). These children will be ill more often (Mayall 1986, Reading 1997) and more seriously than children in more affluent circumstances (Clarke & Hewison 1991, Watson 1991, Wyke et al 1990). Spencer (1984) suggests that these parents are most vulnerable to breakdown of parenting skills and will therefore fail to respond to their child's symptoms, seeking help at a later stage of the child's illness.

IMPLICATIONS OF EXISTING SERVICE PROVISION FOR THE QUALITY OF CARE

Qualifications of healthcare professionals involved in care

Few practice nurses hold a children's nursing qualification, yet 15% of their workload involves children (McCormick et al 1995). Many GPs, health visitors, school nurses and district nurses hold no formal qualification relevant to the care of the sick child, and it is not mandatory for them to do so. It would be unthinkable for a doctor or nurse caring for the adult community not to have a qualification in the care of adults. Clearly children are still considered to be 'little adults' or at least of lesser importance. The quality of care provided for children during acute childhood illness at home has to be less than optimal. As the Health Committee (1997) pointed out: 'as a matter of principle, sick children need and deserve no less (than adults)' (para 49).

Community children's nursing services' involvement in childhood acute illness

In contrast to those currently providing most care to these children at home, children's nurses have access to, and are undertaking in increasing numbers, a course leading to the qualification of specialist practitioner in community children's nursing. This is the equivalent to the district nursing and health visiting qualifications. It would seem to children's nurses that the obvious person to care for the acutely ill child at home is the community children's nurse (CCN). However, where community children's nursing services exist, families are unlikely to be able to access them for help during acute childhood illness. The majority of services are small and as a result focus on the needs of a minority of children who have complex health needs and chronic or terminal illness (Health Committee 1997, Tatman & Woodroffe 1993). Even for these children, only 50% of the country have access to a community children's nursing service and only 10% to a 24-hour service (Health Committee 1997). This situation leaves parents of an acutely ill child with limited choice and access to professional support.

Historically, the early community nursing services for children were designed to care for acutely ill children at home. Their aim was to prevent hospital admissions and therefore reduce the potential for cross-infection (Gillett 1954, Shrand 1965, Smellie 1956). Aspects of this earlier pattern of care are now informing contemporary developments in some areas. These are discussed later in the chapter.

EXPERIENCES OF THE CHILD AND FAMILY WHEN A CHILD IS ACUTELY ILL AT HOME

Children's reactions to acute illness

Most of the research in this area has focused on the child's reaction to hospitalisation rather than to the illness itself. The effects of separation have become confused with the effects of illness. Research from the community setting has found that in the acute phase of illness children are (Mattsson & Weisberg 1970):

- Less active, sleep longer, and lose their appetite
- More irritable with their parents
- Likely to regress to an earlier stage of greater dependency on their carers, particularly in the younger age group

In the convalescent period, separation anxiety reappears in the child aged over 2 years, an effect that many children's nurses would attribute to hospitalisation (Mattsson & Weisberg 1970). Many of the reactions seen in hospital may, in fact, be attributed to the illness, rather than being in hospital (Mattsson & Weisberg 1970, Shrand 1965). Shrand (1965) suggests that illness, separation and hospitalisation act synergistically, supporting the notion that children cared for at home will be less distressed than the hospitalised child, as only one of these three factors will be operating at home – the illness itself.

Whose voice is being heard in this research?

Most of the research that considers the care of the sick child fails to ask children themselves, preferring to research the views of their parents (Alderson 1993, 1995). The assumption made here is that the client is the child's parent, not the child (Alderson 1993). As a result little is known about the influence of the child's characteristics on the family's needs for support during acute childhood illness at home, or of the older child's development of knowledge about self-care. Wilkinson's (1988) review of the literature and report of his own research addresses the child's understanding of what is meant by health and illness, but does not specifically address their experiences or needs during acute childhood illness.

Parental perception of the child's minor illness

Parents develop a sense of what is normal for their child as they develop in their role as parents. They learn about developmental changes with the first child and then apply this knowledge with their subsequent children (Cunningham-Burley 1990, Cunningham-Burley & Maclean 1991, Irvine & Cunningham-Burley 1991, Mayall 1986, Pearson 1995, Spencer 1984). It is from this reference point that the identification of illness is made. For example, parents attribute many symptoms of minor illness to teething (Irvine & Cunningham-Burley 1991, Mayall 1986, Spencer 1984), a process seen as a normal part of child development. It follows, then, that some illnesses are, in themselves, perceived to be normal for an individual child. Likewise, a specific illness such as chickenpox may itself be viewed as a normal childhood illness (McKenna & Hunt 1994). Children with persistent illness were also viewed as essentially healthy, the illness being attributed to an innate predisposition in that child (Irvine & Cunningham-Burley 1991, Mayall 1986). Some symptoms are particularly worrying to parents (Cornford et al 1993, Holme 1995, Hopton et al 1996, Kai 1996a, Mayall 1986, Spencer 1984):

- Respiratory symptoms, particularly a persistent cough
- High temperature
- Vomiting and pain, especially if the pain is severe, unrelieved and unexplained

Altered breathing and/or coughing are the commonest reason for parents to consult a doctor about their child's health (Cunningham-Burley & Irvine 1987, Holme 1995, Wilson et al 1984). This is clearly supported in the statistics presented above.

Parents also fear not recognising serious illness in their children (Kai 1996a). For some parents this was linked to 'past frights', when their child had been diagnosed by doctors to be much more seriously ill than they had thought before seeking medical advice (Hopton et al 1996). This 'fright' reduces the parents' confidence in their own ability to judge the state of their child's health.

Parents' actions in response to illness in their child

Parents constantly monitor the state of their child's health (Cunningham-Burley 1990, Kai 1996a) so that they are able to make a judgement about the normality or abnormality of the child's state of health. When parents notice that there is something wrong with their child, their first action is to wait and see (Cunningham-Burley & Irvine 1987, Spencer 1984). When symptoms persist, their treatment of the child may consist of nursing actions and/or the use of over-the-counter (OTC) remedies (Cantrill et al 1996, Cornford et al 1993, Cunningham-Burley & Irvine 1987, Cunning-Burley & Maclean 1987, Mayall 1986, Spencer 1984). The majority of OTC remedies are already present in the home (Cantrill et al 1996). Generally children are given extra attention and time (Mayall 1986), providing the child with increased emotional support (Spencer 1984). Overall, parents make every effort to treat the child themselves and are reluctant to 'bother the doctor' (Cunningham-Burley & Maclean 1991, Kai 1996a). Difficulties in obtaining an appointment may be one reason for this reluctance (Cantrill et al 1996). Between 59% and 99% of all episodes of acute childhood illness at home are managed without recourse to health professionals (Holme 1995, Mayall 1986).

The role of family and friendship networks

Parents use what is described as a 'lay network' of family and friends to seek information about caring for their child (Kai 1996a, Mayall 1986). This includes suggestions of diagnoses, advice on nursing their child, home remedies and when to refer to the doctor. Where this supportive network is smaller, an increased use of general practice services results (Mayall 1986). Social support for mothers results in better health for their children, an effect that is strongest in families living in poverty (Oakley et al 1994). The importance of a supportive network of family and friends reflects a key theme within the dominant philosophy of children's nursing: the need for children to be viewed and cared for within the context of their families (Royal College of Nursing 1995).

Factors affecting parents' use of health services

The published literature seems to indicate that the family doctor is perceived to be the only source of help available to families once their own resources have been exhausted. Parents' decisions to consult their doctor are based on the following:

- Abnormal symptoms (Cunningham-Burley 1990, Hopton et al 1996)
- Behavioural change (Hopton et al 1996, Kai 1996b)

- Perceived increased severity of illness (Clarke & Hewison 1991, Cornford et al 1993, Wyke et al 1990)
- Feelings of helplessness or of being unable to cope (Kai 1996b, Morrison et al 1991)
- When their own attempts to treat the child have failed (Cunningham-Burley & Irvine, 1987, Hopton et al 1996).

Parents' ability to cope with their child's illness seems to be closely related to their perceptions of the extent to which the illness is a threat to the child's life (Kai 1996a). This logically suggests that the greater the perceived threat to the child's health the more likely it is that a parent will decide to seek professional help and advice.

Parents' perceptions of healthcare services

When parents decide to seek help from health services, the most common desire is for the reassurance that they have not missed anything serious. This is followed closely by their need for information about their child's illness and care (Clarke & Hewison 1991, Cornford et al 1993, Irvine & Cunningham-Burley 1991, Kai 1996b, Mayall 1986, Morrison et al 1991). Such information helps parents to understand their child's illness and the necessary treatment, reducing the perceived threat of the illness to the child's life and, therefore, increasing the parents' ability to continue to manage the episode of illness at home. Parents also seek information from sources other than healthcare professionals, often learning more from the media, in the form of parenting magazines, television dramas and publicity campaigns (Kai 1996b). Parents wish to have their views respected and their competence as a parent recognised. Mothers, in particular, report that they are made to 'feel stupid' or 'silly' by doctors when consulting for a minor illness when all they wanted was reassurance (Cunningham-Burley & Maclean 1991).

Contrary to popular medical opinion, a minority of parents want medication for their child (Clarke & Hewison 1991, Cunningham-Burley & Irvine 1987), yet the majority of parents leave the surgery with a prescription (Wilson et al 1984). There is further conflict between parents and doctors here, as parents also misunderstand the reasons for the prescription of antibiotics. Parents' desire for antibiotics is based on their perception of the severity of their child's illness, rather than on an understanding of bacterial versus viral infection (Kai 1996b). There is an obvious mismatch here between the desires of parents and what GPs provide.

From the doctor's perspective, their practice may be influenced by the necessity to see large numbers of patients in a short period of time, with the average GP consultation time being approximately 8 minutes (Wilson 1991). The extent to which the reassurance and information needs of families can be met in such a short time period must be limited.

At the end of such short consultations, parents may be no clearer about what is wrong with their child, or why they have or have not been given a prescription, and their confidence in their own ability to care for their child may have been reduced. This situation may result in parents resorting to hospitalisation for their child (Meates 1997) or further GP consultations. Clearly the opposite may also occur where parent's needs are met. These parents may feel more confident in their ability to care for their child and reassured that their child is not seriously ill (Cornford et al 1993, Kai 1996a). Consequently their children may be less likely to be admitted to hospital as they feel able to care for them at home.

IMPLICATIONS OF THE EXPERIENCES OF CHILDREN AND THEIR FAMILIES DURING ACUTE CHILDHOOD ILLNESS FOR HEALTHCARE SERVICE DELIVERY

Demand for GP services to children (1–15 years) is increasing (Health Committee 1997, Office of Population Censuses and Surveys 1991). In addition, general practice is facing a recruitment crisis with fewer doctors wanting to move into this field of work. GPs have tried to manage the rising demand for out-of-hours services through the creation of GP cooperatives (Jessopp et al 1997). There appears to be no evidence, however, of consultation of service users in the development of these services. The style of each consultation is unlikely to change, creating even more demand as parents' needs continue to be unmet. Demand also appears to be rising due to the increased accessibility of these services, compared with the individual GPs doing their own on-call. Alternative options for managing the continually increasing demand need to be considered, in particular the role of other health professionals in helping parents to care for the child during acute childhood illness at home.

OPTIONS FOR THE INVOLVEMENT OF CHILDREN'S NURSES IN THE CARE OF THE ACUTELY ILL CHILD AT HOME

Integrated primary care model

This model involves CCNs being based within and integrated into primary healthcare teams (PHCTs). Some of the advantages of this approach are:

- An appropriately qualified professional providing care for children and their families
- Accessibility of services to children and their families at their local health centre
- Ease of communication with the PHCT
- Self-referrals and direct referrals from GPs, practice nurses, health visitors, school nurses and district nurses to the CCN
- Services can be developed in response to the specific needs of the local population, enabling the specific needs of minority ethnic groups to be met more easily.

Minimal research has been conducted which addresses this area. However, a project taking place in Sheffield will provide valuable evidence of the feasibility

BOX 21.1 ***Evaluation of the role and function of a qualified children's nurse within a primary healthcare team***

Two experienced qualified children's nurses were recruited and allocated to two PHCTs. This permitted a comparison of how the two nurses might function and threw further light on the ways in which different types of nursing skills were used. It was important to allow the role to evolve without undue pressure, so that the existing members of the PHCTs could work with them to establish what would be the most useful and relevant care for them to undertake. A formative evaluation process was applied to the study and consisted of the following elements:

- Case studies
- Multiple methods of data collection
- Acknowledgement of the role or influence of evaluators in the evaluation process
- Evaluation as a political process
- Emphasis on utility
- Reflective accounts by each nurse on their role and function as a member of the PHCT

Every child was given a case number. Each time a contact was made, this was recorded on a database and an account was documented within a reflective diary. This yielded the following results:

Number of cases	180
Number of records	721
Average time spent per case =	33.8 min

The data presented in Figure 21.1 indicate that acute childhood illness constituted the largest proportion of cases seen.

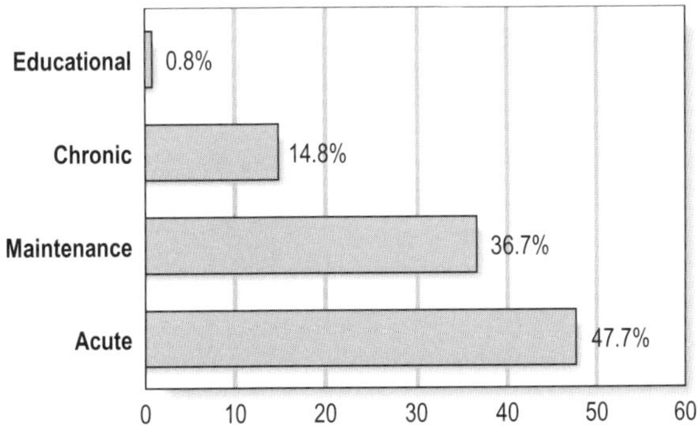

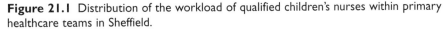

Figure 21.1 Distribution of the workload of qualified children's nurses within primary healthcare teams in Sheffield.

of using children's nurses to care for the acutely ill child at home. Two children's nurses were moved from the children's ward to work within two health centres. For an outline of the project, see Box 21.1. In this project the majority of the work undertaken by these nurses is concerned with acute illness, as can be seen in Figure 21.1. Formal evaluation of the project will provide important information on the feasibility of CCNs working within PHCTs.

BOX 21.2 *Integration of community children's nursing services into primary care*

Integration of community children's nursing services into primary care is a relatively new concept which has become a reality for a Berkshire practice. The CCN is practice based and is employed on a full-time basis to provide nursing care to acutely ill and chronically sick children and their families. The role also incorporates a supportive, educational and teaching element and aims to prevent hospitalisation at all times.

In this setting the CCN works with and has the support of four GPs. This enables the CCN to expand into more specialised areas of practice. One such area is the establishment of a nurse-led minor ailments clinic in which children are examined, assessed and subsequently managed by the nurse or referred to the named GP if indicated. The clinic is offered as an alternative to a GP appointment, rather than a replacement. The advantages include more time to focus on educational aspects of childhood illness and the offer of home visits by the CCN to provide further support.

In summary, a primary care base provides the forum for developing and utilising skills of CCNs that would otherwise be undiscovered, and facilitates the way forward into new areas of practice.

In other areas of the country a few children's nurses are beginning to work with, and be based within, PHCTs. One nurse in this role has developed a minor ailments clinic specifically to address the needs of children with acute childhood illness at home (see Box 21.2). Such initiatives have tremendous potential for the prevention of unnecessary admissions to hospital through enabling parents to cope at home. Parents will receive more detailed information from a children's nurse, whose average consultation time is around 30 minutes (see Box 21.1), compared with 8 minutes with a GP. The increase in information and the accessibility of support will improve parents' personal control and therefore their ability to care for their child (Kai 1996b, Meates 1997), with an accompanying reduction in demand for GP consultations and attendance at accident and emergency departments (Meates 1997). In addition, the reduction of parental anxiety will reduce the child's level of anxiety, potentially facilitating a faster recovery. Examples of the success of a minor ailments clinic combined with home visits is provided in the case studies.

CASE STUDY

James' story

James, a 10-month-old baby with asthma, was seen at the minor ailments clinic. Following an examination and full nursing assessment, he was found to have symptoms that indicated an exacerbation of his asthma and a chest infection. The CCN increased his preventer and reliever treatment, the GP was consulted regarding the chest infection, and antibiotics were prescribed. A review with the GP was arranged for 6 hours later. Follow-up care was arranged at home with the CCN 3 days later and 2 weeks thereafter. The care included adjustment of inhaler doses, inhaler demonstration, asthma management at home, and treatment compliance. James made a full recovery and remains stable on regular preventive treatment.

Alexander's story

Alexander is a 3-year-old boy with a known history of nut allergy and anaphylactic reactions. He presented at the minor ailments clinic following contact with an unknown irritant causing facial urticaria. He had been given oral antihistamine before presenting at the clinic. Following examination he was found to be clinically stable and the urticaria was subsiding. He was given a regimen for oral antihistamine administration over the next 48 hours and follow-up care was discussed. The GP was notified of this incident and confirmed the plan of care. The CCN arranged to see Alexander at home 24 hours later, when the urticaria was found to have resolved. Subsequent management of anaphylaxis and treatment was discussed and a demonstration of injectable adrenaline given. Alexander remains well on a nut-free diet.

Several other initiatives are and have been developed to address the needs of children with acute illness and their families. A few of the generic community children's nursing teams do care for children with acute illness, although this is the exception rather than the rule for the reasons mentioned above. Other services for these children are based around hospital services.

Ambulatory care

This concept has been defined as 'the non-inpatient hospital services and the provision of care to sick children at home or in their local environment' (Meates 1997). This approach includes units such as children's admission units, day-case units, rapid-response outpatient clinics, children's accident and emergency services, and hospital outreach children's nursing services (Glasper & Lowson 1998). Meates (1997) describes the presence of children's nurses in the accident and emergency department as making 'a huge difference to the care of children'. In the best examples, each of these units is able to refer children to a community-based generic CCN for follow-up visits and support.

The ambulatory care approach does prevent some unnecessary admissions, but many of the services delivered under this label do involve hospital attendance (Glasper & Lowson 1998). Consequently, it does disrupt family life as the child has to travel to the hospital, usually at a greater distance from home than the local health centre. Although these units do minimise hospital attendance, this is not community care. Much of the care given in this way could be given at home. Concentrating these services within the hospital environment is convenient for health professionals – not for families. It also reflects the resource constraints within the current climate of the National Health Service.

Inevitably hospital-based services are limited by the nature of their referral system. Referrals usually come from other hospital services. As a result, the service is not accessible to families whose children are not referred to the hospital or who do not attend the accident and emergency department.

CONCLUSION

The majority of childhood illness takes place at home with no recourse to professional care and support. Despite this fact, children with acute childhood illness constitute a significant proportion of the GP's workload. Various professionals are currently involved in the care of these children in the community – most of whom do not hold a qualification in child healthcare. Parents are often dissatisfied with the care provided by GPs, wanting more reassurance and information. The average consultation time with their family doctor is far too short for parents' needs to be met in this way. Rising demand and the non-expansion of GP services means that alternatives to GP care are needed to support children and families during acute illness.

The strategic development of services that integrate CCNs within PHCTs and primary care groups has the potential to meet parents' needs for information and reassurance. In doing so, CCNs are enabling parents to continue to care for their child at home, thus reducing the pressure on both hospital and GP services. The continuing move towards community care and centralisation of tertiary care across the NHS in the UK make the further development of local services, which enable children and families to cope at home, an essential prerequisite for the management of rising demands for services.

FURTHER READING

Health Committee 1997 House of Commons Select Committee. Health services for children and young people in the community: home and school. Third report. The Stationery Office, London

If you only ever read one report about community children's health services, this should be it. It is the most comprehensive review conducted since the Court Report in 1976. If you are looking for evidence to support the need for community children's nursing services, read this.

Mayall B 1986 Keeping children healthy. Allen & Unwin, London

This book gives a comprehensive report of Mayall's research, investigating how children and families manage health and illness. It provides an excellent insight into the parent's perspective.

Wilkinson S R 1988 The child's world of illness. The development of health and illness behaviour. Cambridge University Press, Cambridge

Contains a detailed review of the research on the child's understanding of the concepts of health and illness, addressing each age group in some depth.

Wyke S & Hewison J (eds) 1991 Child health matters. Open University Press, Milton Keynes

This book is a reader containing papers on a variety of subjects related to child healthcare in the community.

REFERENCES

Alderson P 1993 Children's consent to surgery. Open University Press, Buckingham:

Alderson P 1995 Listening to children. Children, ethics and social research. Barnados, Ilford

Balarajan R, Yuen P & Machin D 1992 Deprivations and general practitioner workload. British Medical Journal 304:529–534

Cantrill J A, Johannesson B, Nicolson M & Noyce P R 1996 Management of minor ailments in primary schoolchildren in rural and urban areas. Child: care, health and development. 22(3):167–174

Central Statistical Office 1994 Social focus on children. HMSO, London

Clarke A & Hewison J 1991 Whether or not to consult a general practitioner: decision-making by parents in a multi-ethnic inner city area. In: Wyke S & Hewison J (eds) Child health matters. Open University Press, Milton Keynes, ch 7, p 74

Cornford C S, Morgan M & Ridsdale L 1993 Why do mothers consult when their children cough? Family Practice 10(2):193–196

Cunningham-Burley S 1990 Mothers' beliefs about and perceptions of their children's illnesses. In: Cunningham-Burley S & McKeganey N P (eds) Readings in medical sociology. Tavistock/Routledge, London, ch 4, p 85

Cunningham-Burley S & Irvine S 1987 'And have you done anything so far?' An examination of lay treatment of children's symptoms. British Medical Journal 295:700–702

Cunningham-Burley S & Maclean U 1987 The role of the chemist in primary health care for children with minor complaints. Social Science and Medicine 24(4):371–377

Cunningham-Burley S & Maclean U 1991 Dealing with children's illness: mothers' dilemmas. In: Wyke S & Hewison J (eds) Child health matters. Open University Press, Milton Keynes, ch 3, p 29

Gillam S J, Jarman B, White P & Law R 1989 Ethnic differences in consultation rates in urban general practice. British Medical Journal 299:953–957

Gillett J A 1954 Domiciliary treatment of sick children. The Practitioner 172:281–283

Glasper E A & Lowson S 1998 Innovations in paediatric ambulatory care. A nursing perspective. Macmillan, Basingstoke

Graham H 1994 The changing financial circumstances of households with children. Children and Society 8:98–113

Health Committee 1997 House of Commons Health Select Committee. Health services for children and young people in the community: home and school. Third report. The Stationery Office, London

Holme C 1995 Incidence and prevalence of non-specific symptoms and behavioural changes in infants under the age of two years. British Journal of General Practice 45:65–69

Hopton J, Hogg R & McKee I 1996 Patients' accounts of calling the doctor out of hours: qualitative study in one general practice. British Medical Journal 313:991–994

Irvine S & Cunningham-Burley S 1991 Mothers' concept of normality, behavioural change and illness in their children. British Journal of General Practice 41:371–374

Jessopp L, Beck I, Hollins L, Shipman C, Reynolds M & Dale J 1997 Changing the pattern out of hours: a survey of general practice cooperatives. British Medical Journal 314:199–200

Kai J 1996a What worries parents when their pre-school children are acutely ill, and why: a qualitative study. British Medical Journal 313:983–986

Kai J 1996b Parents' difficulties and information needs in coping with acute illness in preschool children: a qualitative study. British Medical Journal 313:987–990

Leicester City Council 1997 Annual report of the Director of Public Health. Leicestershire 1996/7. Leicester City Council, Leicester

McCormick A, Fleming D & Charlton J 1995 Morbidity statistics from general practice 1991–2. Series MB5. No. 3. Office of Population Censuses and Surveys. HMSO, London

McKenna S P & Hunt S M 1994 A measure of family disruption for use in chickenpox and other childhood illnesses. Social Science and Medicine 38(5):725–731

Mattsson A & Weisberg I 1970 Behavioural reactions to minor illness in preschool children. Pediatrics 46(4):604–610

Mayall B 1986 Keeping children healthy. Allen & Unwin, London

Meates M 1997 Ambulatory paediatrics – making a difference. Archives of Disease in Childhood 76:468–472

Morrison J M, Gilmour H & Sullivan F 1991 Children seen frequently out of hours in one general practice. British Medical Journal 303:1111–1114

Neill S J 1996 Parent participation. Part 1. British Journal of Nursing 5(1):34–40

Oakley A, Hickey D & Rigby A S 1994 Love or money? Social support, class inequality and the health of women and children. European Journal of Public Health 4:265–273

Office of Population Censuses and Surveys 1991 General household survey. HMSO, London

Pearson P 1995 Client views of health visiting. In: Heyman B (ed) Researching user perspectives on community health care. Chapman & Hall, London, ch 6, p 106

Reading R 1997 Poverty and the health of children and adolescents. Archives of Disease in Childhood 76:463–467

Rennick J E 1995 The changing profile of acute childhood illness: a need for the development of family nursing knowledge. Journal of Advanced Nursing 22:258–266

Royal College of Nursing 1995 Paediatric nursing: a philosophy of care. Royal College of Nursing, London

Shrand H 1965 Behaviour changes in sick children nursed at home. Pediatrics 36(4):604–607

Smellie J M 1956 Domiciliary nursing service for infants and children. British Medical Journal i:256

Spencer N J 1984 Parents' recognition of the ill child. In: Macfarlane J A (ed) Progress in child health, vol 1. Churchill Livingstone, Edinburgh, p 100

Tatman M & Woodroffe C 1993 Paediatric home care in the United Kingdom. Archives of Disease in Childhood 69:677–680

Watson E 1991 'Appropriate' use of child health services in East London: ethnic similarities and differences. In: Wyke S & Hewison J (eds) Child health matters. Open University Press, Milton Keynes, ch 8, p 88

Webb E 1996 Meeting the needs of minority ethnic groups. Archives of Disease in Childhood 74:264–267

Wilkinson S R 1988 The child's world of illness. The development of health and illness behaviour. Cambridge University Press, Cambridge

Wilson A 1991 Consultation length in general practice: a review. British Journal of General Practice 41:119–122

Wilson A D, Downham M A P S & Forster D P 1984 Acute illness in infants: a general practice study. Journal of the Royal College of General Practitioners 34:155–159

Wyke S, Hewison J & Russell I T 1990 Respiratory illness in children: what makes parents decide to consult? British Journal of General Practice 40:226–229

22 Collaborative planning for children with chronic, complex care needs

Julia Muir & Sue Dryden

KEY ISSUES

- Sociopolitical influences in meeting the needs of children with chronic, complex care needs
- Impact of the continuing care policy
- Respite care provision
- Joint working – integrating health and social care provision
- Pivotal role of the key worker

INTRODUCTION

Innovations in medical practice and technological advances have meant that children are now surviving once-fatal diseases (Birch et al 1988, Roberton 1993). The prevalence of chronic illness in childhood more than doubled between 1972 and 1991 (Office of Population Censuses and Surveys 1991), and more recently it has been estimated that 14% of under 16 year olds have a chronic illness (Perkins 1996). Often the care of children with chronic illness is complex because of a reliance on technology (Kirk 1998). These combined factors have implications for meeting the continuing care needs of this population. This chapter examines the issues influencing the provision of integrated and appropriate support for these children and their families in the community.

SOCIOPOLITICAL CONTEXT

Government policies and recommendations have continued to advocate for children to be cared for in their own homes and for appropriate services to be augmented accordingly (Department of Health 1991, Department of Health and Social Security 1976, Health Committee 1977, Ministry of Health 1959, National Health Service Executive 1996). For the first time, the Department of Health (1998a) provided funding for the development of community children's nursing teams in memory of Princess Diana. Apart from this recent investment, there has been no other formal strategy, funding or legislation to support this service provision. Rather, the Department of Health has produced guidance documents which require local interpretation and implementation. Indeed, this has been the case with the continuing care policy.

THE CONTINUING CARE POLICY

In 1994 a complaint against a health authority, regarding the provision of long-term care for a patient, prompted the Government to develop the continuing care policy (Department of Health 1995). The aim of this policy was to distinguish nursing (health) care from social care, and to fund nursing care accordingly. Responsibility for the development of eligibility criteria was devolved to local authorities. Some welcomed the ability to interpret and define the policy at a local level while others believed that this contributed to disparity of service provision across the country (Thomas 1996).

The continuing care policy focused primarily on the needs of the elderly with limited reference to the specific needs of children. At the time, a progress review of local policies identified the need for further development of explicit eligibility criteria for children's services (Department of Health 1996). Given the existing inequalities in community children's nursing services within the UK (Health Committee 1997), this policy widened the gulf between the parity of care provision for those who have access to the service and those who do not. Where services exist, community children's nursing teams are uniquely placed to contribute to the development of eligibility criteria for their client group (National Health Service Executive 1998) and to ensure that the total needs of individual children are recognised and met. This is reflected in the example given in Box 22.1.

BOX 22.1 ***Developing continuing care eligibility criteria for children***

In Nottingham, the community children's nursing service worked with the local health authority to create a framework through which continuing care could be resourced. As a result, specific eligibility criteria were produced and a continuing care referral form was designed. This form was developed in collaboration with all the professional groups, including social services, to ensure the documentation reflected their individual requirements and to encourage joint planning. The referral forms could then be circulated for completion by each professional for their assessment of the continuing care needs of identified children. These completed assessments are then presented at a multiprofessional case review at which packages of care are negotiated. In some circumstances it may be agreed that these care packages can be constructed from within current resources. Where additional resources are required, the referral form highlights deficits and helps to ensure that families have knowledge of all the services that may be available to them. A review system is built into every package of care provided.

There were many benefits to this collaborative approach, including:

- The development of effective communication pathways between the community children's nursing service, other professional groups and the health authority
- More efficient referrals to other agencies such as social services and the voluntary sector
- Greater understanding of one another's roles, responsibilities and constraints
- The opportunity to explore more creative solutions to care packages whilst maximising the use of existing resources

Child-specific eligibility criteria provide an ideal framework for either (1) the discharge planning process or (2) a primary care conference. In planning for the continuing care needs of children in the community, aspects that require careful assessment are shown in Box 22.2.

The provision of respite care may be the most difficult to negotiate within the confines of our financially challenged healthcare system and requires further exploration.

RESPITE CARE

Despite the implementation of the continuing care policy, in reality parents are often required to learn complex nursing skills and assume 24-hour responsibility in order to achieve home care (Townsley & Robinson 1999, While et al 1996). This can be socially isolating and leave families virtually housebound (Andrews & Nielson 1988, Kirk 1998, Patterson et al 1994, Teague et al 1993). The consequences of this may be increased parental stress, deterioration of the family structure and marital problems (Andrews & Nielson 1988, Hall 1996, Jennings 1990, Leonard et al 1993, Teague et al 1993). An obvious repercussion has been the expressed shortfall of appropriate respite care provision, particularly where highly specialised care is required (Hall 1996, National Health Service Executive 1998, Townsley & Robinson 1999, While et al 1996).

To meet this need, health and social service provision has been supplemented by the use of voluntary or independent organisations and non-parent carers. The benefits of voluntary services are well recognised as being user led, community based and flexible in their response to need (Cairns et al 1997). However, there has been no national guidance from the Department of Health for the training of such carers, despite being a recommendation of the Health Committee report (1997). As a result, the threat of legal liability has led to

BOX 22.2 ***Points to consider when planning continuing community care for a child***

- The total health needs of the child including social, educational, emotional, spiritual, physical and psychological issues
- The principal caregivers' approach to the child's needs in relation to their:

knowledge	confidence	attitude
understanding	cooperation	competence
compliance	ability	support structure

- The equipment, supplies and medication needs of the child: funding, maintenance and training
- The home and other community environments and their suitability to accommodate the necessary technology, etc.
- Overall level of dependency and nursing input required
- Welfare benefits available to the family
- Respite care needs of the family: the suitability and availability of provision

inconsistent guidance and advice between local authorities and unequal access to respite care for sick children and their families in the community (Townsley & Robinson 1999).

Respite care is most effective when it meets the needs of children and their families and not the needs of those providing it. This was reflected in the surveys undertaken during the 'Evaluation of the pilot project programme for children with life threatening illnesses' (National Health Service Executive 1998). Parents expressed the need for a range of respite care services which:

- Could be accessed as and when necessary
- Were flexible in terms of location
- Allowed them to negotiate the time available from a few hours to a more extended period

The report (National Health Service Executive 1998) proposes that the following recommendations are acknowledged in respite care provision:

1. Families prefer to have a known carer rather than bank staff who may be different for each episode of care.
2. Families require adequate information about the service especially when English is not their first language.
3. Cultural diversity of a local community must be taken into account when planning respite care services.

Within the conclusions it suggests that best practice can be achieved when respite care is provided as part of an integrated children's service. This concurs with the Government's focus on joint working (Department of Health 1998b, c).

JOINT WORKING

The Department of Health (1998b) has finally acknowledged that 'health and social care are often one and the same' (para 2.29). The need to break down existing barriers and to pursue integrated health and social care provision has also been recognised (Department of Health 1998b, c). The 'Partnership in action' discussion document (Department of Health 1998c p 6) states:

'Joint working is needed at three levels:

1. Strategic planning: agencies need to plan jointly for the medium term, share information about how they intend to use their resources toward the achievement of common goals;
2. Service commissioning: when securing services for their local populations, agencies need to have a common understanding of the needs they are jointly meeting and the kind of provision likely to be most effective;
3. Service provision: regardless of how services are purchased or funded, the key objective is that the user receives a coherent integrated package of care and that they, and their families, do not face the anxiety of having to navigate a labyrinthine bureaucracy.'

These recommendations seek to overcome the current challenges faced by sick children and their families. It is hoped that legislation will facilitate joint commissioning opportunities. This may be achieved by pooling budgets so that 'staff from either agency can put care packages together best suited to particular individuals without worrying whether it was health or social services money they were using' (Department of Health 1998c p 18). Townsley & Robinson (1999) acknowledge that this legislation could radically improve the lives of children with complex health needs and their families, but stress the urgency for national guidelines that explicitly address the requirements of non-parent carers within education, social services or independent sectors.

THE KEY WORKER ROLE

A number of documents have described the essential role of a named key worker for these families (Association for Children with Life-threatening or Terminal Conditions and their Families & Royal College of Paediatrics and Child Health 1997, English National Board for Nursing, Midwifery and Health Visiting & Department of Health 1999, National Health Service Executive 1998). Whilst definitions vary slightly, all note the important elements of the role as being an advocate, a single point of reference, a source of support and a coordinator of services on behalf of the family.

Sadly, a key worker is rarely nominated on a formal basis for many of these families (Hall 1996, Kirk 1998, National Health Service Executive 1998). Where services exist, the community children's nurse is in a prime position to fulfil this role (National Health Service Executive 1998). However, the role is time consuming and potentially stressful. It therefore requires formal recognition and the provision of appropriate support mechanisms in the form of supervision (Association for Children with Life-threatening or Terminal Conditions and their Families & Royal College of Paediatrics and Child Health 1997, National Health Service Executive 1998).

In the absence of community children's nursing services, parents frequently adopt the work undertaken by the key worker (Hall 1996, Kirk 1998). This inevitably leads to dissatisfaction on behalf of the family (Hall 1996) and contradicts the aim of providing optimum quality of patient care.

CONCLUSIONS

It is clear that the maintenance of good health and treatment of ill health is the responsibility of many agencies, not just the health service (Green & Thorogood 1998). Whilst the continuing care policy was divisive in its approach, it has provided a potential framework from which to coordinate the complex care packages so often needed by children with chronic, complex care needs and their families. The involvement of community children's nursing services in this process significantly improves the quality of care provision for these families. The model outlined in Box 22.1 provides a useful benchmark to take forward the joint working initiative, now seen as essential by the Government. Furthermore, the recently formed Diana, Princess of Wales Community Children's Nursing Teams have a clear remit to facilitate such practice (English National Board & Department of Health 1999). These nurse-led teams provide community children's nurses with a unique opportunity to influence and shape future models of collaborative practice.

FURTHER READING

National Health Service Executive 1998 Evaluation of the pilot project programme for children with life threatening illnesses. The Stationery Office, London

This document provides some exceedingly good examples of good practice in meeting the needs of sick children in the community. It is usefully supplemented by practical examples, such as eligibility criteria and training protocols for carers. Both new and existing community children's nursing teams will benefit from its contents.

English National Board for Nursing, Midwifery and Health Visiting & Department of Health 1999 Sharing the care. Resource pack to support Diana, Princess of Wales Community Children's Nursing Teams. English National Board, London

This resource pack offers practical advice on the following five themes: (1) developing a shared vision and values, (2) working in partnership, (3) leading and managing a team, (4) developmental needs and (5) Flexible, responsive and creative. It will be an essential asset to both new and existing community children's nursing teams.

Department of Health 1998 Partnership in action. A discussion document. The Stationery Office, London

This document clearly outlines the future plans for integrated health and social services. It offers good examples which can easily be translated into clinical practice.

REFERENCES

Andrews M M & Nielson D W 1988 Technology dependent children in the home. Pediatric Nursing 12(2):111–114

Association for Children with Life-threatening or Terminal Conditions and their Families & Royal College of Paediatrics and Child Health 1997 A guide to the development of children's palliative care services. Association for Children with Life-threatening or Terminal Conditions and their Families, Bristol

Birch J M, Marsden H B, Morris Jones P H, Pearson D & Blair V 1988 Improvements in survival in childhood cancer: results of a population-based study over 30 years. British Medical Journal 296:1372–1376

Cairns B, Nicholson J & Webb W 1997 Buying quality. HIV volunteering in the age of contracting. National Aids Trust, Oxford

Department of Health 1991 The welfare of children and young people in hospital. HMSO, London

Department of Health 1995 NHS responsibilities for meeting continuing health care needs. HSG(95)8 LAC(95)5. HMSO, London

Department of Health 1996 Progress in practice: initial evaluation of the impact of the continuing care guidance. EL(96)89 CI(96)35. The Stationery Office, London

Department of Health 1998a A proposal to develop a national children's community nursing service. Department of Health, London

Department of Health 1998b Our healthier nation. The Stationery Office, London

Department of Health 1998c Partnership in action. A discussion document. The Stationery Office, London

Department of Health and Social Security 1976 Fit for the future. Report of the committee on child health services (chairman Professor S D M Court). HMSO, London

English National Board for Nursing, Midwifery and Health Visiting & Department of Health 1999 Sharing the care. Resource pack to support Diana, Princess of Wales Community Children's Nursing Teams. English National Board, London

Green J & Thorogood N 1998 Analysing health policy. A sociological approach. Addison Wesley Longman, Harlow, UK

Hall S 1996 An exploration of parental perception of the nature and level of support needed to care for their child with special needs. Journal of Advanced Nursing 24:512–521

Health Committee 1997 House of Commons Select Committee. Health services for children and young people in the community: home and school. Third report. The Stationery Office, London

Jennings P 1990 Caring for a child with a tracheostomy. Nursing Standard 4(30):24–26 & 4(32):38–40

Kirk S 1998 Families' experiences of caring at home for a technology-dependent child: a review of the literature. Child: Care, Health and Development 24(2):101–114

Leonard B J, Dwyer Brust J & Nelson R P 1993 Parental distress: caring for medically fragile children at home. Journal of Pediatric Nursing 8(1):22–30

Ministry of Health 1959 The welfare of children in hospital. Report of the committee (chairman Sir Harry Platt). HMSO, London

National Health Service Executive 1996 A patient's charter: services for children and young people. HMSO, London

National Health Service Executive 1998 Evaluation of the pilot project programme for children with life threatening illnesses. The Stationery Office, London

Office of Population Censuses and Surveys 1991 OPCS surveys of disability in Great Britain. HMSO, London

Patterson J M, Jernell J, Leonard B J & Titus J C 1994 Caring for medically fragile children at home: the parent–professional relationship. Journal of Pediatric Nursing 9(2):98–106

Perkins E 1996 Community children's nursing: generalist or specialist? NHS Executive, Leeds

Roberton N R C 1993 Should we look after babies less than 800 g? Archives of Disease in Childhood 65:1076–1081

Teague B R, Fleming J W, Castle A, Lobo M L, Riggs & Wolfe J G 1993 'High-tech' home care for children with chronic health conditions: a pilot study. Journal of Pediatric Nursing 8(4):226–232

Thomas B 1996 Continuing care needs for the elderly mentally ill. British Journal of Nursing 5(10):622–624

Townsley R & Robinson C 1999 What rights for disabled children? Home enteral tube feeding in the community. Children and Society 13:48–60

While A, Citrone C & Cornish J 1996 A study of the needs and provisions for families caring for children with life-limiting incurable disorders. King's College, London

23 Meeting the palliative care needs of children in the community

Anna Sidey & Andrea Lambert

KEY ISSUES

- Who needs palliative care?
- Clinical responsibility for the child receiving palliative care
- The role of the community children's nurse
- Respite care and support services
- Emotional and bereavement support

INTRODUCTION

Misconceptions can occur when the term palliative care is used. It can conjure images of a child in the last days or hours of their life. However, the Association for Children with Life-threatening or Terminal Conditions and their Families (ACT) and the Royal College of Paediatrics and Child Health (RCPCH) (1997 p 7) provide the following definition:

> 'Palliative care for children and young people with life-limiting conditions is an active and total approach to care, embracing physical, emotional, social and spiritual elements. It focuses on enhancement of quality of life for the child and support for the family and includes the management of distressing symptoms, provision of respite and care through death and bereavement.'

Similarly, Sutherland et al (1993) offer the following definition:

> 'care which is provided when curative treatment is not possible or not appropriate, and which personalises the care of the whole child and family, focusing on the relief of physical, emotional, social and spiritual distress and aiming for the best possible quality of life.'

The number of children with life-limiting illness who may require palliative care is relatively small. Conditions from which they suffer are often rare and the length of time for which a child requires palliative care may vary from days to years. ACT and RCPCH (1997), in their guide to the development of children's palliative care services, estimated that in a health district of 250 000 people five children will die each year from a life-limiting condition, and three of these will be from non-malignant disease. In addition, approximately 50 children will actively require palliative care in any one year.

BOX 23.1 *Groups of children who may require palliative care*

1. Where a cure may be possible but treatment may fail (e.g. cancer or organ failure)
2. Where there may be intensive treatment to prolong and improve quality of life but premature death is probable (e.g. cystic fibrosis and human immunodeficiency virus infection)
3. Where the condition is progressive and degenerative and care is required for a number of years (e.g. Batten's disease)
4. Where severe neurological damage causes disability that will impact on health and may cause rapid deterioration (e.g. severe cerebral palsy)

It is generally recognised that children with cancer or leukaemia have access to charitable funds and relatively well-established services provided by outreach care from tertiary and local hospitals. However, services to children with non-malignant disease are under-developed (Liben 1998). Community children's nurses (CCNs) are frequently involved in caring for children with life-limiting illnesses. A child may be visited on only one occasion, or care and support for the child and family may span many years. The CCN is able to optimise and personalise the package of care received by each family.

WHO NEEDS PALLIATIVE CARE?

ACT and RCPCH (1997) define life-limiting conditions as those 'for which there is no reasonable hope of cure and from which children will die'. The report categorises children who may require palliative care and their conditions into four groups (Box 23.1).

CLINICAL RESPONSIBILITY FOR THE CHILD RECEIVING PALLIATIVE CARE

The stage at which palliative care commences may be dependent on the type of disease and on choices made by the family, the child and the multiprofessional care team. There may be a slow transition from curative treatment to palliative care, or palliative care may start suddenly when it is realised that a cure is not possible. The decision as to which professional assumes clinical responsibility, and at which stage of the illness, can be complex. Parents are often unsure as to who, exactly, is clinically responsible (Read 1998, While et al 1996).

During active, curative, treatment at a regional centre, families and professionals often assume that clinical responsibility is maintained by the paediatrician. General practitioners (GPs) may see very few children with life-limiting conditions throughout their time in practice. This lack of experience may contribute to the family and members of the primary healthcare team losing contact with one another during acute illness and long periods of hospitalisation. However, the GP may be the most appropriate physician to provide clinical responsibility during the palliative stages of the illness when care has been transferred to the community (Goldman 1998). It is essential, therefore, that contact is maintained and positively encouraged throughout the illness trajectory.

Appropriate primary healthcare involvement will reduce or prevent the need for a child to return to hospital. The GP and health visitor may be among the few professionals to have known the family before the child's illness. This can be comforting to the parents and help them to relate to the care team as individuals as well as the parents of a sick child. A CCN may be able to facilitate the ongoing involvement of the GP by coordinating effective liaison between members of the care team at all stages of the child's illness.

ROLE OF THE COMMUNITY CHILDREN'S NURSE

Most children will require nursing support at home. The ACT and RCPCH report (1997) recommends that every family should have a named key worker who is responsible for the coordination of care and that 'care' should be interpreted as both health and social care. The report also recommends that families should not be caught up in disagreements between the roles of the different sectors involved and that services need to be flexible in their approach to ensure this.

The family and the community children's nursing team may have developed a trusting relationship which commenced at the onset of the child's illness and in some congenital conditions at the child's birth. Because of this, the role of key worker is most frequently designated to the CCN. However, the identification of a key worker must be made in collaboration with the child and the family, who need to identify the person whom they feel able to trust and communicate with freely (National Health Service Executive 1998, English National Board for Nursing, Midwifery and Health Visiting & Department of Health 1999). Children with life-limiting conditions frequently have complex medical, nursing and social needs, and are the recipients of numerous services and professionals' attention. The number of professionals and services involved can be overwhelming and leave families feeling isolated and unsupported (Stein and Woolley 1990). Many childhood conditions are extremely rare, and this can increase a sense of isolation. Without the support and coordination of a key worker (See Box 23.2), input and care can be disorganised and inappropriate (Goldman 1998).

BOX 23.2 ***Responsibilities of the key worker (ACT & RCPCH 1997)***

To ensure that:

- Services do not overlap
- Gaps in service provision do not exist
- Communication between agencies is accurate and speedy
- Equipment is available
- The care plan is followed
- The package of care is appropriate and meets the needs of the child and family

To provide:

- Emotional support
- Access to a range of required resources

To act:

- as a link and an advocate ensuring that total care is available

The Diana, Princess of Wales Memorial Committee (Department of Health 1998) recognised that only three health authorities employed community children's nursing teams specialising in palliative care. However, all community children's nursing teams should have the available resources to offer care and support to children and their families who require palliative care (Health Committee 1997). The CCN plays a crucial role in empowering the family to care for their child and to optimise the child's quality of life. The functions within the role may be dictated by the needs and coping mechanisms of the family and child (ACT and RCPCH 1997).

Access to education that is suitable for their health status remains important for the personal and social development of children with life-limiting illness. This may be gained through mainstream or special needs school or home tuition. The CCN can offer advice and support to teaching and care staff within the school and address concerns that the child or their peers may demonstrate (Liben 1998).

EMOTIONAL SUPPORT

Families require emotional support from the time of diagnosis. The CCN may not have been introduced to the family at this point, but from their first meeting this type of support is an important part of the relationship between nurse and family. Grieving begins from the time a family is told that their child will die (Goldman 1998); their lives are in turmoil and the whole family is disrupted. Many children still have their grandparents living and this may be the first loss that the parents have had to face. Most families are incredibly resilient and continue to function; however, the CCN needs to be able to recognise the factors that may indicate families are finding it difficult to cope. Children and parents may benefit from the support of a clinical psychologist or from talking to families who have experienced a similar situation (Goldman 1998).

Looking towards the death of their child is immeasurably painful. After the death, parents recount how helpful it was to have planned what they would do when their child died. The CCN can help parents to explore a range of options. For example, it can be a relief to families to know that they can keep their dead child at home for as long as practically possible (Liben 1998).

The CCN will often continue to visit the family for many months after their child's death. Every family's grief is unique and bereavement support will be led by the needs and wishes of the family. They can be offered choices concerning support in their bereavement and who they wish to be involved in the support (Goldman 1998).

RESPITE CARE AND SUPPORT SERVICES

The following case study highlights the provision of respite care for a child with a life-limiting condition.

CASE STUDY

Mary was the youngest of three sisters. She was well until aged 5 months, when she started to experience convulsions. These resulted in periods of illness requiring intensive care and long episodes of admission to the children's ward. No diagnosis was made but Mary continued to have poorly controlled seizures and eventually failed to respond to any stimuli. Her parents took her home with the knowledge that she would die in the near future and the family was referred to the community children's nursing team. Initially the CCN planned visits to complement those of the health visitor. Mary's mother looked to her health visitor for support and had a well-established relationship with her. The relationship with the CCN developed over many weeks and, as Mary's condition deteriorated, the CCN became the trusted key worker in her care.

The parents had never left their children with anyone and found respite care a difficult concept to embrace. The CCN arranged for a children's nurse from the local respite care team to visit weekly; however, it was many weeks before they felt able to use and enjoy the offered respite care. In the early stages of palliative care, the CCN suggested introducing the family to the local children's hospice, but they did not want to consider this at the time. The hospice was able to offer a much needed holiday to the elder girls, which was a great success. Following this, the parents agreed to Mary receiving respite care at the hospice. This proved to be the beginning of a wonderful and supportive relationship. The hospice offered a home from home environment in which the family felt very comfortable.

As Mary's condition deteriorated, she frequently required suction, nebulisation and continuous feeding. The CCN provided the necessary equipment and liaised closely with the GP and neurologist for advice on symptom control. It was not until this time that her parents felt able to talk about her death. Mary died cuddled up in bed with her mother. As planned, support was provided by the respite care nurse and the CCN. Mary stayed at home until the next day when the whole family went to the hospice and stayed there with her until the day of the funeral. Ongoing bereavement support was provided by the counsellor from the hospice.

The strain of caring for a sick child at home is immense. Parents may suffer physical, psychological and emotional exhaustion and can become isolated. Unfortunately few families have access to adequate or suitable respite care facilities (ACT & RCPCH 1997, Hall 1996, National Health Service Executive 1998, While et al 1996). Respite care provision varies greatly across the country and may be provided by a variety of services providers, as shown in Box 23.3.

BOX 23.3 ***Examples of providers of respite care***

- Health service-funded nursing teams
- Charitably funded teams
- Hospices
- Hospice outreach services
- Social services homecare
- Social services residential care
- Learning disabilities residential and outreach care
- Short-term fostering
- Family and friends

Providing palliative care can be challenging and distressing for all professionals involved and it is recognised that staff require support (ACT & RCPCH 1997, National Health Service Executive 1998).

The CCN is able to explore with the family which of the available services is best able to meet their needs. Introductions at an early stage of palliative care will avoid the possible need for unknown carers to be introduced to the child and family at a time of crisis. Respite care provision must be flexible to meet the changing needs of the child and family, and the parent should not be forced to relinquish the care of their child – however tired or desperate they appear to be (Dominica 1990, Farrell and Sutherland 1998). Having suitable respite care enables families to cope through what may be many years of their child's illness and can allow them to decide where they would like to be at the time of their child's death.

CONCLUSION

In most areas of the country, palliative care services for children are underdeveloped. Models of care may be disparate or non-existent. In 1992, a number of pilot projects to provide care for children with life-threatening illnesses were established. The evaluation of these projects was very positive, and a report on them was published by the Department of Health (National Health Services Executive 1998). The report noted that demand for palliative care is unpredictable and therefore service provision needs to be flexible. The ACT and RCPCH report (1997) produced comprehensive recommendations for future provision of care for children with life-limiting and life-threatening conditions. One of the main recommendations was that 'community children's nursing teams are essential for the management of children with palliative care needs' and that commissioners should facilitate their establishment or development to address the needs of this group of children. In addition, this report recognised that children and families who need palliative care require access to 24-hour nursing support. The Diana, Princess of Wales community children's nursing teams aim to meet the needs of this distinct group of children (English National Board & Department of Health 1999).

This chapter has explored some of the key issues in children's palliative care and the associated role of the CCN. The recommendations of the ACT and RCPCH report (1997) provide comprehensive guidance to enable the CCN to ensure that families receive appropriate care and support.

FURTHER READING

Association for Children with Life-threatening or Terminal Conditions and their Families & Royal College of Paediatrics and Child Health 1997 A guide to the development of children's palliative care services. Association for Children with Life-threatening or Terminal Conditions and their Families, Bristol.

This guide provides an overview of the measures that can help families to meet the emotional, therapeutic, spiritual and psychological needs of children who are always in the shadow of pain, physical deterioration and premature death.

Goldman A (ed) 1998 Care of the dying child, 2nd edn. Oxford University Press, Oxford

The second edition, written by the consultant in paediatric palliative care at the Hos-

pital for Sick Children, London, identifies the medical, social, psychological and practical issues of caring for children dying from life-limiting illness and their families.

World Health Organization 1998 Cancer pain relief and palliative care in children. World Health Organization, Geneva:

A pocket-sized book that provides information on best practice in holistic and comprehensive relief of pain within the practice of palliative care. It also addresses issues such as education of health workers, public awareness of the special problems for children who require palliative care, and the regulations concerning the distribution and prescribing of opioid analgesics.

REFERENCES

Association for Children with Life-threatening or Terminal Conditions and their Families & Royal College of Paediatrics and Child Health 1997 A guide to the development of children's palliative care services. Association for Children with Life-threatening or Terminal Conditions and their Families, Bristol.

Department of Health 1998 Diana, Princess of Wales Memorial Committee. Preliminary advice. The Stationery Office, London

Dominica F 1990 Hospices: a philosophy of care. In: Baum J, Dominica F & Woodward R (eds) Listen my child has a lot of living to do. Oxford University Press, Oxford, p 3

English National Board for Nursing, Midwifery and Health Visiting & Department of Health 1999 Sharing the care. Resource pack to support Diana, Princess of Wales community children's nursing teams. English National Board, London

Farrell M & Sutherland P 1998 Providing paediatric palliative care: collaboration in practice. British Journal of Nursing 7(12):712–716

Goldman A 1998 Palliative care for children. In: Fauld C, Carter Y & Woof R (eds) Handbook of palliative care. Blackwell Science, London

Hall S 1996 An exploration of parental perception of the nature and level of support needed to care for their child with special needs. Journal of Advanced Nursing 24:512–521

Health Committee 1997 House of Commons Select Committee. Health services for children and young people in the community: home and school. Third report. The Stationery Office, London

Liben S 1998 Home care for children with life threatening illness. Journal of Palliative Care 14(3):33–38

National Health Service Executive 1998 Evaluation of the pilot project programme for children with life threatening illness. The Stationery Office, London

Read S 1998 The palliative care of people with learning disabilities. International Journal of Palliative Nursing 4(5):246–251

Stein A & Woolley H 1990 An evaluation of hospice care for children. In: Baum J, Dominica F & Woodward R (eds) Listen my child has a lot of living to do. Oxford University Press, Oxford, p 67

Sutherland R, Hearn J, Baum D & Elston S 1993 Definitions in paediatric palliative care. Health Trends 25(4):148–150

While A, Citrone C & Cornish J 1996 A study of the needs and provision for families caring for children with life-limiting incurable disorders. King's College, London

24 Meeting the mental health needs of children and young people

Kath Williamson

KEY ISSUES

- The provision of child and adolescent mental health services for children and young people
- The role of a specialist children's nurse in meeting the mental health needs of children and young people in practice
- The use of a family systems approach

INTRODUCTION

This chapter examines the role of the specialist children's nurse in mental health (CNMH) liaison and consultation. Issues related to meeting the mental health needs of children and young people in both acute and community services are considered. The chapter focuses specifically on the role of the specialist children's nurse in working directly with children, young people and families. It also considers the facilitation of communication across the interface of services such as:

- Hospital children's services
- Community children's nursing services
- Child and adolescent mental health services
- Social services
- Education services
- Voluntary agencies

The CNMH is based within a community children's nursing team in a hospital-based service. The role is considered within the context of a model for the provision of child and adolescent mental health services.

INCIDENCE OF MENTAL HEALTH PROBLEMS AND DISORDERS

Kurtz (1992 p 6) defines mental health problems in children and young people as:

> 'abnormalities of emotions, behaviour or social relationships sufficiently marked or prolonged to cause

- suffering or risk to optimal development in the child
- distress or disturbance in the family or community.'

There are difficulties in measuring the overall prevalence of mental health problems in the child population. Estimates vary between 5% and 40% (Wallace et al 1997). The prevalence of diagnosable mental health disorder in the child population has been estimated as up to 25%, with 7–10% having moderate to severe problems (NHS Health Advisory Service 1995). The House of Commons Health Committee (1997) concluded that there is compelling evidence to suggest some increase in mental health problems in children.

There is an increased rate of mental health and adjustment problems in children with chronic health problems. Children with a chronic medical condition and associated disability which limits usual childhood activities are at more than threefold risk of developing mental health disorders compared with their healthy peers (Wallace et al 1997). Furthermore, Taylor and Eminson (1994) assert that the research measures commonly employed to identify increased rates of disorder in children often fail to reveal generally increased levels of distress and dysfunction within these families.

A national review of services for the mental health of children and young people in England (Kurtz et al 1994) estimated that 5–15% of children were referred to paediatric departments primarily because of emotional and behavioural problems. Paediatricians estimated that 15% (median) had an underlying or additional emotional or behavioural disorder in addition to the main presenting condition. Some 70% of paediatric departments said they needed more support and training for staff in responding to these types of problem (Kurtz et al 1994). The remainder of this chapter will consider how a CNMH can contribute to meeting this need.

PROVISION OF CHILD AND ADOLESCENT MENTAL HEALTH SERVICES

Currently there are large discrepancies in the provision of mental health services for children and young people across the UK (Wallace et al 1997). A four-tier model of service provision for child and adolescent mental health services (CAMHS) has been endorsed by the NHS Health Advisory Service (1995) (Box 24.1).

BOX 24.1 ***Four-tier model for provision of child and adolescent mental health services***

Tier 1

Primary or direct contact services, including interventions by:

- GPs
- Voluntary workers
- School nurses
- Health visitors
- Teachers
- Social workers
- Juvenile justice workers

BOX 24.1 *Continued*

who are in a position to:

- Identify mental health problems early in their development
- Offer general advice, and in certain cases treatment for less severe mental health problems
- Pursue opportunities for the promotion of mental health and the prevention of mental health problems

Serving a population of about 250 000.

Tier 2

Interventions offered by individual specialist CAMHS professionals, including:

- Clinical child psychologists
- Educational psychologists
- Psychotherapists
- Child psychiatrists
- Community child psychiatric nurses
- Occupational therapists

offering:

- Training and consultation to other professionals (who might be within Tier 1)
- Consultation for professionals and families
- Assessment which may trigger treatment at a different tier

Serving a population of about 250 000.

Tier 3

Intervention offered by teams of staff from specialist CAMHS, including:

- Specialist assessment teams
- Psychotherapy supervision team
- Substance misuse teams
- Family therapy teams
- Day unit teams

A specialist service for the more severe, complex and persistent disorders, usually a multidisciplinary team or service working in a community child mental health clinic or child psychiatry outpatient service, offering:

- Assessment and treatment of child mental health disorders
- Assessment for referrals to Tier 4
- Contributions to the services, consultation and training at Tiers 1 and 2
- Participation in research and development projects

Serving a population of about 250 000.

Tier 4

Very specialised intervention and care, using highly specialised teams, including:

- Patient services for young people with very complex and/or refractory problems
- Inpatient child and adolescent mental health services
- Special units for sensorily impaired young people
- Specialised neuropsychiatric services

This tier comprises infrequently used but essential tertiary-level services such as day units, highly specialised outpatient teams, and inpatient units for older children and adolescents who are severely mentally ill or at suicidal risk. These services serve a population of about 750 000 and may need to be provided on a supra-district level.

The House of Commons Health Committee (1997), in its fourth report, endorsed this model. It also recommended that provision should be made at Tier 1 'for securing access to more specialised services for a group of children whose needs are currently neglected: children with a life threatening or chronic illness who also suffer from mental health problems' (para 105). Whilst the committee envisaged that a combined and integrated children's health service might address this issue, moves to implement this have been slow. A further recommendation was that the Government support and monitor local initiatives that attempt to bring children's health services closer together. Liaison posts, such as the one described in this chapter, have an important role to play in strengthening the interface between child health services and professionals at Tiers 1, 2 and 3. They can facilitate partnership and joint working, to meet the mental health needs of children being treated in both acute and community children's services.

Traditionally psychiatric liaison and consultation services in paediatrics have been provided by child psychiatrists and psychologists (Lask 1994). Reference to children in the literature on liaison mental health nursing is limited and often describes the provision of services by mental health nurses to paediatric units (Tunmore 1997a). However, children's nurses have developed expertise in this area and the roles of specialist nurses have been developed to meet local need.

ROLE OF THE SPECIALIST NURSE: CNMH

The community children's nursing service began to develop in the early 1980s. At that time it was apparent that some children with chronic medical conditions were spending time in hospital as a result of unresolved family dynamic or mental health problems in the child. It was considered that a children's nurse with training in child and adolescent psychiatric nursing, working with the liaison child psychiatrist, could address some of these issues in the hospital and community.

Within the context of the four-tier model described above, the role of the CNMH is located within Tier 2. The purposes of Tier 2 services have been described by the NHS Health Advisory Service (1995) (Box 24.2).

BOX 24.2 ***Purpose of Tier 2 services (NHS Health Advisory Service 1995 para 449 p 141)***

- To enable families to function in a less distressed manner
- To enable children and families to overcome their mental health problems
- To diagnose and treat disorders of mental health
- To increase the skill level of all those working with children, young people and families
- To enable children, young people and their families to benefit from their home, community and education
- To enable children, young people and their families to cope more effectively with their life experience

BOX 24.3 *Role of the children's nurse in mental health (CNMH)*

1. Provides consultation and support to professionals in Tier 1
2. Accepts referrals to assess and undertake direct work with children, young people and families, as part of a holistic approach
3. Maintains strong links with the child and adolescent mental health services. This is achieved through: (1) consultation and clinical supervision with a child and adolescent mental health team and (2) joint working
4. Liaises with other services involved in the family's care
5. Is involved in development work, research and training

The role of the CNMH can achieve the objectives of a Tier 2 service (Box 24.3).

Fundamental to the role of the CNMH is a systemic approach, which goes beyond seeing the child in the context of the family to viewing the family as the unit of care. Whyte (1997), drawing on the work of Wright & Leahey (1994), defines this approach as family nursing, acknowledging that within this approach there is potential for the nurse to intervene at a systems level or at individual and interpersonal levels. Consideration of the culture, environment and wider social systems within which the family is operating is an integral part of this approach.

The availability of the CNMH within the children's service facilitates the identification of concerns about children and adolescents at an early stage. This is important for intervention to make a difference (Eiser 1993). In addition, if following an assessment it is agreed that the problems could be better addressed at another tier, the CNMH can act as a bridge between services. Initial contact with and assessment by the nurse can overcome the reluctance of some families to seek help from the child and adolescent mental health services and enable them to go on to receive appropriate intervention.

CONSULTATION

The term consultation is used here to describe a form of collaborative work where one person helps another with a particular problem 'without taking on responsibility for the solution' (Tunmore 1997a p 207). The CNMH provides consultation for other professionals within the paediatric service. For example:

- A colleague in the community team might discuss their concerns about a young person with a chronic illness who is not adhering to treatment
- Members of the ward team may seek support in managing the difficult behaviour of a child or young person on the ward

Professionals who already know the family are often the most appropriate people to undertake the work with them. They can be enabled to do this by having the opportunity to reflect on the problem and explore different possible interventions. The CNMH is accessible to colleagues and can offer continuing support by being based in the paediatric service and attending ward and team meetings.

LINKS WITH THE CHILD AND ADOLESCENT MENTAL HEALTH SERVICE

There are formal channels for liaison with the child and adolescent mental health service, and these are essential to the framework of the role. They include individual consultation for the specialist nurse, group supervision and a monthly joint consultation meeting with professionals from the paediatric team and child and adolescent mental health service. Joint work is undertaken with workers from this service when their expertise is required, or when they believe they can benefit from the CNMH's experience of working with children with physical illness.

LIAISON

Effective liaison requires workers to develop good relationships and respect for one another's professional practice. Liaison with other workers in health, education, social services and voluntary agencies, within both the hospital and the community, is endorsed by current policy (Department of Health 1997, 1998). This multiagency approach facilitates a broader understanding and perspective to the child or young person's problem, and leads to care and treatment strategies being redesigned where and when appropriate (NHS Health Advisory Service 1995).

WORK WITH CHILDREN, YOUNG PEOPLE AND FAMILIES

Referrals to the CNMH are accepted from all members of the multiprofessional team. However, it is important that the referral is discussed and agreed within the team to ensure that the referral is appropriate and to prevent duplication of the work, which could have adverse effects on the family. Reasons for referral of children and young people are shown in Box 24.4.

The CNMH is not involved in the assessment of children and young people who deliberately self-harm as this service is provided by the child and adolescent mental health service.

ASSESSMENT, INTERVENTION AND EVALUATION

Following a referral for direct work, an assessment is arranged on the ward, in the outpatient department or at home, as appropriate. When possible the assessment will involve meeting all the members of the child's immediate family. A systemic approach is used which includes gathering information about the family structure, family history and family beliefs. These must be considered within the context of the family's culture. Drawing a genogram is useful as part of this process (Burnham 1986, Wright & Leahey 1994). Information about the

BOX 24.4 *Reasons for referral to the children's nurse in mental health.*

Emotional and behavioural problems in addition to a physical problem, for example:
- a preschool child who has asthma and a sleep problem
- a school-age child who has recently been diagnosed as having Type I diabetes and has become anxious about attending school
- a young person with a chronic illness who has become withdrawn following a deterioration in their condition

Emotional and behavioural problems as the primary reason for referral to the paediatric service, for example:
- a child with behavioural difficulties that might be diet related

Psychosomatic complaints, for example:
- recurrent abdominal pain when an organic cause has been excluded

Difficulties associated with adapting to and coping with chronic and life-threatening illness, treatments and procedures:
- includes bereavement work with carers and siblings

child's development, education, medical history, current treatment and interaction with systems providing health, education and social care is gathered. How the child and family perceive the problem and what issues they feel they need help with are very important, and these may differ from the opinions of the referrer. The nurse must be alert to child protection issues that may arise. The assessment may take more than one session and, with permission from the family, involve liaison with other professionals who are working with them.

The assessment process can be therapeutic in itself, enabling families to explore their perception of the difficulties and reflect on their experience. This can enable them to identify their own problems and mobilise their own coping resources (Whyte 1997). A care plan is then formulated with the family.

The role of the specialist nurse requires an eclectic approach and the ability to offer a variety of approaches according to the needs of the child and family (Sharman 1997). Interventions might involve working with the family together, or individually with a child or parent. A plan for a child who has difficulties with constipation and soiling might include a combination of behavioural and family work. In this work, self-awareness and the ability to recognise the limitations of one's practice role is essential. Clinical supervision is important in this process. In some cases it is more appropriate to refer to another service (e.g. child psychiatry team, psychologist or social services). This may lead to the nurse working jointly with another professional.

Evaluation is undertaken with the family and considers the impact of actions undertaken or changes within the family. It can provide an opportunity to emphasise further the family's strengths and highlight small changes that have taken place over a period of time. Key issues where further work is needed can be clarified or it may be decided that it is appropriate for the intervention to end (Whyte 1997).

It is important that professionals undertaking psychological work with children who have physical illness have some knowledge and understanding of that illness, its current treatment and the impact it can have on children, siblings, parents and other carers. This understanding is particularly helpful when initially engaging the family in the therapeutic process and when exploring the family and child's perception and understanding of the illness. Equally important is the ability to listen to children and find ways to communicate effectively with them. This requires creativity, imagination (Sharman 1997) and a range of techniques, which the worker must be able to adapt according to the needs of the child or young person. This is demonstrated in the following case study.

CASE STUDY

David is 8 years old and has cystic fibrosis which was diagnosed at 6 weeks of age. His brother, aged 10, does not have the condition. David's treatment includes physiotherapy and nebulisers twice a day, vitamin, enzyme and dietary supplements, and frequent courses of antibiotics. He was referred to the CNMH during an admission to hospital for his first course of intravenous antibiotics and to commence overnight nasogastric feeding.

Practitioners working within the cystic fibrosis team were concerned at David's reluctance to communicate with them. He was not cooperating fully with treatment. One doctor described him as 'clinically depressed'. Initially, the team discussed together how far David's behaviour was a reaction to the deterioration in his condition and his admission to hospital and what intervention, if any, was appropriate to help him adjust to his changed circumstances. Through discussion, it was decided that he did not meet the diagnostic criteria for clinical depression.

An initial assessment was carried out between the CNMH, David and his mother in hospital. Throughout this assessment David was willing to play table football but reluctant to talk about his illness. He simply expressed a strong desire to go home as soon as possible. His mother thought that David saw himself as 'no different to any one else' and he considered his admission to hospital to be an imposition which prevented him getting on with his life. Anger and resentment about his illness were perhaps part of the origins of David's difficult behaviour in hospital. His parents were not as anxious about his mental health as the hospital staff. They did not feel they experienced the same difficulties with treatment at home and reported that he was doing well at school and socialised with his peers. They addressed questions about cystic fibrosis as David raised them, but they had not talked about it recently. They agreed that it might be appropriate to address the issues raised by the deterioration in David's condition and the need for more treatment. A home visit was arranged to continue to build a relationship with David and to try to engage him in thinking about this.

Close liaison with the community children's nurse and physiotherapist was maintained by the CNMH throughout the course of home visits. Initially David would engage only in talking about football. It was therefore decided that this could be a useful metaphor for talking about cystic fibrosis and a way of externalising his illness. David was encouraged to create his own football team of all the players who were helping him to beat cystic fibrosis. He drew cartoon figures of the people he saw as being on his side. This included friends, family, teachers and health professionals. A football pitch poster was designed to stick the drawings on (Figure 24.1). David decided to call the team C.F.F.C. or Cystic Fibrosis Football Club. As he stuck the pictures to the pitch it provided an opportunity to explore with him how these individuals were helping him, and the different tactics he and the team could use. This yielded information about how David perceived his condition and understood his treatment. It revealed some gaps in his knowledge and understanding which were discussed with him and, with his permission, passed on to members of the cystic fibrosis team. Subsequently, David was encouraged to think about the opposing team, which he called the Illness Football Club or I.F.C. He chose a black marker, wrote directly on the pitch

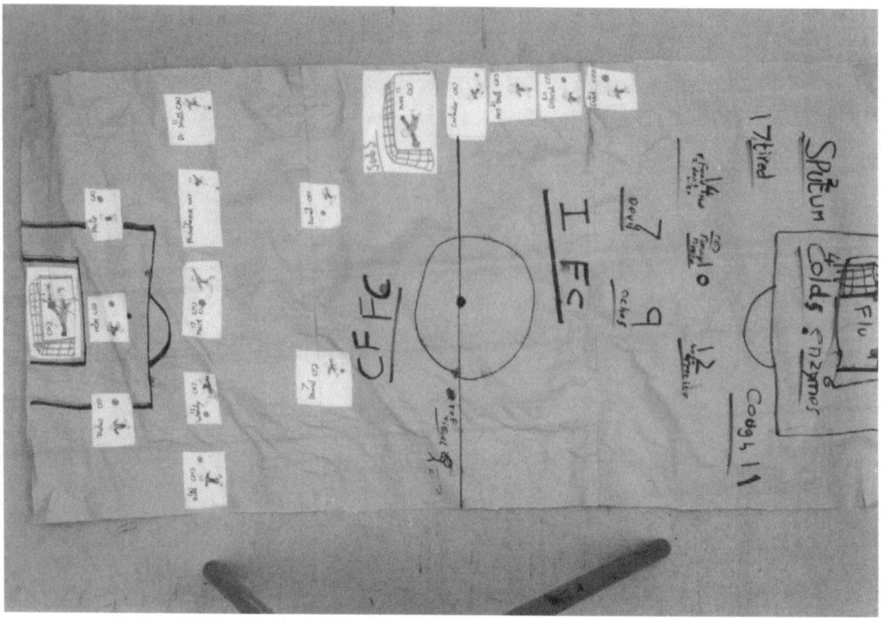

Figure 24.1 Cystic Fibrosis Football Club (C.F.F.C.) versus Illness Football Club (I.F.C.). Reproduced with permission.

and was able to express some of his anger. He felt this team was winning. He was encouraged to think about why he might feel like that and how the C.F.F.C. might get back into the lead. It was important to do this without David feeling that his negative feelings were unacceptable or had been dismissed.

A few weeks later David required a further admission to hospital. He took his football poster with him and put it up in his cubicle. The hospital staff reported that David appeared more relaxed and communicative, and was cooperating better with his treatment. On follow-up, he reported that the C.F.F.C. was winning 2–1 because his Dad was on his team and they were 'going to rip the legs off' the opposing team. It appeared that he had been able to channel some of his anger in a more positive way. David now appears to have adapted to the need for regular intravenous antibiotics and overnight nasogastric feeding, which are administered at home.

TRAINING FOR CHILDREN'S NURSES IN CHILD AND ADOLESCENT MENTAL HEALTH

The knowledge, skills and experience of children's nurses provide a firm foundation for further training in working with children and young people with mental health problems who have physical illness. Undertaking training in child and adolescent mental health and acquiring expertise in family work can lead to specialist practice and working in partnership with established child and adolescent mental health services. This would provide community children's nurses with an opportunity to expand their holistic approach to family-centred care. This has been shown to be effective and is supported by Whyte et al (1997 p 80), who suggest that 'a fuller understanding of family transitions and interaction, and the development of therapeutic skills in working with families, is a logical expansion of the role of paediatric nurses'.

CONCLUSIONS

CNMHs have a valuable role within the paediatric service working directly with children, young people and families, and offering consultation and support to colleagues in the multiprofessional, multiagency team. They can help to detect and address mental health difficulties at an early stage, prevent the development or consolidation of mental health problems, and facilitate appropriate referrals to other agencies, working with them to address mental health needs.

Tunmore (1997b) has suggested that nurses working at the traditional boundaries of different clinical services, or on clinical problems at the interface of mind and body, have the potential to identify new and evolving specialisms and shape the future delivery of nursing care.

FURTHER READING

Edwards E & Davis H 1997 Counselling children with chronic medical conditions. BPS Books, Leicester

An important book for all healthcare workers who come into contact with children. Includes detailed information about the practical skills necessary to promote supportive and facilitative communication.

Sharman W 1997 Children and adolescents with mental health problems. Baillière Tindall, London

An excellent introduction to the mental health difficulties experienced by children and young people, written from a nursing perspective.

Whyte D A 1997 Explorations in family nursing. Routledge, London

Examines a systemic approach to nursing care which can be applied widely in both hospital and community settings.

REFERENCES

Burnham J B 1986 Family therapy: first steps towards a systemic approach. Routledge, London

Department of Health 1997 The new NHS. Modern, dependable. The Stationery Office, London

Department of Health 1998 Partnership in action. A discussion document. The Stationery Office, London

Eiser C 1993 Growing up with a chronic disease: the impact on children and families. Jessica Kingsley, London

Health Committee 1997 House of Commons Select Committee. Child and adolescent mental health services. Fourth report. The Stationery Office, London

Kurtz Z 1992 With health in mind. Action for Sick Children. In association with South West Thames Regional Health Authority, London

Kurtz Z, Thornes R & Wolkind S for South West Thames Regional Health Authority 1994 Services for the mental health of children and young people in England: a national review. Report to the Department of Health. The Stationery Office, London

Lask B 1994 Paediatric liaison work. In: Rutter M, Taylor E & Hersov L (eds) Child and adolescent psychiatry: modern approaches, 3rd edn. Blackwell, Oxford, ch 58, p 996

NHS Health Advisory Service 1995 Together we stand: the commissioning role and management of child and adolescent mental health services. HMSO, London

Sharman W 1997 Children and adolescents with mental health problems. Baillière Tindall, London

Taylor D C & Eminson D M 1994 Psychological aspects of chronic physical sickness. In: Rutter M, Taylor E & Hersov L (eds) Child and adolescent psychiatry: modern approaches, 3rd edn. Blackwell, Oxford, ch 42, p 737

Tunmore R 1997a Liaison mental health nursing and mental health consultation. In: Thomas B, Hardy S & Cutting P (eds) Mental health nursing: principles and practice. Mosby, London, ch 15, p 207

Tunmore R 1997b Mental health liaison and consultation. Nursing Standard 11(50): 46–53

Wallace S A, Crown J M, Cox A D & Berger M 1997 Child and adolescent mental health: health care needs assessment. Radcliffe Medical Press, Oxford

Whyte D A 1997 Explorations in family nursing. Routledge, London

Whyte D A, Baggaley S E & Rutter C 1997 Chronic illness in childhood. In: Whyte D A (ed) Explorations in family nursing. Routledge, London, ch 4, p 54

Wright L M & Leahey M 1994 Nurses and families: a guide to family assessment and intervention, 2nd edn. F A Davis, Philadelphia

25 Meeting the nursing needs of children with learning disabilities

Kirsty Read

KEY ISSUES

- Children with profound learning disabilities and associated healthcare needs in the community
- Historical context
- The needs of the child and family, and the associated stressors
- Integration of services to meet the needs of these children and their families

INTRODUCTION

This chapter focuses on the issues surrounding care of children with profound learning disabilities and their associated healthcare needs in the community. After briefly setting the historical context, sources of stress for the prime caregivers will be considered. The final section considers the potential for the integration of services to meet these needs using a case study.

HISTORICAL CONTEXT

The disciplines concerned with nursing children have experienced dramatic changes during the past 50 years. A profound revolution has occurred in the field of learning disability nursing. Social conscience and an analysis of human values preceded, and indeed informed, the theory and implementation of normalisation in the 1960s (Hughson & Brown 1992). Implementing the concepts of normalisation in practice led to the de-institutionalisation movement and eventually to community care (Brown 1992, Department of Health and Social Security 1976, 1981). Political reform also initiated the term 'learning disability' as less socially stigmatising than 'mental handicap' (Ayer & Alaszewski 1984). These changes in ethos have led to increased numbers of children with learning difficulties being cared for by parents at home (Elfer & Gatiss 1990, Orr et al 1991).

Recent advances in medical knowledge, together with technological interventions, appear to have preceded detailed legal or ethical guidance as to the 'reasonable effort' involved in preserving life (Youngblut et al 1994).

Consequently, more children are surviving birth with increasingly complex needs and medical dependence (Fradd 1994, Teague et al 1993). The emphasis on home care appears to have coincided with this (Heaman 1995, While 1991).

THE NEEDS OF THE CHILD AND FAMILY

A major brain insult will affect not only a child's cognitive and psychological abilities but also their physiological functioning. Children with profound learning disabilities are increasingly entering the caseload of the community children's nurse (CCN) for specialist knowledge, skills and support to meet their healthcare needs. However, the assessment and provision of care is complicated due to the child's altered cognitive function or restricted communication abilities associated with their learning disability.

This situation is further complicated by the lack of integrated service provision for these children and their families, who clearly require the skills of both CCNs and learning disability nurses. These services are under-resourced nationally (Health Committee 1997). Families may be required to open their home to a number of professionals and, for mothers particularly, to conduct complex nursing care.

Within the current political arena of healthcare provision, resource rationing, clinical governance, dependency scoring systems and eligibility criteria are essential. However, such requirements should not overwhelm one of the core philosophies of community nursing, that of 'client centredness' (Barr 1995). In the context of community children's nursing, together with learning disability nursing, the 'client' is invariably the whole family. Having a child with learning disabilities within the family is associated with an increased risk of stress, irrespective of the degree or detail of the disability (Beresford 1994, Keeley et al 1995). To maintain these children in their own homes, the needs and stressors of the primary carers, who are the mothers in the majority of cases (Gallagher et al 1984), should be considered.

STRESSORS

For this purpose stressors are defined as 'stimuli which threaten survival or emotional needs' (Totman 1990). The quantity and quality of stressors exerted on an individual are believed to carry major influence on the person's subsequent stress experience (Gallagher et al 1981). The literature identifies a range of stressors, from which four themes arise:

1. Diagnosis
2. Developmental milestones
3. Daily burden of care
4. Future concerns

Diagnosis

Poor or inadequate diagnostic information is a recurring theme in the literature (Maxwell 1993, Waisbren 1980). This is associated with immediate distress and carries long-term implications such as affecting parental adjustment to the situation, childcare and attitude to subsequent service provision (Richards & Reed 1991). This may provide a number of challenges for the CCN including the need to:

- Recognise and sensitively defuse hostility or apathy towards healthcare professionals
- Present clear accessible information about the child's condition
- Consider realistic and available options for childcare
- Understand the family dynamics, for example:
  - Personality influences, the effect of an individual's attitude to disease and their normal interpretation of the meaning of illness
  - Social variables, the possible threat to family status, socioeconomic class and cultural pressures
  - Possible feelings of 'genetic guilt'

There are, however, a proportion of children who have no diagnosis and the family may need support with 'the unknown'.

Developmental milestones

The attainment of certain skills or the reaching of socially significant ages represent normal transition points for a child and require family adjustment. Severe delay or failure to meet such developmental achievements is reported to be a stressor to parents, who are again reminded of their child's difference (Cullen et al 1991, Keeley et al 1995).

Arguably, this is not a specific area of responsibility for the CCN, but within the realms of 'holism' there is a duty to work with other professionals to provide appropriate family support. The multiprofessional team may include the:

- Learning disability nurse
- General practitioner
- Social worker
- Health visitor
- Child development centre (or equivalent)

Daily burden of care

Research has recognised the stressors associated with increased time input and physical 'workload' when mothering a child with learning disabilities (Dyson 1993, Quine & Pahl 1991). Fatigue is commonly reported, as simple daily tasks take on an increased complexity and energy requirement (Taanila et al 1996). The number of additional and abnormal care-giving tasks appear to also be stressors, for example having to change the nappy of an adolescent (Beckman 1991). For children with complex nursing needs, the CCN may be required to coordinate support to the family and teach other staff to deliver this care within or outside the home.

Future concerns

Future concerns are consistently reported as a parental stressor, irrespective of the child's developmental stage or the parent's age. Where concerns relate to the child's survival and physical health, these were reiterated with regard to child welfare when parents were unavailable or unable to care (Dyson 1993, Heaman 1995). The latter is perhaps of more concern to social workers. The child's physical health and well-being is the primary concern of the nurse. However, it could be suggested that in comprehensively meeting the child's nursing needs the experienced CCN would address and support the parents in their concerns, and subsequently empower them to identify appropriate strategies for meeting their child's needs.

WHO IS THE 'APPROPRIATE NURSE'?

Clearly this group of children, who have a host of divergent health, social and nursing needs, together with the associated stress faced by their parents, demand the knowledge, skills and expertise of a range of professionals. It is imperative to consider who is best equipped to meet their nursing needs.

Political recommendations and social influence have provided clear guidance that all children benefit from being cared for in their own home (Health Committee 1997). However, no regulation is imposed as to who should meet their nursing needs. The Allitt Enquiry (Department of Health 1994) provided an opportunity to address this, but avoided it by simply recommending an 'appropriately qualified nurse'.

These children have obvious physiological needs, to be addressed by the CCN, and cognitive or behavioural aspects, to be considered by the learning disability nurse. For example, in the assessment of pain the expression of a physiological experience may be severely frustrated by a learning disabled child's immense restrictions on communication – no speech or signing, inability to use a physical communication aid or to point to the affected area. In addition, there may be an altered behavioural response, such as aggression or withdrawal rather than crying. These issues provide evidence of each nursing group's complementary, but not comprehensive, ability to meet all the needs of the child with profound learning disability and associated medical dependency. Either their skill-mix has to merge to become comprehensive in one dually qualified nurse, or the two teams of nurses must provide integrated nursing care.

Although input via one nurse may be preferable to avoid an invasion of professionals into the family home, it does seem unreasonable to expect to staff a community children's nursing team with multiqualified nurses. Perhaps the pragmatic response would be an integrated children's trust, where the CCNs and learning disability nurses could work closely with natural links and fewer funding issues. These concepts may be appreciated more practically by considering a case study.

CASE STUDY

Paul's story

Paul had suffered postnatal hyperbilirubinaemia and associated jaundice, due to ABO incompatibility and kernicterus. He had profound learning difficulties and developmental delay. He also had multiple associated problems, including:

- Visual impairment with an alternating convergent squint
- Spastic quadriparesis and epilepsy, episodes of severe spasms and seizure activity with increased muscle tone
- Inability to mobilise independently or weight-bear
- Breathing difficulties requiring a tracheostomy, oxygen and suction
- Several episodes of pneumonia with a tendency to recurrent chest infections
- Apnoeic attacks
- Feeding difficulties
- Intermittent diarrhoea and vomiting
- Gastrostomy for administering medications
- Jejunostomy used for nutrition
- Allergy to Sunset Yellow colouring (e.g. Calpol 6+)

Despite his complex health needs, Paul was aware of his surroundings, could eye-point, use facial expressions and had normal hearing. His parents had strong feelings against resuscitation. The following synopsis demonstrates how a collaborative and integrated package of care was identified and developed.

Paul received home-based respite care from the community children's respite team and residential respite from the learning disability nurses. The respite care provision between the two services, located in different Trusts, was coordinated by phone and was extremely time consuming. Fortuitously, Paul's named learning disability nurse undertook a post-registration children's nursing course which included a placement with the community respite care team.

Following a home visit to Paul, during which a full assessment was completed, discussion between the two nurses revealed fundamental differences in each other's nursing approach. From a learning disability perspective, allowing Paul to experience normal childhood activities through play and social interaction is essential. However, the importance of a thorough systems assessment to meet his physical needs had not previously been realised. Conversely, the community respite nurse began to see the need to integrate play with Paul's complex nursing care. She was able to explore the meaning of respite care for a medically dependent learning disabled child compared with that of a chronically sick child.

Over a period of months Paul's health deteriorated. The frequency of apnoeic attacks increased and Paul suffered unconscious episodes related to increased brainstem damage. He also experienced repeated chest infections. These increased care needs demanded further collaborative work between both nursing teams.

At this time, Paul's mother had a car accident and seriously damaged her neck, leaving her unable to carry out practical care. Compounding this was the fact that Paul's father, the only other non-childcarer in the home, worked six nights per week. Therefore on six days per week nursing support was needed to bath and dress Paul, attend to his stoma site dressings and conduct chest physiotherapy. In addition everyone recognised that Paul's lifespan appeared to be severely limited and wished to promote optimum quality of life.

These complex circumstances taxed even the combined resources of the teams. Paul not only required intensive home care but his family needed time to rest. Effective planning, coordination and liaison were of paramount importance, as was the recognition of the others' skills and limitations. It required careful negotiation with managers, as the demands of other clients using the two services had to be considered and balanced. This situation continued for 6 months until Paul died in his sleep. Both teams supported the family throughout this time.

Paul's total needs had been met and his family supported through the good will and professional commitment to the family above each organisation's idiosyncratic approaches. The effective communication and liaison between the two teams overcame the inherent funding issues. However, had these services been situated within an integrated and combined Trust, this nursing experience could have been much easier and smoother for both the nurses and the family.

CONCLUSION

The child in the community with a profound learning disability has multiple needs. Research suggests that the medical aspect of this picture is increasing with the advance of technology (Teague et al 1993). Therefore, the CCN has an essential role to play as a member of a multiprofessional team. Perhaps this is a team of players who now need to wear the same strip, have the same sponsor and who need a player-manager.

In conclusion, it should be argued that this cohort of children represents a special challenge to nursing. It is not the breadth of the knowledge base nor the proficiency of skill-mix that counts, but the commitment to perceiving each child as a whole individual and interacting with them and their families with integrity. This involves not only the communication of humility, honesty, sensitivity and respect, but the recognition of professional limitations and the seeking of answers through communicating with other experts who may be a resource or become directly involved with the family.

FURTHER READING

Read K 1997 Sources of parenting stress in mothers of children with learning disabilities. A literature review. Dissertation, School of Health Care Studies, Oxford Brookes University, Oxford

Although unpublished this provides a comprehensive review of the stress experience for mothers of children with learning disabilities briefly touched upon within the chapter. It applies a family stress model and identifies useful implications for nursing practice development.

Sines D 1995 Community learning disability nursing In: Sines D (ed) Community health care nursing. Blackwell Science, Oxford, ch 14, pp 288–309

This contemporary text focuses clearly on the philosophies of learning disability nursing transcribed to community care. However, it is not child focused so is best read alongside other chapters in the text, especially Chapter 11 'Competence for community health care nursing' (children) by Anna Sidey.

Thompson T & Mathias P (eds) 1992 Standards and mental handicap: keys to competence. Baillière Tindall, London

This is a broad, easily readable, text which provides a good introduction to the issues surrounding the care of people with learning disabilities.

REFERENCES

Ayer S & Alaszewski A 1984 Community care and the mentally handicapped. Croom Helm, Beckenham, UK

Barr O 1995 Normalisation: what it means in practice. British Journal of Nursing 4(2):90–94

Beckman P J 1991 Comparison of mother's and father's perceptions of the effect of young children with and without disabilities. American Journal on Mental Retardation 95(5):585–595

Beresford B A 1994 Resources and strategies: how parents cope with the care of a disabled child. Journal of Child Psychology and Psychiatry 35(1):171–209

Brown J 1992 The residential setting in mental handicap: An overview of selected policy initiatives 1971–1989. In: Thompson T & Mathias P (eds) Standards and mental handicap: keys to competence. Baillière Tindall, London

Cullen J C, Macleod J A, Williams P D & Williams A R 1991 Coping, satisfaction, and the life cycle in families with mentally retarded persons. Issues in Comprehensive Pediatric Nursing 14:193–207

Department of Health 1994 The Allitt Enquiry. HMSO, London

Department of Health and Social Security 1976 The Court Report. Fit for the future: the report of the committee in child health services. HMSO, London

Department of Health and Social Security 1981 Care in the community: a consultative document on moving resources for care. HMSO, London

Dyson L L 1993 Response to the presence of a child with disabilities: parental stress and family functioning over time. American Journal on Mental Retardation 98(2):207–218

Elfer P & Gatiss S 1990 Charting child health services. National Children's Bureau, London

Fradd E 1994 Whose responsibility? Nursing Times 90(6):34–36

Gallagher J J, Beckman P & Cross A 1981 Families of handicapped children: sources of stress and its amelioration. Exceptional Children 50:10–19

Gallagher J J, Scharfman W & Bristol M 1984 The division of responsibilities in families with pre-school handicapped and non-handicapped children. Journal of the Division for Early Childhood 2:3–10

Health Committee 1997 House of Commons Health Select Committee. Health services for children and young people in the community: home and school. Third report. The Stationery Office, London

Heaman D J 1995 Perceived stressors and coping strategies of parents who have children with developmental disabilities. Journal of Pediatric Nursing 10(5):311–319

Hughson E A & Brown R I 1992 Learning difficulties in the context of social change: a challenge for professional action. In: Thompson T & Mathias P (eds) Standards and mental handicap: keys to competence. Baillière Tindall, London

Keeley D, Dennis J & Hart C 1995 The parents of a severely dependent child. The Practitioner 239:505–512

Maxwell V 1993 Look through the parent's eyes: helping parents of children with a learning disability. Professional Nurse December: 200–202

Orr R R, Cameron S J & Day D M 1991 Coping with stress in families with children who have mental retardation: an evaluation of the double ABCX model. American Journal on Mental Retardation 95(4):444–450

Quine L & Pahl J 1991 Stress and coping in mothers caring for a child with severe learning difficulties. Journal of Community and Applied Psychology 1: 57–70

Richards C & Reed J 1991 Your baby has Down's syndrome. Nursing Times 87(46):60–61

Taanila A, Kokkonen J & Jarvelin M 1996 The long-term effects of children's early-onset disability on marital relationships. Developmental Medicine and Clinical Neurology 38:567–577

Teague B R, Fleming J W, Castle A, Kiernen B A, Lobo M L & Riggs S 1993 'High tech' home care for children with chronic health conditions. Journal of Pediatric Nursing 8:226–232

Totman R 1990 Mind stress and health. Souvenir Press, London

Waisbren S E 1980 Parents' reactions after the birth of a developmentally disabled child. American Journal of Mental Deficiency 84:345–351

While A 1991 An evaluation of a paediatric home care scheme. Journal of Advanced Nursing 16:1413–1421

Youngblut J M, Brennan P F & Swegart L A 1994 Families with medically fragile children: a study. Pediatric Nursing 20:463–468

26 Young carers

June Hutt

KEY ISSUES

- Defining the term and role of young carers
- Assessing young carers' needs
- Valuing the uniqueness of family membership and roles alongside children's rights
- Multiagency care planning

INTRODUCTION

The vulnerability and support needs of carers has been recognised by the Government in its 'National strategy for carers' (Department of Health 1999). This report complements the focus on multiagency working and collaborative approaches to community care as outlined in the White Paper 'Modernising health and social services' (Department of Health 1998).

Children with complex healthcare needs are increasingly being cared for at home, yet with inadequate community children's nursing and respite care provision. The current philosophy of family-centred care aims to involve all family members in the care of the sick or disabled child. Whilst it is assumed that adult members of the family provide the care, it could be argued that siblings are being prepared to become carers, with either primary or secondary responsibilities. According to Dearden and Becker (1998) approximately 3–6% of the child population (0–18 years) in the UK are carers.

The realisation that children and young people act as carers is relatively new to those involved in social policy formation and seems to have surfaced in explicit thought in the 1990s. This realisation was informed by the collaborative research undertaken in the 1980s by local authority social services departments in conjunction with the education department and the Carers National Association (O'Neill 1988, Page 1988). Further work, funded by the Department of Health, built on the previous research and recognised the complexity of the issues faced by such children (Meredith 1990, 1991, 1992). These studies were mainly descriptive and quantitative, whilst later work attempted to expose the life experiences of young carers through qualitative studies by profiling those who care and those who are cared for (Aldridge & Becker 1993, 1994, Becker et al 1995).

DEFINING THE CARERS

The children and young people recognised by Dearden and Becker (1995) as carers have a wide range of experiences, as identified in Box 26.1.

BOX 26.1 ***Some facts about young carers***

- Children aged 2–18 years act as young carers with an average age of 12 years
- 60% of young carers are from a lone parent family
- 60% of young carers care for their mother
- 17% of young carers care for a sibling
- 60% of illnesses and conditions that generate the need for care relate to physical health
- 29% of illnesses and conditions relate to mental health issues
- One in three young carers of compulsory school age experience educational difficulties
- 61% are girls
- One in ten young carers care for more than one person
- 60% are involved in general care such as assisting with mobility and giving medication

Given the range of experiences outlined in Box 26.1, it is not surprising that there are inconsistencies in the definition of the term 'young carer'. Some commentators restrict this within an age limit, for example 'Any child or young person under 18 years whose life is restricted by the emotional or physical dependence or care of another family member/s' (Advisory Group on Young Carers 1999). Similarly, according to the Carers National Association (1995), young carers may be defined as 'Children and young people under the age of eighteen years whose lives are in some way restricted because of the need to take responsibility for the care of a person who is ill, has a disability, is experiencing mental distress or is affected by substance misuse or HIV/AIDS'. Conversely, the Department of Health (1995) offers the following: 'A child or young person who is carrying out significant caring tasks on a regular basis and assuming a level of responsibility for another person which would usually be taken by an adult'. This definition, which removes an age limit, allows for the inclusion of the young person whose transition into a higher education or training experience is contained and/or limited by the caring activities, which may affect the attainment of adulthood opportunities and potential.

There is a need for an agreed definition in order to ensure consistency and commonality. This may then provide opportunities for the access of equitable and appropriate services. A definition that is inclusive and non-restrictive, recognising the actual and potential extent and nature of caring, is needed to clarify and permeate boundaries between adult, child and carer legislation. This should ensure the achievement of integrated family assessments. A recent study found that only 11% of young carers received any form of assessment (Dearden & Becker 1998).

CASE STUDY

Lisa's story

When Lisa was 13 years old her mother was discovered to have a malignant condition. This diagnosis was made when she had her fifth child. Consequently, Lisa became 'mum' for her four younger siblings. Her mother developed cerebral metastasis and had seizures. Lisa assumed her mother had epilepsy and the professionals assumed that she knew about her mother's condition. As a result she did not realise that her mother was dying until a few weeks before her death. She cared for her mother and the children as there was no other adult family member. As an adult, Lisa felt angry by the lack of information given to her and her siblings about her mother's illness: 'I was expected to take on the role of the carer but had no rights, only responsibilities'. Even though she was just 13, Lisa needed to know the facts and to be told the truth. Her sister, 2 years younger, said: 'I pretended there was nothing wrong, so I could be like my friends. Looking back I wish that I had told my teachers. The school must have wondered why I kept having days off but no one asked'. Although Lisa felt very alone and that life was chaotic in her attempts to remember to do everything and also to study, she would never regret looking after her mother. Somehow she and her siblings have remained together.

Lisa's needs were for:

- Assessment
- Recognition of the service she gave
- Information relevant to her cognitive level and situation
- Support
- Assumptions to be eliminated

Thomas's story

As the elder child and only son Thomas, aged 11 years, feels very protective of his three sisters, especially Emma aged 7 with autism. She has social and behavioural difficulties and often becomes noisy and destructive. Emma requires constant supervision. Sophie, aged 10, and Sally, aged 9, are great friends and help to look after each other as both parents are fully occupied, either caring for Emma or working. On return from school Thomas helps with household chores, goes to the shops and watches over Emma to give his mother a break. His mother is receiving treatment for depression and his father treatment for hypertension. Thomas loves his sister Emma. He feels guilty when her behaviour is beyond his control and she has to return to the protective environment of her specially adapted, padded playroom. He rarely invites schoolfriends home. On occasion, Thomas feeds Emma, changes her incontinence pads and administers her medicines. He does not really understand what autism is and wonders about her future.

Thomas's needs are for:

- Assessment
- Peer support
- Information relevant to his cognitive level
- Freedom to be a child and brother to Emma
- Counselling support

Both Lisa's and Thomas's childhoods have contained many responsibilities usually undertaken by adults. Concepts of childhood have varied throughout times and throughout the world (Aries 1973, Wozniak 1993). Childhood is now acknowledged as a period of development in its own right, and experiences within this time period contribute to the development of the adult (While 1991). The pathway from birth to adulthood reflects a complex interaction of 'nature and nurture' factors within a cultural and historical period (Wozniak 1993).

ASPECTS OF ASSESSMENT

The children's nurse will have explored the theory and practice of promoting optimum growth and development for his or her client population throughout their education. Registered nurses are required to act within the United Kingdom Central Council (UKCC) Code of Professional Conduct (UKCC 1992), namely to 'Act always in a manner as to promote and safeguard the interests and well being of patients and clients'. As a children's nurse, this professional conduct is practised alongside the concept of family-centred care, a 'knotty phrase' under much deliberation (Darbyshire 1992). Campbell and Glasper (1995) identify a number of components of family-centred care:

- Acceptance of the family's own definition of what constitutes family
- Recognition of the family's strength
- Respect for their uniqueness and approaches to coping

These factors may challenge the beliefs and values of the individual nurse, especially where siblings play a primary role in the care-giving process.

CHILDREN

Children are autonomous members of our society, as acknowledged by the Children Act (Department of Health 1989) and the United Nations declaration of children's rights (United Nations General Assembly 1959). They have the right to be respected, express their own wishes and be able to maximise their health and developmental potential. Tucker and Taturn (1999) identify a lack of a culture in the UK which listens to children who, as a consequence, have difficulty in making their needs known.

Defining health from a child-centred perspective is challenging. Edlin and Golanty (1992) describe holistic health as having three components:

1. Being as free from disease and pain as is possible
2. To be able to be active and do what one wants to do
3. To be in good spirits most of the time

Brykczynska (1989) goes on to argue that health is more to do with lifestyles and ways of being, and suggests that professionals involved in health promotion may also be using coercion and persuasion. In relation to children as carers, ethical issues begin to emerge which involve the concepts of free will, choice and advocacy. Do children and young people act as carers of their own free will, and are they given a choice as to whether they undertake such duties or not? Aldridge and Becker (1993) suggest that they have little choice in commencing the role and are in fact socialised into the caring act. They recognise that the care receivers, similarly, also have little choice.

The ethos of the Code of Professional Conduct (UKCC 1992) is to do no harm. Not only should we avoid doing harm but we should actively try to prevent harm continuing. The primary goal should be to try to prevent it occurring in the first place. Where siblings are acting as carers, embracing these concepts could cause confusion and conflict for the community children's nurse (CCN), who is required to act as advocate for the sick or disabled child. There is the need to balance the roles of family members alongside the freedom of childhood and the components of holistic health.

During the 1990s researchers, campaigners, local authorities, health and social services alike have all focused on ways to recognise and meet the conspicuously unmet needs of children who act as carers. The profile of such young people has been raised by many local and national initiatives. Multimedia approaches have heightened awareness of the emotional and physical impact of caring and the associated responsibilities placed on these young people. The implementation of the Carers Act 1995 demonstrates political recognition. As a result more than 100 'young carers' projects have mushroomed across the UK. These have been funded from a variety of sources including social services, charitable organisations, lottery awards and innovative local initiatives.

Through these projects, young carers and their families have been supported in a number of ways, including the provision of information, opportunities to network and other support mechanisms such as counselling and leisure activities. Collaborative projects with schools have also encouraged a multiagency approach to the issues that frequently occur for young carers. Bullying and teasing by peers, attrition or aggressive behaviour, and insensitive reaction by peers and adults to the consequences of the demanding role are frequently reported (Aldridge & Becker 1993). An example of such a project is in Surrey where caring and disability issues have been incorporated into the personal, social and health education (PSHE) curriculum (Arnot 1998). A resource pack has been developed which contains case studies, background information and ideas regarding support approaches. Lesson plans have been developed for use in the national curriculum, and the pack is available nationally.

THE WAY FORWARD

The needs of young carers can, and do, easily fall between organisational divisions and agency boundaries. They may be recognised as a priority only when a family crisis point is reached. It is essential, therefore, that a multiagency approach is used to assess the needs of young carers and to implement such projects as identified above. Communities need to establish a formal interagency network within which there is equal ownership. Strategies could then be developed which take into account local and national policies, existing resources and current service provision. Such a multiagency approach requires professional practitioners to have the expertise, enthusiasm and commitment to ensure that the needs and rights of young carers are constantly examined. Formal evaluation is essential for the effective management of these projects. The development of health action zones and health improvement programmes (see Box 26.2) may facilitate this process (Department of Health 1997).

CONCLUSION

To meet the needs of young carers effectively it is essential that assessment is performed at a number of levels:

BOX 26.2 ***A health roadshow***

In Oxfordshire a group of school nurses, in conjunction with educational services, have developed and implemented a health roadshow which incorporates the recognition and support needs of young carers. A scholarship award allowed for the development of visual and media tools to explore health issues of concern. This programme is taken to young people, aged 12–15 years, to provide a proactive approach in raising awareness. All children involved in the event complete a workbook which then becomes a personal resource book. A young carers' project worker uses this show as an opportunity to inform young carers, peers, teachers, classroom assistants and school nurses. This illustrates a health improvement programme in action.

- Micro – the individual
- Meso – the family
- Macro – the community

In this process, cultural, religious and social diversity must be acknowledged and respected alongside the development of multiagency and multiprofessional provision.

All professionals who recognise that a young person or child is acting as a carer need to ensure that the young carer and family are aware of and understand their rights to assessment within the Carers Act (Department of Health 1995) and the Children Act (Department of Health 1989).

FURTHER READING

Department of Health 1999 Caring about carers: a national strategy for carers. The Stationery Office, London

Chapter 8 summarises the situation for young carers and endorses the Government's belief in multiagency work.

Dearden C & Becker S 1998 Young carers in the UK. Carers National Association, London

This book discusses the incidence of assessment for both children and young people, and reflects upon the process and outcomes. It offers the current profile of children with care-giving responsibilities.

Tucker S & Taturn C 1999 On small shoulders. The Children's Society, London

This research was initiated by the Open University and the Children's Society. It examines some long-term effects of being a young carer, which include social exclusion alongside health problems such as backache, nutritional problems and depression.

REFERENCES

Advisory Group on Young Carers 1999 Report on young carers in Oxfordshire: Where are we? What is needed? A way Forward. Children's Strategy Group, Oxford

Aldridge J & Becker S 1993 Children who care – inside the world of young carers. Loughborough University, Leicester

Aries P 1973 Centuries of childhood. Penguin, Harmondsworth

Arnot J 1998 Information pack for teachers. Surrey Education Service, Kingston-on-Thames

Becker S, Aldridge J, Brittain D, Clasen J, Dietz B & Gould A (eds) 1995 Young carers in Europe: an exploratory cross-national study in Britain, France, Sweden and Germany. Loughborough University, Leicester

Brykczynska G 1989 Ethics in paediatric nursing. Chapman & Hall, London

Campbell S & Glasper E A 1995 Whaley and Wong's children's nursing. Mosby, London
Carers National Association 1995 Debate on definition of young carers. Carers National Association, London
Darbyshire P 1992 Parenting in public: a study of the experiences of parents who live-in with their hospitalised child and their relationships with paediatric nurses. PhD thesis, University of Edinburgh
Dearden C & Becker S 1995 Young carers: the facts. Reed Business Publishing, Sutton, Survey
Dearden C & Becker S 1998 Young carers in the UK: a profile. Carers National Association, London
Department of Health 1989 The Children Act. HMSO, London
Department of Health 1995 The Carers Act. HMSO, London
Department of Health 1997 The new NHS. Modern, dependable. The Stationery Office, London
Department of Health 1998 Modernising health and social services: national priorities guidance. The Stationery Office, London
Department of Health 1999 Caring about carers: a national strategy for carers. The Stationery Office, London
Edlin G & Golanty E 1992 Health and wellness, 4th edn. Cited in: Fatchett A 1995 Childhood to adolescence: caring for health. Baillière Tindall, London, p 195
Meredith H 1990 A new awareness. Community Care February: 9
Meredith H 1991 Young carers. Contact Summer: 4
Meredith H 1992 Supporting the young carer. Community Outlook May: 12
O'Neill A 1988 Young carers: the Tameside research. Tameside Metropolitan Borough Council, Tameside
Page R 1988 Report on the initial survey investigating the number of young carers in Sandwell secondary schools. Sandwell Metropolitan Borough Council, Sandwell
Tucker S & Taturn C 1999 On small shoulders. The Children's Society, London
UK Central Council for Nursing, Midwifery and Health Visiting 1992 Code of professional conduct for nurses, midwives and health visitors. UKCC, London
United Nations General Assembly 1959 Declaration of the rights of the child. UNICEF, Geneva
While A 1991 Caring for children: towards a partnership with families. Edward Arnold, London
Wozniak R 1993 Worlds of children. Harper, New York

27 Play therapy within community children's nursing

Helen Shipton

KEY ISSUES

- The developing role of the community play specialist integrated within a community children's nursing team
- Parameters of the role
- A consideration of the types of therapeutic play

INTRODUCTION

The benefits of play have been recognised within the Save the Children Fund report (1989) as a fundamental part of helping a child cope during an illness. The report recommends that on admission to hospital a child's emotional and psychological needs should be addressed through play. This aims to provide the child with a medium in which to deal with the often threatening and unfamiliar experience of hospitalisation. In support of these recommendations Peterson (1989) suggests that play can be used as an indirect factor in removing the formality of the medical experience.

Traditionally the role of the play specialist has been limited to the hospital setting. However, with the increasing number of children with complex health needs being cared for at home, a more focused and specialised play therapy role is required which extends beyond the acute setting.

This chapter examines the development and some components of the community play specialist (CPS) role, as developed at Stoke Mandeville Hospital.

DEVELOPMENT OF THE COMMUNITY PLAY SPECIALIST ROLE

The need for this role was highlighted through a specific case review. Having gained managerial support and agreement for the role, a pilot project was developed with the community children's nursing team. It was agreed that the focus of the project was to provide therapeutic play for individual children and their families in the safe environment of their own home. The role was to complement that of community children's nurses (CCNs) by working collaboratively with them and the multidisciplinary team. The aim was to encourage the

BOX 27.1 *Components of the community play specialist's role*

- Preparation for children and their families
- Developmental play
- Play therapy and chronic illness
- Play therapy in adolescence
- Distraction therapy
- Play therapy and phobias
- Play therapy in bereavement

BOX 27.2 *Parameters of the service*

- Acknowledgement of boundaries, including the length of each session and the anticipated number
- Confidentiality issues
- Identification of objectives and evaluation mechanisms
- Recognition of ending the relationship
- Future open access to the service if required

integration of the knowledge and skills of different disciplines in order to provide the most effective care for the child and their family within the community setting (Knott 1999). The main components of the CPS role were agreed and are illustrated in Box 27.1.

Throughout this pilot project, it was important to audit the service delivered in order to secure funding for its effective development. This was achieved, and the remainder of this chapter outlines some components of the role.

REFERRALS

As an integral member of the community children's nursing team, the CPS is accountable to the team leader, with whom criteria for referral to the CPS were developed which included children with life-threatening illness, neonates, siblings and adolescents.

Following referral, the CPS undertakes an initial assessment either before discharge from hospital or in the child's home. Where appropriate, this assessment involves the child in order to gain an understanding of their feelings about play support. Time taken with the family, to identify both actual and potential problems, enables individual and effective play programmes to be developed. These would highlight and focus on the needs of the siblings as well as those of the sick child. At this stage, issues in relation to the parameters of the service are discussed and mutually negotiated (Box 27.2).

After this initial assessment, joint visits with associated healthcare professionals are undertaken as appropriate. Mutual trust and respect within the healthcare team should facilitate awareness of one another's roles and responsibilities, and increase the quality of the service provided. This is reflected in the following case study.

CASE STUDY

Jane, a 3-year-old girl diagnosed with cystic fibrosis, objected to all aspects of her treatment. Following referral to the CPS, twice weekly home visits were agreed. Objectives were negotiated with the family which focused on teaching Jane and her younger sister about the condition and the treatment. Evaluation was to take place after 2 weeks.

Role play was implemented using an adapted doll who was given pretend medicines and physiotherapy. Alongside this, a simple and achievable star chart was used to encourage Jane to comply with her own treatment. These play therapy techniques enabled Jane to work through her feelings and comply with treatment.

This case study illustrates how therapeutic play activities can increase a child's sense of control over new situations which they perhaps do not understand and may perceive as threatening. Involving the family also helps them to become more informed and relaxed, which has a positive impact on all family members. In this case, a collaborative approach with the CCN and physiotherapist was essential. Through negotiation, their services were withdrawn whilst the intensive play programme was in operation. This overall strategy resulted in the child's increased confidence with other healthcare professionals. Her subsequent cooperation ensured that the treatment was delivered quickly and effectively.

PREPARATION

The safe and familiar environment of home provides ideal surroundings to implement play therapy in preparation for planned treatment and care. Taylor (1991) logically suggests that the presence of the parents is important during preparation as they know their child intimately. Over time the CPS is able to develop a relationship with the child and family, and therefore be aware of the most appropriate methods of preparation in each individual case. This is captured in the following case study.

CASE STUDY

Three-year-old Christie was due to receive a course of radiotherapy. A play programme was designed to prepare her for the experience, which involved Christie lying on a large sheet of paper on which her outline was drawn. The purpose of this was to explain the importance of lying still during the radiotherapy session. To emphasise this, a water spray was used to show that when she moved it was difficult to spray the correct part of her body. A family game, of sleeping lions, was also used to reinforce the concept. Christie's mother was taught a visualisation exercise which she audio-taped and used during the radiotherapy, allowing Christie to hear her mother's voice whilst focusing on a favourite image. Her mother became involved with the treatment and both acquired a sense of control.

Whitting (1993) comments that simply telling a child a story about their procedure is no indication that the child has understood what is involved, and this may result in misconceptions. As children are used to accepting information through their play, this kind of preparation, as described above, can only be a positive experience for all involved (Reid 1988). Enabling the child to play out the experience provides the professional with a window of vision into the child's thoughts.

BOX 27.3 *Distraction techniques*

Bubbles	Breathing techniques give the child a sense of control over a situation
Counting	Using number games to count up, down, backwards and forwards
Imagery	Using imagery to guide a child through a previously agreed subject
Music	Relaxation and music tapes may develop a sense of repose
Puppets and dolls	Allow a child and the carer to talk through a third person

DISTRACTION THERAPY

The importance of distraction therapy following preparation provides an effective combination of play therapy techniques to ensure a child's confidence in the nursing or medical experience remains intact. Distraction focuses the attention away from what is happening. The professional or parent can be actively involved in the distraction whilst the child remains passive; this can be important when a child is required to lie still. Conversely, the child may be actively involved in the distraction (Box 27.3).

DEVELOPMENTAL PLAY

Children with developmental delay are encouraged to reach their maximum potential through the provision of different types of play. Honeyman (1994) showed that careful planning and knowledge of a child's capabilities are essential to ensure that the type of play offered is not only challenging to the child, but also gives pleasure. The CPS aims to empower the parents to have fun with their child and treat the child as normally as possible. Close liaison with relevant professionals ensures that a unified outcome is achieved through collaboration. The following case study demonstrates the effectiveness of developmental play.

CASE STUDY

Fourteen-month-old Lottie was chronically ill with a progressive muscular disorder. She was referred because of difficulties in manipulating and playing with objects. Twice-monthly visits, with evaluation at 3 months, was agreed upon. A play programme was designed with the dietitian and physiotherapist. This included the introduction of messy play using food, such as jelly, pasta and yogurt, which helped Lottie to have a greater awareness of her hands whilst developing skills in feeding herself. Her parents were actively involved in promoting her development in this playful way.

SUPPORT FOR ADOLESCENTS

Adolescents with ill health may experience reduced self-confidence and self-esteem alongside developmental regression at an already turbulent time of life.

Respecting their needs and taking time to listen can provide opportunities for emotional space and personal growth. Referral to the CPS may give the adolescent permission to play games or be involved in activities that may normally be associated with a younger child. This provides opportunities for an undemanding escape. Alternatively, others may feel the need to be more creative through artwork or do constructive activities to enhance the medical experience for others.

PLAY THERAPY AND PHOBIAS

Children, for example those requiring growth hormone replacement therapy, often experience needle phobias. This may be associated with the fact that they are not physically ill and find it difficult to understand why they need treatment. A collaborative approach by the CCN and CPS can provide age-appropriate information alongside a play programme to help the child comprehend the nature of their disorder and necessary treatment. The use of real equipment for play purposes can help familiarise children with the planned treatment. Play can be in the form of syringe painting or involve injecting water into oranges.

CLINICAL SUPERVISION

Clinical supervision should be an integral part of professional practice under the clinical governance agenda (Royal College of Nursing 1998). The aim is to sustain and develop practice through a formal process with a chosen colleague. Jones (1988) states that supervision is designed to explore issues related to the effectiveness of professional practice. However, in order ultimately to ensure the delivery of safe and effective care, respect and trust must be gained by all involved.

The role described here may be viewed as an extension of the hospital play therapist's role which, at times, involves delicate and distressing situations on a long-term basis. At Stoke Mandeville Hospital, clinical supervision for the CPS took place monthly and was facilitated by a child psychotherapist. This provided the opportunity to reflect upon the therapeutic programme of care for each child.

CONCLUSION

An audit of this role revealed that all families were satisfied with the service. However, 30% requested more frequent support and, of those, 20% requested support through group work. This resulted in an increase in CPS hours and the development of a more extensive role.

The CPS is in a unique position to draw upon the knowledge and skills of the multiprofessional team in supporting children and families who require their specialist intervention. The availability of a CPS to focus on the play and development needs of children provides space within the under-resourced community children's nursing team, allowing the CCN to concentrate on other priorities.

FURTHER READING

Garvey C 1977 Play. Openbooks, London

This book gives a basic, but full, account of the differing types of play. With imagination, these kinds of play can be drawn upon and adapted to suit the needs of the sick child in the hospital environment.

Axline V 1964 Dibs in search of self. Penguin, London

Using play therapy during psychotherapy sessions, Dibs, who is a young boy, is able to work through difficult experiences in his life. This book shows the powerful communication aspect of play.

Save the Children Fund 1989 Hospital; a deprived environment for children. Save the Children Fund, London

This Government report looks at the history of play in hospital and provides recommendations for the role of the play specialist in ensuring that the emotional needs of the child are met at all times during their hospital experience. The report states that failure to provide play 'constitutes a neglect of the child's basic developmental needs, and also deprives the child of a medium through which they can successfully cope with the whole experience'.

Ward B et al 1993 Good grief 1 & 2. Jessica Kingsley, London

These comprehensive guides provide the reader with exercises and background reading to explore feelings of loss and death with children and adults. The books are broken up into two age ranges: under 11 years and over 11 years, enabling an age-appropriate holistic approach to be achieved. They are a good resource, with a variety of exercises and worksheets covering all areas of bereavement. Children's own work on their individual experiences is published, along with articles from professionals. Some of the suggested activities may be used more appropriately in group form, although with a little imagination they could all be adapted to individual support. There is a valuable section on good listening skills in the over 11s book.

REFERENCES

Honeyman L 1994 Play for children with special needs. Paediatric Nursing 6(3):18–19

Jones A 1988 Building professional relationships. Nursing Times Learning Curve 2(4):12–13

Knott M 1999 Integrated nursing teams: developments in general practice. Community Practitioner 72(2):23–24

Peterson G 1989 Let the children play. Nursing 3(41):22–25

Reid J 1988 Playing away the pain. Nursery World 7 April:10–11

Royal College of Nursing 1998 Guidance for nurses on clinical governance. RCN, London

Save the Children Fund 1989 The case for hospital playschemes. Save the Children Fund, London

Taylor D 1991 Prepare for the best. Nursing Times 87(31):64–66

Whitting M 1993 Play and surgical patients. Paediatric Nursing 5(6):11–13

SECTION

4 ADVANCING COMMUNITY CHILDREN'S NURSING

Community children's nursing is evolving at an astounding rate. The need to support and inform this evolution through creative thought and research-based evidence is essential. This final section provides stimulating accounts of the potential and very real opportunities that lie ahead. Each of the contributions offers a cutting-edge approach to the advancement of community children's nursing practice.

SECTION CONTENTS

28 Opportunities and challenges for community children's nurses

Pat Ludder-Jackson

KEY ISSUES

- The arena for changes in community children's nursing practice in the UK
- Advanced nursing practice in the United States: clinical nurse specialists, nurse practitioners, advanced practice nurses and pediatric nurse practitioners
- Comparing experiences in the United States with the current situation in the UK: the opportunities for community children's nursing

INTRODUCTION

Community children's nurses (CCNs) in the UK have an opportunity to be the nursing leaders in the movement towards advanced practice nursing and in the delivery of primary healthcare and preventive health services to children with special healthcare needs. The political leadership in the UK has identified the 'super-nurse' as a health professional who will be able to help the National Health Service (NHS) meet the healthcare needs of a population with chronic health conditions and with a growing awareness of the benefits of preventive healthcare services (Tindall 1998). Children's nurses can make great changes in child healthcare through advanced nursing practice. This can occur if the nursing leadership, including educators, administrators and clinicians, is able to seize the opportunities for change. These opportunities are provided by the current destabilisation of the healthcare system, the budget deficit, changing roles and education of both nurses and physicians, and the national recognition of the need for primary healthcare services exemplified by the recent proliferation of private health plans focused on preventive care.

These are exciting and challenging times for children's nursing and will require nursing leadership, in both the clinical and educational arenas, and the willingness to look at new ways of providing nursing care to children across institutional and community settings. The changes occurring in the NHS and the budget deficits for healthcare services can be viewed as great reductions in health benefits and services to children and families, which should be resisted at all costs. Alternatively, they could be seen as an opportunity to reflect on why service is delivered the way it is, what services are cost-effective and result in improved health, and how nursing care to children could be provided more effectively.

Unfortunately, the current system of nursing education and practice appears to limit children's nurses from working towards a holistic plan of care by compartmentalising nurses into narrow roles with competing budgets. The practice nurse, district nurse, school nurse, health visitor, hospital nurse, learning disabilities nurse and specialist nurse all provide healthcare services to children but with varying scopes of practice, skill levels and educational training. Is this the most cost-effective and efficient way to provide children's health services? If children's nurses were educated for a broad-based nursing role, with emphasis on children's health maintenance and preventive health services, health assessment and the care of children with acute and chronic conditions both in the community and hospital, would the healthcare needs of children and families be better served? Is providing care in the child's home a cost-effective nursing service? If there was only one budget for children's nursing services, which had to include all hospital and community-based services, what would be the most effective way to provide those services?

THE ADVANCED PRACTICE NURSE IN THE UNITED STATES

Briefly reviewing the evolution of the advanced practice nurse in the United States may provide some ideas for expansion of the role of children's nurses in the UK. In the US, roles in advanced practice children's nursing have existed for over 30 years and have dramatically altered the delivery of children's healthcare.

Clinical nurse specialists

There have always been 'specialist' nurses who acquired special skills and knowledge in a particular practice setting. However, the evolution of the current clinical nurse specialist (CNS) dates to the early 1960s when it was recognised that nurses with advanced levels of competence and clinical judgement were needed to keep abreast of the knowledge explosion both in technology and behavioural sciences (Stafford & Appleyard 1994). From the outset, CNSs were identified as nurses with graduate education at the master's or doctorate level with expertise in a specific area of practice. The American Nurses' Association (ANA 1996 p 3) currently describes the CNS as:

> 'an expert clinician and client advocate in a particular specialty or subspecialty of nursing. The clinical nurse specialist provides direct client care, including assessing, diagnosing, planning, and prescribing pharmacologic and non-pharmacologic treatment of health problems, health promotion and preventive care within a specialized area of practice. In addition to direct practice, the sub-roles of the clinical nurse specialist role include education, research, and consultation.'

CNSs work primarily in institutional settings, usually acute care hospitals, frequently acting as a nursing resource and expert for nursing staff, physicians and families. As more and more medical care is provided outside of the hospital, CNS positions are also moving into ambulatory care and home settings, providing services to children and families with chronic health conditions. CNSs frequently participate in research projects related to their area of specialisation and are involved in hospital administrative committees. The current number of children's CNSs practising in the US is unknown.

Pediatric nurse practitioners

During the mid 1960s, Loretta Ford and Dr Henry Silver were developing an educational training programme in Denver, Colorado, for baccalaureate nurses to expand their role in providing healthcare for children in areas where there was limited access to physician care and primary healthcare services (Silver et al 1967). This first nurse practitioner programme was developed to meet:

- Healthcare needs created by a shortage of doctors, especially in low-income and rural areas
- An increase in the demand for healthcare services because of the expansion of medical knowledge and resultant treatable conditions
- The growing awareness of the public of the benefits and availability of preventive healthcare services such as immunisations

In 1930, children averaged only two visits to a physician in their childhood. By 1967, the average child saw a physician five times during childhood, and today the American Academy of Children recommends that children be seen for preventive children's healthcare 28 times from birth to the age of 21 years (Committee on Practice and Ambulatory Medicine 1995, Stone 1995).

Unlike the CNS, the early nurse practitioner role was centred in the community, providing children's health screening, comprehensive well-child care, assessment and management of common acute conditions, and management of children with chronic conditions in collaboration with physician specialists. In 1998, there were approximately 10 000 nationally certified pediatric nurse practitioners (PNPs) in the United States, and 82 master's degree PNP educational programmes that met certification criteria (Hoekelman 1998).

The ANA (1996 p 4) currently defines the nurse practitioner as:

> 'a skilled health provider who utilizes critical judgment in the performance of comprehensive health assessments, differential diagnosis, and the prescribing of pharmacologic and non-pharmacologic treatments in the direct management of acute and chronic illness and disease. Nurse practitioners practice promotes wellness and prevents illness and injury. Nurse practitioners function in various settings for individuals, families, and communities. This includes working autonomously and in interdisciplinary teams as resources and consultants. The role of this provider may include conducting research, providing education, and impacting public policy.'

The similarities between the definition of a CNS and a nurse practitioner are striking. During the last decade, the classical roles of the children's CNS and PNP began to overlap as the healthcare system changed. The growing emphasis on preventive healthcare, shortened hospital stays for all surgical and medical conditions, and advances in medical technology used in the home has resulted in the employment of CNSs in tertiary care centres and their involvement in health promotion and disease prevention activities. Nurse practitioners working in the community must now be knowledgeable in the care of individuals with complex health conditions. This blurring of roles has resulted in much confusion regarding titling and educational requirements for recognition as a children's CNS or PNP (Jackson 1995) and a growing recognition that there is a common body of knowledge and skills required of nurses practising in advanced roles.

Advanced practice nurses

The ANA has tried to acknowledge these similarities in education and practice by recognising both the CNS and the PNP as examples of advanced practice nursing. The ANA now identifies clinical nurse specialists, nurse practitioners, nurse anesthetists, and nurse midwives as all advanced practice nurses. As advanced practice nurses they:

> 'manifest a high level of expertise in the assessment, diagnosis, and treatment of the complex responses of individuals, families, or communities to actual or potential health problems, prevention of illness and injury, maintenance of wellness, and provision of comfort. The advanced practice registered nurse has a master's or doctoral education concentrating in a specific area of education, and has ongoing clinical experiences.' (ANA 1996 p 2)

There are estimated to be approximately 100 000 advanced practice nurses across all specialities and age groups (Mundinger 1994).

In 1996 the ANA identified standards of advanced practice registered nursing. These standards are listed in Box 28.1. The breadth of expectations identified under standards of care and standards of professional performance reflect the ANA's professional stance that advanced practice nursing is:

BOX 28.1 ***Standards of advanced practice registered nursing (American Nurses' Association 1996 p 9)***

Standards of care

Assessment
Diagnosis
Outcome identification
Planning
Implementation
- Case management and coordination of care
- Consultation
- Health promotion, health maintenance, health education
- Prescriptive authority and treatments
- Referral

Evaluation

Standards of professional performance

Quality of care
- Self-evaluation

Education
Leadership
Ethics
Interdisciplinary process

- Not just the ability to perform a task *not* done by most nurses or previously under the domain of medicine
- Having a knowledge level in a special area of practice above and beyond that of most nurses
- Having graduate education in nursing

It is an integration of these factors into a nursing role that enables the nurse to provide a greater depth and breadth of nursing care. This is due to their ability to synthesise and analyse complex data, perform complex clinical tasks, and function as a professional leader. Their focus is on quality care that is evidence based and delivered to clients and families in an ethical and culturally sensitive manner that supports the partnership between nursing care provider and client/family – in other words, the 'super-nurse'. Competencies of advanced practice nursing are further delineated in the National Organization of Nurse Practitioner Faculties Curriculum Guidelines Task Force's report (Boodley et al 1995). Educational programme guidelines have recently been established by the American Association of Colleges of Nursing (1995) in its document on the essentials of master's education for advanced practice nursing.

Advanced practice nurses have been shown to provide quality care equivalent to physician care which is also more cost-effective and acceptable to clients and families (Brown & Grimes 1993, Stone 1995, US Congress Office of Technology Assessment 1986). Although the initial nurse practitioner programme was co-founded by a physician to help serve the healthcare needs of under-served children, physician support over the past 30 years has varied (Kassirer 1994, Mundinger 1994, Stone 1995). Of particular concern are the issues of physician supervision versus physician collaboration in the care of children, direct reimbursement for services and full prescriptive authority (Anderson et al 1996, Finocchio et al 1996, Kassirer 1994, Mundinger 1994). Additional regulatory constraints on expanded practice roles have limited the full utilisation of advanced practice nurses (Safriet 1992). The inconsistency in State regulations on the scope of practice for advanced practice nurses has further complicated this matter (Pearson 1998).

The need for child health services will continue to expand, in part due to the growth and recognition of the 'new morbidities' identified in children (Haggerty et al 1975), such as unintentional injuries, secondary complications of medical interventions, acquired immune deficiency syndrome, behavioural and learning problems, early initiation of sexual behaviour, reactions to divorce, physical or sexual abuse, community or domestic violence, and substance abuse including alcohol and tobacco (American Academy of Pediatrics Committee on Pediatric Workforce 1998). In addition, children with chronic health conditions are living longer, requiring not only speciality care services, but health maintenance and disease prevention services to enable them to reach their full productive potential (Jackson & Vessey 1995). To meet these needs for additional healthcare services, recommendations have been made to double the number of nurse practitioners by the year 2000 (Pew Health Professions Commission 1994).

HOW DOES THE US NURSING EXPERIENCE RELATE TO COMMUNITY NURSING OF CHILDREN IN THE UK?

Even though the healthcare systems in the US and the UK are fundamentally different, many of the same issues are present, and hopefully children's nurses in the UK can benefit from the successes and challenges already experienced by American children's nurses. First, both systems of healthcare are undergoing tremendous changes brought about by the need to reduce, or at least control, the cost of healthcare. Healthcare costs are growing more rapidly than any other sector of government expenditures and, with the ageing population and increased cost brought about by advanced technology, these costs will continue to rise. Whether we like it or not, evaluating healthcare services from a cost–benefit ratio must be done, and done by nurses.

Second, as healthcare technology continues to grow and science expands the knowledge base for healthcare, doctors' roles will change. They will be required to take on more complex condition management and procedures. Other health professionals will need to assume roles previously under medicine. In addition, junior doctors' hours are being cut or restricted in both countries. These changes open up the opportunity for nurses to expand practice. Every opportunity to learn new knowledge, new skills, new roles and responsibilities should be seen as an opportunity to expand nursing practice.

Third, there is a growing recognition among healthcare providers of the need for preventive healthcare services, and a greater demand from the public for these services so they can lead full productive lives. This increased demand for preventive healthcare cannot be met by the physicians alone, and the 'new morbidity' currently having the greatest impact on child health can be assessed and managed effectively by nurses with advanced education and training in these areas.

Fourth, the number of children with chronic conditions continues to grow as they live longer, healthier lives. They need specialised care during acute exacerbations of their condition, but during periods of stability need well-child care and preventive health services not found in speciality clinics. Advanced practice children's nurses, with knowledge and training in children's healthcare maintenance and preventive health services, working in speciality practices can integrate well-child care and thereby reduce the fragmentation of care given to these children and promote wellness (Jackson & Vessey 1995).

Nursing in the UK has a strong and proud sense of tradition, which can sometimes stand in the way of change and advancement in the profession. Nursing is not static, and never has been. It is a dynamic profession and, as such, will need continually to change. At the beginning of the century, nurses did not take vital signs. That was a physician's responsibility. Thirty years ago, nurses in America used a stethoscope only to take blood pressures. Now all hospital-based nurses use them to assess lung and bowel sounds on their patients, and advanced practice nurses use the stethoscope to evaluate cardiac function and diagnose illness. Advanced practice nurses in speciality areas are now performing many procedures, such as suturing, biopsying, bone marrow aspiration and lumbar punctures, and ordering and administering complex pharmacological treatments under nursing protocols as part of their nursing position. They are doing this as nurses because it allows them to provide more coordinated comprehensive services to children under their care.

Nurses in advanced practice roles must be clinically skilled in all procedures performed. But clinical expertise is not the hallmark of advanced practice (Jackson 1995). Nurses can learn to do technical procedures without ever assuming additional responsibility or autonomy for client care. True advanced practice assumes nursing leadership. Just because a nurse applies a cast, withdraws arterial blood from central lines or provides medication to a child using protocols does not make her or him an advanced practice nurse. Leadership in nursing is reflected in the nurse's ability to provide culturally sensitive care, comprehensive assessments, develop management plans, evaluate care, develop new roles, educate staff, families and clients, integrate research into practice, work independently and collaboratively, consult and be a consultant.

The United Kingdom Central Council has not established educational and training credentials for nurses calling themselves 'specialist nurses', 'nurse practitioners' or 'advanced practice nurses'. No clear role has been developed and accepted by the nursing leadership. Maybe it is time for the rank and file nurses in focused areas of practice, such as community children's nursing, to organise and determine what their speciality practice 'super-nurses' will be? What are the opportunities presenting now due to the restructuring of the healthcare system? How could CCNs provide more comprehensive services to children? Is there a need for additional children's preventive health services for all children and for children with special healthcare needs? How are the 'new morbidities' in children being addressed in the UK? What educational standards or criteria should be developed to assure consumer safety and professional integrity when a nurse is called an advanced practitioner? What partnerships can be forged with other nursing specialities and health professionals, so that comprehensive care can be assured to all children?

From the outside looking in, there would appear to be great opportunities for children's nurses to expand their role. Because of the high costs of hospital care and the advances in home-care technology, children are being discharged earlier from the hospital and require more complex healthcare in the community. This requires enhanced community nursing services with greater nursing ability to assess and manage problems in the outpatient arena. Community nurses are accustomed to working independently, even if plans need to be approved by a physician. Greater autonomy of practice could come with greater skills and education in comprehensive assessment, diagnosis and management of common conditions or associated conditions in speciality practice. Home visits are not a cost-effective use of nursing time and should be reserved for initial home assessments and for those children whose condition precludes them from attending a community clinic. But this does not mean the values of community health need to be compromised. Concerns regarding resource needs in the home, family adaptation to the condition, reintegration into school and education of the family can continue in a clinic setting where families come to 'see the nurse'.

Community nurses could also provide cost-effective comprehensive health maintenance and preventive healthcare services for children from birth through to adolescence. Some assessment services are now provided by the health visitor, but these are limited in scope, only for children from birth to age 5 years, and may be provided by a nurse with limited children's education or experience. General practitioners may also have limited training in paediatrics and see their role as diagnosing and managing illness, most often focused on the older population. The treatment of common illnesses in essentially healthy children, symptom management for children with stable chronic conditions, and triage and treatment of minor injuries in children are all services that nurses could provide above and beyond well-child care. Community health issues such as drug use by children (including smoking and alcohol), violence, both community and domestic, communicable diseases, and injury prevention could all be addressed by the community health nurse. Nursing's assumption of these roles could greatly expand and enhance the fragmented services currently offered, and free physicians for the diagnosis and management of individuals with more complex health needs. Community health clinics could be established to provide these services, with a physician as consultant for complex management and a second opinion in situations where the nurse considered this advisable.

CONCLUSIONS

CCNs have already established their role in providing nursing services to children with special healthcare needs and are recognised for their expertise in an identified speciality. With additional knowledge and skill development, they could provide even greater services to these families. In addition, they could identify the special well-care needs resulting from the chronic health condition. Hopefully, through good preventive care, re-hospitalisations would be reduced, complications from common childhood illnesses minimised, and the child's full potential realised.

Standards for education and training of advanced practice community nurses must be established to assure the professionalism of this expanded role and to assure the public of quality care. Children in the UK deserve no less than the children in America from their nurses. Degree and master's level programmes of nursing education are now well established in the UK. Nurses should set high standards for themselves. Some nurses have scoffed at the 'super-nurse' title, but this can also be seen as an opportunity to demand the educational and practice resources needed to develop nurses to this level. Changes in regulations regarding practice often follow actual success in practice, which has proved that nurses can perform certain functions safely and effectively. Promoting the 'super-nurse' can only bring all of nursing to a higher plane of professionalism. The time is ripe for the advancement of community children's nursing in the UK. Will community children's nurses provide the leadership?

FURTHER READING

Gibson F 1998 The development of advancing clinical practice roles within paediatric nursing. The Florence Nightingale Foundation, London

Faith Gibson provides a stimulating analysis of the emerging specialist and advanced practice roles in the UK in comparison with her experiences in America. The work derived from her Florence Nightingale award and offers an extremely comprehensive debate around this complex area.

REFERENCES

American Academy of Pediatrics Committee on Pediatric Workforce 1998 Pediatric workforce statement. Pediatrics 102(2):418–427

American Association of Colleges of Nursing 1995 Report from the task force on the essentials of master's education for advanced practice nursing. American Association of Colleges of Nursing, Washington, DC

American Nurses' Association 1996 Scope and standards of advanced practice registered nursing. American Nurses Publishing, Washington, DC

Anderson A L, Gilliss C L & Yoder L 1996 Practice environment for nurse practitioners in California: identifying barriers. Western Journal of Medicine 165:209–214

Boodley C A, Harper D C, Hanson C, Jackson P, Russell D D, Taylor D & Zimmer P A 1995 Advanced nursing practice: curriculum guidelines and program standards for nurse practitioner education. National Organization of Nurse Practitioner Faculties Curriculum Guidelines Task Force, Washington DC

Brown S A & Grimes D E 1993 Nurse practitioners and certified nurse-midwives: a meta analysis of studies on nurses in primary care roles. American Nurses' Association, Washington, DC

Committee on Practice and Ambulatory Medicine 1995 Recommendations for preventive pediatric health care. Pediatrics 96(2):373–375

Finocchio L J, Coffman J M, Dower C M & O'Neil E H 1996 Physician and nurse practitioners – old conflicts and new opportunities. Western Journal of Medicine 165:246–248

Haggerty R J, Roghmann K J & Pless I B 1975 Child health and the community. John Wiley, New York

Hoekelman R A 1998 Commentary on a program to increase health care for children. The pediatric nurse practitioner program. Pediatrics June supplement:245–247

Jackson P L 1995 Advanced practice nursing – Part 2: Opportunities and challenges for PNPs. Pediatric Nursing 21(1):43–46

Jackson P L & Vessey J A 1995 Primary care of the child with a chronic condition. Mosby Year-Book, St Louis

Kassirer J P 1994 What role for nurse practitioners in primary care? New England Journal of Medicine 330(3):204–205

Mundinger M O 1994 Sounding board: advanced practice nursing – good medicine for physicians? New England Journal of Medicine 330(3):211–213

Pearson L J 1998 Annual update of how each state stands on legislative issues affecting advanced nursing practice. Nurse Practitioner 23(1):14–66

Pew Health Professions Commission 1994 Nurse practitioners – doubling the graduates by the year 2000. UCSF Center for the Health Professions, San Francisco

Safriet B J 1992 Health care dollars and regulatory sense: the role of advanced practice nursing. Yale Journal of Regulation 9:417–488

Silver H K, Ford L C & Stearly S G 1967 A program to increase health care for children: the pediatric nurse practitioner program. Pediatrics 39:756–760

Stafford M & Appleyard J 1994 CNSs and NPs: who are they, what do they do, and what challenges do they face? In: McCloskey J C & Grace H K (eds) Current issues in nursing. Mosby, St Louis, p 19

Stone E L 1995 Nurse practitioners and physician assistants: do they have a role in your practice? Pediatrics 96(suppl):844–850

Tindall B 1998 One stop to the best patient care. Nursing Standard 12(52):2–30

US Congress Office of Technology Assessment 1986 Nurse practitioners, physician assistants and certified nurse-midwives: a policy analysis. US Government Printing Office, Washington, DC

29 Opportunities for the development of nurse-led clinics in community children's nursing

Julia Muir & Clare Burnett

KEY ISSUES

- The development of nurse-led initiatives in the UK
- Characteristics of nurse-led services
- Issues to consider in the creation of nurse-led services
- Maintaining the values of nursing in the development of nurse-led services
- Potential opportunities for community children's nursing practice

INTRODUCTION

The concept of nurse-led services originated from America with the advent of the nurse practitioner role in the early 1960s (Stillwell 1988). In the UK it is a relatively recent initiative. Whilst nurse-led services in primary care are more established (Fulton & Phillips 1998), the implementation within community children's nursing is quite a new phenomenon. This chapter outlines the underpinning influences in the development of nurse-led services in the UK and briefly analyses the fundamental issues that need to be considered in the creation of such services. The chapter concludes with a summary of the potential opportunities for community children's nursing practice.

DEVELOPMENT OF NURSE-LED SERVICES IN THE UK

The growth of nurse-led services in the UK is increasing. This growth has been informed by a number of influences, which may be summarised as political, professional and educational.

Political

The healthcare reforms of the early 1990s were perhaps of greatest influence in the rise of nurse-led clinics in primary care. Changes in the contracting process

(Department of Health 1989a), alongside the Health of the Nation targets (Department of Health 1992a), gave general practitioners the incentive to consider more effective and efficient means of providing services for their clients. Subsequent to this, the report on the reduction of junior doctors' hours (Calman 1993) provided the impetus for similar opportunities in ambulatory and acute care settings. The potential for nurse-led initiatives has been supported further by the present Government, which wishes to strengthen the contribution of nurses to healthcare delivery (Department of Health 1998). The culmination of these changes has been fundamental to the development of nurse-led services in the UK.

Professional

The United Kingdom Central Council (UKCC) (1992) embraced the political perspective with the publication of the 'Scope of professional practice'. The document describes autonomous practice as the expansion and enhancement of nursing roles according to locally identified needs, whilst recognising the limitations of one's own practice. In tandem, nurse prescribing and the administration of medication by nurses under group protocols (Department of Health 1989b, 1991, National Health Service Executive 1998) have gained momentum and provided a much-needed professional basis to develop nurse-led initiatives even further.

Educational

Concomitant to both professional and political influences, educational establishments have seized the opportunity to develop new programmes in preparation for, and response to, the numerous 'new roles' emerging (Gibson 1998). The drive towards an all-graduate nursing profession in the UK has provided the foundation for the upsurge in postgraduate educational programmes.

Whilst the above synopsis provides a logical rationale for the growth in nurse-led initiatives, a number of issues have been highlighted within the literature which require careful attention in the creation of such services.

THE CREATION OF NURSE-LED SERVICES

The lack of a standardised or uniform approach to nurse-led development is a recurrent theme in the literature (Campbell et al 1999, Garbett 1996, Gibson 1998). Garbett (1996) notes that there appear to be no consistent or exact criteria in existence to identify a service as being nurse-led. Consequently, a logical fear would be that this will dilute, rather than strengthen, the potential contribution of nursing. Before developing such a service it is necessary, therefore, to clarify what this means. Characteristics of nurse-led services are shown in Box 29.1.

BOX 29.1 *Characteristics of nurse-led services (Campbell et al 1999, Fulton & Phillips 1998, Garbett 1996, Guerrero 1994).*

- Responsibility of the nurse for the consultation process with the client
- Nursing autonomy in the planning, implementation and evaluation of care from referral to discharge
- Decision-making authority within the remit of the service

BOX 29.2 *Key issues in the development of new nursing roles*

1. Liability and accountability
2. Education and competence
3. Management and support
4. Motivation to provide a patient-centred service
5. Public and interprofessional confidence
6. Orientation to the caring values of nursing

The obvious autonomy and responsibility, necessary for the delivery of nurse-led care, gives rise to many other factors that require examination. Read (1995) has identified these as six key issues that need to be considered in the planning and development of new nursing roles. These will provide a framework for the ensuing debate (Box 29.2).

LIABILITY AND ACCOUNTABILITY

Liability and accountability are related to taking personal responsibility for one's professionalism and practice within the realms of the UKCC (1992) 'Scope of professional practice' and the law. As yet, however, the relationship between the two is unclear and requires legal clarification (Wilson 1996). Consequently, many support the development of clearly defined protocols that outline the boundaries of nurse-led practice (Campbell et al 1999, Fulton & Phillips 1998, Guerrero 1994, Muir 1999, Murray 1997). However, whilst these strategies do not necessarily ensure legal protection, they do provide some support for nurse-led initiatives during this time of rapid evolution.

Some nurse-led services incorporate the notion of 'shared care', in which the nurse provides a follow-up service after an initial medical consultation (Guerrero 1994, McKinnon 1997, Muir 1999, Murray 1997). This provides an opportunity for community children's nurses (CCNs) who either specialise in a particular clinical area or work closely with identified consultants to develop follow-up services. For example, the CCN may offer a follow-up clinic for children with chronic constipation seen first by a gastroenterologist (Muir 1999).

EDUCATION AND COMPETENCE

There remains much confusion and debate around the level of education required for those offering nurse-led services, which is exacerbated by inconsistencies in grading, activities, titles, etc. (Gibson 1998). Campbell et al (1999) stress that, in relation to nurse-led clinics, the level of expertise 'should be debated, clarified and standardised before this model is extended'. The discrepancy in educational preparation is evident, with some services being offered by degree-level nurses (Hyett 1997) and others educated to master's level (Hill 1997). Given the level of autonomy and decision making required, it is not surprising that some commentators advocate master's level education to fulfil the requirements of these new roles (Castledine 1996, Fulton & Phillips 1998). These master's level outcomes could then provide a framework for ongoing competency assessment in practice (Manley 1996). For CCNs who have completed their degree in specialist practice, this would mean identifying a specific programme that reflects their unique needs in practice. An alternative may be for institutions to consider offering current specialist practice programmes at different exit points.

MANAGEMENT AND SUPPORT

Given the different models of community children's nursing services in the UK (Eaton & Thomas 1998), the scope clearly exists for a variety of nurse-led initiatives to emerge. Logically, the management of potential developments would also be complex. Developing standards for clinical supervision could perhaps provide some consistency in the management and support offered to practitioners. This process should provide 'professional support and learning which enables individual practitioners to develop knowledge and competence, assume responsibility for their own practice and enhance consumer protection and safety in complex clinical situations' (National Health Service Management Executive 1993). To maximise the benefits, it is essential that the supervisory role is fulfilled by the 'right' person whilst ensuring that nursing values are upheld. However, it should not be assumed that this 'right' person is a nurse.

MOTIVATION TO PROVIDE A PATIENT-CENTRED SERVICE

A patient-centred service is designed to minimise disruption to patients' lives and provide the optimum quality of care that is considerate to patient lifestyle and commitments. In the light of the UK patient's charter (Department of Health 1992b) and, more recently, clinical governance (Department of Health 1997), the aim is continuously to improve quality, safeguard standards of care, and deliver healthcare that is cost-effective with maximum benefit to the consumer.

Patient satisfaction is a measurable outcome of service provision (Hill 1997, Murray 1997). Patient satisfaction is closely correlated to compliance (Ley 1993), to patient well-being and quality of life (Hill 1997). It is also linked to the provision of information and continuity of care (Hill 1997, Murray 1997). Studies have suggested satisfaction in a nurse-led service to be at least equivalent to that in a medical one (Hill 1997, Murray 1997), although this needs further evaluation (Fulton & Phillips 1998). This may be related to longer consultation times (Kincey et al 1975), more effective communication in terms of listening and understanding (Stillwell 1988) and a greater opportunity for continuity of care and ongoing support by nurses. Within community children's nursing, patient-centred services are provided to the child and the family. The potential for nurse-led initiatives within this field is strengthened by the recognition that sick children should be cared for at home. In addition, close liaison between the acute and ambulatory setting promotes effectiveness both in terms of cost and clinical outcome.

PUBLIC AND INTERPROFESSIONAL CONFIDENCE

Recent years have seen advances in nursing roles and, in accompaniment, public and interprofessional confidence. Nurse-led services in primary healthcare are already established. Some of these are in the form of health visitor drop-in clinics, which have continued to grow with clear public support (McKinnon 1997, Murray 1997). Primary healthcare teams enthusiastically support the advances in nurse-led care (Hyett 1997). Within the healthcare system as a whole, there has been a distinct change in attitude towards combining the skills of doctors and nurses. Confidence in nurse-led services is growing alongside the recognition and appreciation of nursing skills. Consequently, shared-care philosophies, either where nurse practitioners work alongside the consultant (McKinnon 1997) or where partnerships in care are developed, are realistic options to consider. These principles concur with those outlined in the clinical governance agenda (Department of Health 1997).

ORIENTATION TO THE CARING VALUES OF NURSING

Nursing is an exciting and challenging profession. Currently, the profession is experiencing great changes, especially with advances in nursing practice where there are associated increased responsibilities (Hyett 1997) and autonomy in decision making (Guerrero 1994). To nurse is to care for, and caring is a skill. This is fundamental to nursing practice. Advancing nursing roles and advocating nurse-led services are means to provide holistic care to the consumer whilst utilising expert knowledge and skills to determine and evaluate their care. CCNs have specific 'caring' skills that are complementary to those of acute and ambulatory care: effective communication, providing a relaxed atmosphere for consultation, ongoing support, education and the provision of time for the unravelling of often-complex family concerns. Within community children's nursing, nurse-led services may provide a quality service to children and families that proves cost-effective. It is cost-effective, in that CCNs utilise skills to promote family health and well-being, and prevent hospital admission.

CONCLUSION

The development of nurse-led services in community children's nursing is a challenging enterprise. Considering the current political and professional climate, there are a number of factors encouraging the formation of nurse-led services within acute, ambulatory and primary care. Support exists in the public sector and amongst professional colleagues with the motivation being to provide the optimum quality of care to children and families. Considerations need to be given to the issues of liability and accountability, especially with regard to the administration and prescribing of medication, clinical decision making, continuing education and formal support frameworks. The development of a nurse-led service requires personal and professional motivation and ambition. It is a highly rewarding experience, generating great role satisfaction. The opportunities for the development of nurse-led services are abundant in community children's nursing and may prove a significant landmark in the evolution of nursing as a whole.

FURTHER READING

Fulton Y & Phillips P 1998 Nurse-led clinics in ambulatory care. In: Glasper E A & Lowson S (eds) Innovations in paediatric ambulatory care. Macmillan, London, p 115

This chapter offers interesting background reading into the development of nurse-led initiatives in the UK. It then provides a useful practical example and goes on to describe the setting up of an enuresis clinic.

Gibson F 1998 The development of advancing clinical practice roles within paediatric nursing. The Florence Nightingale Foundation, London

Faith Gibson provides a stimulating analysis of the emerging specialist and advanced practice roles emerging in this country compared with her experiences in America. The work derives from her Florence Nightingale Award. It offers an extremely comprehensive debate around this complex area.

REFERENCES

Calman K 1993 Hospital doctors: training for the future. HMSO, London

Campbell J, German L & Lane C 1999 Radiotherapy outpatient review: a nurse-led clinic. Nursing Standard 13(22):39–44

Castledine G 1996 The role and criteria of an advanced nurse practitioner. British Journal of Nursing 4(5):264–265

Department of Health 1989a Working for patients. HMSO, London

Department of Health 1989b Report of the advisory group on nurse prescribing. (Crown report). HMSO, London

Department of Health 1991 Nurse prescribing. Final report: a cost benefit study. (Touche Ross report). HMSO, London

Department of Health 1992a The health of the nation: a strategy for health in England HMSO, London.

Department of Health 1992b The patient's charter HMSO, London

Department of Health 1997 The new NHS. Modern, dependable. The Stationery Office, London

Department of Health 1998 Our healthier nation. The Stationery Office, London

Eaton N & Thomas P 1998 Community children's nursing: an evaluative framework. Journal of Child Health Care 2(4):170–173

Fulton Y & Phillips P 1998 Nurse-led clinics in ambulatory care. In: Glasper E A & Lowson S (eds) Innovations in paediatric ambulatory care. Macmillan, London, pp 115

Garbett R 1996 The growth of nurse-led care. Nursing Times 92(1):29

Gibson F 1998 The development of advancing clinical practice roles within paediatric nursing. The Florence Nightingale Foundation, London

Guerrero D 1994 A nurse-led service. Nursing Standard 9(6):21–23

Hill J 1997 Patient satisfaction in a nurse-led rheumatology clinic. Journal of Advanced Nursing 25:347–354

Hyett J 1997 A health visitor surgery. Community Nurse September: 28–29

Kincey J, Bradshaw P & Ley P 1975 Patient satisfaction and reported acceptance in general practice. Cited in: Murray S 1997 A nurse-led clinic for patients with peripheral vascular disease. British Journal of Nursing 6(13):726–731

Ley P 1993 Communicating with patients: improving communication, satisfaction and compliance. Chapman Hall, London

McKinnon K 1997 Going it alone. Health Service Journal 3 April: 31

Manley K 1996 Advanced practice is not about medicalising nursing roles. Nursing in Critical Care 1(2):56–57

Muir J 1999 Advancing practice in the community. A nurse-led clinic for children with chronic constipation. Presented to the conference 'Advancing practice in children's nursing', Institute of Child Health, London, 19 February 1999

Murray S 1997 A nurse-led clinic for patients with peripheral vascular disease. British Journal of Nursing 6(13):726–731

National Health Service Executive 1998 Report on the supply and administration of medicines under group protocols. Health Service Circular 1998/051 Department of Health, London

National Health Service Management Executive 1993 A vision for the future. NHSME, London

Read S 1995 Catching the tide: new voyages in nursing? Sheffield Centre for Health and Related Research, Sheffield

Stillwell B 1998 The origins and development of the nurse practitioner role – a worldwide perspective. In: Bowling A & Stillwell B (eds) The nurse in family practice. Scutari Press, London, p 3

UK Central Council for Nursing, Midwifery and Health Visiting 1992 The scope of professional practice. UKCC, London

Wilson J 1996 A look up the scope. Nursing Management 2(8):16–17

30 Nurse prescribing: a new opportunity for community children's nursing

Mark Jones

KEY ISSUES

- Overview of the 20-year quest for nurse prescribing rights
- Summary analysis of the Crown I and Crown II reports
- Future models for nurse prescribing
- Challenges facing community children's nurses should they wish to prescribe

INTRODUCTION

Over 20 years ago the quest toward achieving prescribing rights began when a group of district nurses put their case to the Royal College of Nursing (RCN 1978). The case was a logical and reasonable one, in that the nurses believed they had the knowledge base required to make prescribing decisions for a range of wound care products they used, and that time would be saved for both patients and the general practitioners they had to harangue into signing off prescriptions for items that they did not really understand too well.

These basic tenets – knowledge base and competency, time saving, and improved patient care – have been at the centre of the nurse prescribing debate. A range of 'official' reports have supported the original stance that nurses who are competent should be able to prescribe from a specific formulary to meet their patients' care needs. The Cumberlege report (Department of Health and Social Security 1987) notably recommended to ministers that community nurses with a district nursing or health visiting qualification should be able to prescribe from a limited formulary. This was followed by the report of a Government review group specifically charged with the task of determining whether prescribing by nurses was a viable concept. The so-called 'Crown report' (Department of Health 1989) once more endorsed the concept of prescribing by competent nurses with health visiting and district nursing qualifications. Crown suggested that these nurses should be able to 'prescribe' in three ways, as outlined in Box 30.1.

Encouraged by these reports and ongoing examples of how nurses might benefit from prescribing, the RCN lobbied the Government to introduce

BOX 30.1 ***Proposals on nurse prescribing in the Crown report***

- Nurses could prescribe from a limited formulary as a medical practitioner would.
- Nurses could alter the timing and dosage of administration of a medicine that had already been prescribed.
- Nurses would be able to use a protocol to select medicines for administration from a list agreed with a medical practitioner prescriber.

legislation to allow nurses to prescribe. There was a problem, though, in that in the early 1990s, as the nurse prescribing case was being proven the Treasury was particularly keen to reduce the National Health Service (NHS) drugs budget. A number of initiatives (e.g. Department of Health 1990, 1993) were put in place to cap the prescribing habits of general practitioners (GPs), and in this climate the Government was not keen to be seen supporting further prescribing by nurses. Faced with this situation the RCN used its political influence to encourage the then Conservative member of parliament (MP) for Chislehurst, Roger Sims, to put forward a private member's bill to facilitate nurse prescribing when he was given the opportunity to do so by Parliament (Gardener & Sims 1999).

Before Sims presented his Bill, the RCN had primed MPs through an opinion poll and distribution of information supporting the nurse prescribing argument. Together with covert Government support, this lobby activity ensured the Sims Bill passed through Parliament, receiving Royal assent and entering the statute books as the Prescription of Medicinal Products by Nurses Etc. Act 1992.

PILOT SITES AND THE CURRENT MODEL

Even though the law had now been changed to allow nurses to prescribe, it was not until Baroness Julia Cumberlege, a champion of nurse prescribing as discussed above, became junior minister for health that a series of pilot or 'demonstration' projects were set up. These pilots evaluated well, and proved that nurses with appropriate education and training could prescribe effectively for their patients without increasing the drugs budget. The next move, therefore, was to have the Government extend the pilot projects to all eligible health visitors and district nurses.

Using the Government's own analysis of the pilot sites, the RCN argued that the ability of health visitors and district nurses to prescribe from their formulary without problem warranted extension of the scheme. Consequently, just before the Secretary of State for Health was to make a keynote address to the 1998 RCN congress, his office telephoned the author to ask how much this would cost and how many health visitors and district nurses would be involved. Time was pressing and a 'back of an envelope' calculation led to an insertion into the speech agreeing a budget of £14 million to extend the current model of prescribing.

WHY JUST DISTRICT NURSES AND HEALTH VISITORS?

It is worth taking time here to discuss why nurse prescribing had, until this point, been concerned only with health visiting and district nursing. As mentioned above, the original case had been made by district nurses and a key factor was the time wasted having to hassle GPs into signing prescriptions. The general feeling was that community nurses would be best advantaged if allowed to prescribe, given that they did not have the same access to medical colleagues as nurses working in acute-care environments. The Cumberlege report, with a remit only for community nursing, picked up on this theme (Department of Health and Social Security 1987). When Crown's team reported in 1989, they too considered prescribing only for community-based practitioners (Department of Health 1989). Both Cumberlege and Crown believed that prescribing should be reserved for nurses with post-basic qualifications. At the time their work was carried out, the only such qualifications existing in community practice were those of health visiting and district nursing. This is now recognised as being anachronistic, especially as there are now a range of specialist recordable qualifications in community practice, such as community children's nursing and practice nursing, in addition to those for health visiting and district nursing. Although supporting the extension of the health visitor–district nurse scheme nationally, the RCN is of the opinion that any specialist nurse who has been appropriately trained, and can demonstrate competence, should be able to prescribe products required to meet the nursing care needs of their patients (RCN 1997).

The area of 'hot debate' is, of course, whether nurses should be able to prescribe in their own right, without the sanction of another healthcare professional (i.e. medical practitioner). The second Crown review team considered this issue in some detail, and agreed with the evidence presented to it by the RCN (1997) that there was a case for competent nurses to be able to prescribe products to meet their patients' nursing care needs (Department of Health 1999).

So, having examined the current system, what of the future? Will the day eventually come when community children's nurses (CCNs) will be able to prescribe more than a bandage and a dose of Calpol for their patients? To answer this, several steps need to be considered.

TYPES OF PRESCRIBER

The future starts with the recommendations of Crown's team in the final report of the second review considering prescribing by nurses (Department of Health 1999). Crown acknowledges that competent and suitably trained nurses should be able to prescribe. Furthermore, she suggests two forms of prescribing which will be applicable to nurses in the future: 'independent' and 'dependent' prescribing.

An *independent prescriber* is described as someone:

> 'who is responsible for the assessment of patients with undiagnosed conditions and for decisions about the clinical management required, including prescribing.' (Department of Health 1999 para 6.19)

It is pointed out that, at present, only doctors and dentists and those nurses prescribing from the nurse formulary are legally authorised prescribers. As stated above, they fulfil the criteria of being able to assess patients with undiagnosed conditions and make a prescribing decision, and they should continue to do so. However, Crown states that 'certain other health professionals may also become newly legally authorised independent prescribers' (Department of Health 1999 para 6.19).

Crown goes on to define the *dependent prescriber* as someone:

> 'who is responsible for the continuing care of patients who have been clinically assessed by an independent prescriber. This continuing care may include prescribing, which will usually be informed by clinical guidelines and will be consistent with individual treatment plans; or continuing established treatments by issuing repeat prescriptions, with the authority to adjust the dose or dosage form according to the patients' needs. There should be provision for regular review by the assessing clinician.' (Department of Health 1999 para 6.19)

The basic difference in the type of prescriber is that a dependent prescriber will not have the diagnostic and assessment ability to make a decision about an initial prescription, but will have sufficient knowledge to determine whether that prescription should be continued, or whether to alter the dosage. Furthermore, a dependent prescriber may still be able to prescribe a drug for the first time, but this would be within the parameters of clinical guidelines for a given condition and the care plan of a patient. This system differs from the supply and administration of medicines using group protocols in that the dependent prescriber will be able to provide patients with a prescription form which they can take to a pharmacy to have their medicines dispensed. This cannot happen with protocol arrangements.

HOW DOES THIS APPLY TO THE COMMUNITY CHILDREN'S NURSE?

The challenge for all nurses wishing to prescribe will be to demonstrate the competencies required to justify either independent or dependent prescribing rights. Aside from the need to be equipped with prescribing skills *per se* (pharmacological knowledge, ethics and accountability in prescribing, legal aspects of prescribing, etc.), which will be considered below, CCNs will need to identify the attributes their particular speciality of nursing has, to underpin their prescribing practice. Only those nurses who can demonstrate diagnostic and assessment ability will be considered for independent status. No doubt some CCNs fall into this category, but not all. Perhaps many more will qualify as dependent prescribers as they find themselves in situations where they are sufficiently *au fait* with the drugs used to treat children in their care on a regular basis. In addition, they need to demonstrate the ability to alter dosages or prescribe an alternative medicine within the same therapeutic category as that originally prescribed by an independent prescriber, be that a medical practitioner or nurse. Identifying the criteria by which some nurses (1) are independent prescribers, (2) are dependent prescribers, and (3) have no prescribing rights at all, is a significant challenge for community healthcare nurses. It is essential that this process is completed in a coordinated way, leading to a high degree of consensus. If we cannot agree amongst ourselves, there will be little chance of convincing those who will determine our prescribing rights in the future.

PRESCRIBE WHAT?

As discussed above, the RCN has campaigned for all specialist nurses who have completed a prescribing course to be able to prescribe any product required for the nursing care of their patient. This point acknowledges the potential to redefine 'nursing' as developments within the profession widen the scope of practice. However, it underlines the fact that nurses seek prescribing rights to do their job as a nurse, not to substitute for another professional group. In its evidence to the Crown review (RCN 1997) the College suggested that by virtue of their registration with the United Kingdom Central Council for Nursing, Midwifery and Health Visiting, as professionals accountable for their own actions, nurse prescribers should have access to a wide formulary, with their prescribing habits defined by virtue of their competence base. For example, an independent prescriber – a CCN – may well have access to the majority of the British National Formulary but would not be prescribing treatments for adults. Similarly an independent prescriber who happens to be a diabetes specialist would not, as a rule, prescribe pain control for a terminally ill child. This commonsense approach acknowledges nurses' ability to judge the boundaries of their competence and realise that inappropriately exceeding those boundaries leaves one open to de-registration and legal action.

The Crown review team acknowledged this proposal (Department of Health 1999 para 8.13), yet failed to endorse it (RCN 1999). Rather they suggested that the extension of prescribing rights should be based on a system of formularies restricted to the particular practitioner's field of expertise or speciality (Department of Health 1999 para 6.10). We may envisage a situation, therefore, whereby a CCN who works primarily with patients having respiratory problems is limited to a 'respiratory' formulary, whereas a colleague who is a diabetes specialist may have access only to a formulary containing insulins and other blood glucose stabilising medications. How the regulation of such formularies could occur in practice is questionable, with so many different highly specialised groups of nurses in practice. It seems a logistical nightmare to propose many different specialist formularies and to expect dispensing pharmacists to know which prescriber can access which formulary.

HOW WILL IT ALL WORK?

The Crown team proposed a whole new system, separate from any existing bodies with responsibility for regulating medicines, for the extension of prescribing rights to nurses and other health professionals who do not currently have them. At the centre of the proposals is the New Prescribers Advisory Committee (NPAC), which would consider submissions from professional organisations seeking powers for suitably trained members to become independent or dependent prescribers (Department of Health 1999 para 6.27). It is not clear who would sit on the NPAC and to what extent it would be proactive in setting criteria for submissions. However, the good news is that nursing will have access through its own membership organisations. Crown expects that proposals for new professional groups, to be considered as potential prescribers by the NPAC, will come from 'nationally recognised organisations'; those relevant national organisations must be able to confirm that the professional group is formally recognised by the appropriate regulatory body. As such, it would seem that nursing organisations such as the RCN, the Community Practitioners and Health Visitors Association (CPHVA) and the Community and District Nursing Association (CDNA) would be able to put proposals to the NPAC as to why groups of their members should have dependent or independent prescribing rights. Once CCNs have determined their own competency framework, as described above, their proposal could be submitted to the NPAC by one of these organisations.

TIMESCALE

The quest for prescribing rights for nurses has continued for over two decades. The consultation period for the second Crown report continued until June 1999. In reality, it is unlikely that CCNs will be prescribing in the near future. The logistics of determining competency base, training requirements, calming Treasury fears about overspend on the drugs budget, and enacting enabling legislation, are probably without precedent so far as health service changes are concerned, but, then again, nurses always relish a challenge ...

CONCLUSION

Health visitors and district nurses currently equipped with the skills thought necessary to prescribe from the existing nurse formulary, as recommended in the first Crown report (Department of Health 1989), complete a 3-day taught programme with approximately 15–20 hours of self-directed study. This may be adequate considering the limited product range available to these prescribers; however, it is inevitable that, if we seek prescribing rights from a wider formulary, nurses will be required to undertake a more in-depth training programme. With increased prescribing powers comes increased accountability for this significant new role. As the range of skills available to nurses is expanded, so the expectations of the consumer will increase.

The securing of prescribing rights for CCNs cannot be guaranteed, but at last there is an opportunity to pursue this expanded role, which should enhance the overall quality of care to children and their families. Some of the questions that still remain to be answered are highlighted in Box 30.2.

BOX 30.2 ***Questions for consideration***

- How will CCNs demonstrate the competencies required for independent or dependent prescribing practice?
- If able to prescribe, what products should be included in the formulary?
- Will patients and their carers accept prescribing by CCNs?
- What challenges might face the 'would be' prescriber?

REFERENCES

Department of Health 1989 Report of the advisory group on nurse prescribing (Crown report). Department of Health, London

Department of Health 1990 Improving prescribing. Department of Health, London

Department of Health 1993 Prescribing incentive scheme 'will benefit patients' says Dr Brian Mawhinney. Press Release H93/620. Department of Health, London, 11 March 1993

Department of Health 1999 Review of prescribing, supply and administration of medicines. Final report (Chair Dr June Crown). Department of Health, London

Department of Health and Social Security 1987 Neighbourhood nursing – a focus for care (Cumberlege report). HMSO, London

Gardener E & Sims R 1999 Nurse prescribing – the lawmakers. In: Jones M (ed.) Nurse prescribing – politics to practice. Baillière Tindall, London, p 67

Royal College of Nursing 1978 District nurses dressings. Report to the Community Nursing Association. RCN, London

Royal College of Nursing 1997 Review of prescribing, supply and administration of medicines. Update on the evidence submitted by the Royal College of Nursing. Unpublished evidence to the Crown II review. RCN, London

Royal College of Nursing 1999 RCN response to the review of prescribing, supply and administration of medicines. Final report. RCN, London

31 Alternative practice and complementary therapies in community children's nursing

Sue Spurling

KEY ISSUES

- Increasing numbers of people are using complementary therapies
- There are moves to integrate allopathic and complementary medicine
- Supporting the internal environment
- Complementary therapies applied to community children's nursing

INTRODUCTION

The French use the term 'terrain' to describe the status of our internal environment, one in which the seeds of healing can be sown and nurtured. Creating such an environment is an important aspect of care in helping children to be comfortable and develop insights into their own needs and future coping strategies. There are rigorous psychoimmunological studies to support the thesis that healing can be enhanced by reducing stress within our environment, for example through relaxation (Pert 1998), massage, visualisation and eating healthy foods (Null 1997).

This chapter is concerned with identifying ways in which community children's nurses (CCNs) may use complementary therapies to help support the child's internal and external terrain, for example by reducing anxiety, pain and stressors to their immune systems. Complementary therapies can support a child's ability to heal and maintain inner equilibrium (Pert 1998). The therapies discussed in this chapter include aromatherapy, reflexology, massage, visualisation, guided imagery and Bach flower remedies. Case studies will be used to illustrate points made.

There is a growing movement towards an integrated healthcare system, which encourages individuals to take some responsibility for their own health and well-being. His Royal Highness, The Prince of Wales, addressing the Foundation for Integrated Medicine's international congress in 1998 (HRH The Prince of Wales 1998), suggested that it is a movement in which it is hoped that complementary and allopathic medicine can come together to offer choice and appropriate treatments for each individual. The Foundation's membership comprises healthcare professionals from allopathic and complementary medicine, as well as input from a wide range of official bodies including the Royal College of Nursing and institutes of higher education.

Interest in complementary medicine has increased steadily over the past 10 years, as indicated by the numbers of people who attend complementary practitioners. Barnes and Ernst (1997) suggested that one-third to one-half of the population uses some form of complementary medicine.

Nurses who undertake complementary therapy courses will develop their knowledge and skill base, and should also develop their reflective skills, as part of their own personal and professional development. It is essential that nurses ensure the therapies are appropriate for the children they are caring for and not administered on the basis that they think it will be good for them. They must be guided in their practice by the United Kingdom Central Council for Nursing and Midwifery (UKCC) codes of practice in terms of accountability, professional conduct and practice (UKCC 1992, 1996, 1997). Nurses should be rigorous and analytical in assessment of the quality of their work and of the literature they may use to argue for the benefits of their chosen therapies.

Providing therapeutic practice for children should be underpinned by knowledge of child development in order to take account of children's cognitive abilities at any given age. It is also important for nurses to understand family needs and dynamics to ascertain stresses within their lives that may impact upon the child's ability to recover fully. By working empathetically with and supporting a child and family, nurses may be able to assist them to gain knowledge and learn techniques that will help them manage their own life stressors more effectively.

As children are increasingly cared for in the community (Health Committee 1997) CCNs are in an advantageous position to create a therapeutic environment, because of the close contact they have with children and their families. As the general public becomes more conversant with different therapies, it is incumbent upon nurses to gain a deeper understanding of complementary therapies and to develop networks with complementary practitioners. By doing so, parents will be helped to make informed decisions about the most effective care for their child.

Complementary medicine is not new. Some of the principal therapies used today have their roots in ancient times. Some, such as aromatherapy, go back 5000 years or more (Harrison 1995). But, in spite of the relative antiquity of some therapies, assumptions should not be made about their effectiveness, and nurses must be rigorous in their understanding of chosen therapies in order to ensure efficacy. This is particularly pertinent with the move towards evidence-based practice.

For CCNs it is important that they evaluate their practice, and a mechanism for evaluation, supervision and support for practitioners should be established with specialists in the field of complementary medicine (Nicoll 1995). Within that process, a range of issues that arises from practice can be explored, such as consent (Stone & Matthews 1996) and clinical effectiveness, as well as daily practice issues.

Detailed descriptions of specific therapies can be found elsewhere. Here, brief descriptions of some therapies will be offered and illustrated with case studies.

AROMATHERAPY

Aromatherapy involves the use of concentrated aromatic or essential oils extracted from botanical sources, such as leaves, flowers, bark, berries and roots, for therapeutic effects. Whilst René Gattefosse coined the term 'aromatherapy' at the beginning of this century, essential oils and herbs have been used for thousands of years for medicinal purposes (Rankin-Box 1995). The oils are used to treat the 'whole' person as they work on many levels through the senses of smell, touch and direct application. They can be applied in a variety of ways including massage, inhalation, compresses, creams, lotions, in baths. Because essential oils are very concentrated, they should be diluted before administration to the skin.

When working with children, blends need to be much more dilute than for adults, and even more so in neonates and preterm infants, as highlighted by Tisserand & Balacs (1995). Neonates and preterm infants have fewer layers of epidermis than older children or adults. The choice of oils is somewhat limited for children, because of the possibility of adverse reactions to some of the constituents of particular oils and different rates of absorption and excretory pathways, and because of immature physiological systems. Safe application must be ensured (Fowler & Wall 1997).

Essential oils can be very useful to enhance conventional care. Two examples illustrate how essential oils can not only help support children and families in the short term, but can also have implications in the long term when considering, for example, body image.

CASE STUDY

A 3-month-old baby, who had a $1\frac{1}{2}$-inch keloid scar along the medical aspect of her left foot to which pressure dressings were being applied, was treated with essential oils. Both parents were distressed by the accident, the resulting scar and the length of time expected for healing to occur.

A 1% solution of neroli and lavender essential oil in grapeseed base oil was used. This was massaged into the scar by the baby's parents for about 10 minutes twice a day. The parents elected to apply the pressure dressing at night only, to allow and encourage the baby's mobility. After a week, the scar line began to soften. The blend was well tolerated and so a small amount of wheatgerm oil and vitamin E was added to aid healing. Wheatgerm is thought to be an effective anti-scarring oil with some vitamin E content (Buckle 1997).

Gradually over the next few weeks the scar softened, greatly reduced in size and become pale pink. After 3 months they visited their consultant, who was apparently greatly impressed as he had expected the scar to take at least a year to reach this state. The scar all but disappeared, except for a small point at the centre, which had suffered the greatest depth of tissue damage.

CASE STUDY

A 2-year-old child had undergone open heart surgery and had been left with a keloid scar along the sternum. Again, the child's parents were concerned by the nature of the scar. A blend of rose and lavender essential oils with wheatgerm and vitamin E mixed into a vegan base cream was used. All three siblings helped with the massage, as they liked the smell! The scar reduced and softened, but took some time to reduce because it was extensive in size and depth. Positive results were nevertheless

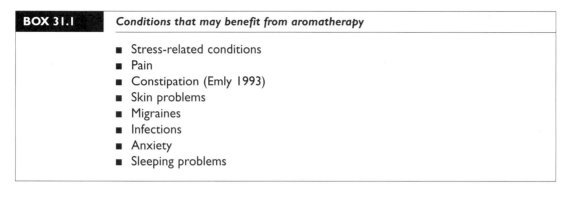

BOX 31.1 ***Conditions that may benefit from aromatherapy***

- Stress-related conditions
- Pain
- Constipation (Emly 1993)
- Skin problems
- Migraines
- Infections
- Anxiety
- Sleeping problems

achieved and had long-term implications for the child's body image in later years. Her parents were glad to have been able to use a pleasant and effective treatment for their daughter.

In both these cases it was noted how calm the children and parents became when giving the massage. In personal experience of working with children, applying oils through massage can result in a marked reduction in anxiety; this finding is supported by Acolet et al (1993). Aromatherapy offers the opportunity to develop a different and more positive relationship between child and parents/carers, who often choose to learn massage. It can also enhance the relationship between child and nurse. Inducing a relaxation response and encouraging enjoyment and fun may promote stimulation of the child's immune responses (Pert 1998) and hence healing.

Carrier oils are also of considerable importance, not least because of their varied therapeutic qualities and varying dermal uptake (Price & Price 1995). Where nut allergies are suspected, a grapeseed oil may be used.

Shenton (1996) identified the conditions in Box 31.1 as benefiting from aromatherapy.

However, essential oils should be used with caution and by appropriately qualified practitioners. It is important, for example, that the recipient likes the 'smell', because, by virtue of their action on the limbic system, the oils may evoke memories or emotional reactions or put in place future memories – either positive or negative. This is an important consideration in such areas as haematology and oncology, where smells may be negatively associated with, for example, chemotherapy and may cause problems for the child and carers if they come into contact with the same smell at a later stage.

THERAPEUTIC MASSAGE

Massage is probably one of the oldest therapies known to humankind, but it is only in the past 150 years that it has become more formalised into the methods we know today. Massage offers a means of communicating through caring touch, which is very different to the 'clinical' touch associated with much of nursing (Estabrooks 1992). It can be used to bring about changes in soft tissues and the circulation, and to promote a range of physiological and psychological effects such as reduction in anxiety (Paterson 1990) and problems such as constipation, relief of muscle tension and pain relief (Fritz 1995).

The beneficial effects of massage are well researched and recognised (McCormack 1991), although the research tends to be adult oriented. When implementing massage for children in the community, children should always be approached with respect and openness and with an understanding of verbal and non-verbal cues to ensure that the contact is appropriate and respected. It is also important that a parent or carer is present during the massage, unless the child is able to give consent to therapy in their own right and would be embarrassed at having a parent or carer present. In the main, children enjoy physical contact, but Horgan et al (1996) stress the importance of careful assessment of need, their body language and the relevant history. Children cannot usually tolerate long sessions and so a massage treatment, as with most other therapies, should be given over a short time, such as 30 minutes.

CASE STUDY

A boy aged 13 months, with profound global developmental delay as a result of a genetic abnormality, was offered massage. His mother gave permission and was very much a part of the therapy, staying close by as contact was made with him. As the massage proceeded, the child started to make very specific eye contact and demonstrated non-verbally his pleasure and seeming contentment with the contact (Harrison 1995). Particular attention was paid to his hands to encourage stretching of tight muscles.

The child's mother was shown how to carry out the massage, which she performed several times a week. She was asked for her assessment of her son's responses to the massage. He responded very well and she found it to be therapeutic and relaxing for both of them. Her son's hands relaxed sufficiently to allow him to pick up and grip toys, which benefited his overall development.

REFLEXOLOGY AND REFLEX ZONE THERAPY

In reflexology, gentle pressure is applied to different parts of the body, particularly the hands and feet, to stimulate different systems and organs of the body. It is suggested that there are reflex zones, running in specific lines through the body, which are reflected on the surface of the hands and feet, and that by stimulating them through specific touch health and well-being can be promoted (Griffiths 1995). Reflexology can be used very successfully in inducing a state of relaxation in an anxious person, lowering blood pressure, or in relieving distressing complaints such as constipation.

Children cannot tolerate the same length or depth of treatment as an adult (Bayly 1982), and any contraindications should be understood by the practitioner.

CASE STUDY

A 4-year old boy's mother requested help for her son who suffered from severe epilepsy which became much more unstable when he was constipated. Laxatives had little or no effect. The boy had recently been discharged home following a hospital admission for severe uncontrolled seizures. He was constipated and his mother was distressed as she could envisage the cycle repeating itself, but felt unable to help her son.

The child was offered a reflexology treatment, after which his mother reported a good bowel response on that same day. His mother was taught how to work on his bowel reflex points, and this treatment seemed to help keep the constipation more manageable.

BACH FLOWER REMEDIES

During the early part of this century, Dr Edward Bach, a physician and bacteriologist, identified 38 flower remedies, one for each of the most common negative moods or states of mind. Bach flower remedies derive from non-poisonous wild flowers and act as a form of supportive therapy used to establish equilibrium and harmony through the personality, addressing such feelings as fear, envy, jealousy, guilt, self-recrimination, rigidity of attitude, intolerance, impatience, procrastination and self-pity (Challoner 1990).

Brandy is used to preserve the essences. They should be taken in non-carbonated spring water, although they can be taken neat. Dilution applies particularly to children, who would probably find the effect of alcohol on their tongue too strong and unpleasant. Parents must be aware of the alcohol content of the remedies, but since only two to four drops are used at a time it should not be a problem for most parents to accept. Rescue Remedy, a combination of five remedies which offsets the effects of shock and severe anxiety and distress, calming the individual by 'quietening' the autonomic nervous system in response to shock, is probably one of the most useful of all the remedies.

These remedies have been used to help children, particularly in supporting them when they are anxious and/or have poor self-esteem and confidence, and in helping to overcome disharmony within themselves. They have been shown to have a gentle but observable benefit. More rigorous studies should be undertaken to demonstrate their effectiveness.

VISUALISATION AND GUIDED IMAGERY

Visualisation is the technique of using the imagination to create pictures of a desired outcome (Grant 1993). We all do this in daily life, but in this context it is carried out in a very focused way. Visualisation can be used as a means of handling a difficult situation more easily (Ryman 1995), such as before an intervention. It is a form of relaxed, focused concentration and is a natural and powerful coping mechanism. Visualisation can easily be learned and used as an adjunct to the care of toddlers and pre-school children, as well as older children who are experiencing anxiety and pain (Bullock & Shaddy 1993, Ott 1996).

Preparation for visualisation is important to enable the therapist to be very relaxed, 'centred' and focused on the child and their needs. The parents should be informed of goals, and permission for the visualisation obtained. The therapist should have an open and honest relationship with the child about the visualisation, listen to any expressed concerns and then help the child to re-focus anxiety to the goals and images. However, Ott (1996) has suggested that visualisation should not be used for those who are experiencing emotional instability. It can be harmful to those who are freely disassociating or acutely psychotic.

Visualisation can be used to teach the child and parents relaxation techniques and enable the child to cooperate with treatment, for example immunisations, venepuncture, bone marrow aspirations, biopsies and radiotherapy (Decker & Cline-Elsen 1992). Self-esteem may be improved by enabling a child to see how they have coped positively with a difficult situation.

CONCLUSION

CCNs can use complementary therapies to encourage trust and coping behaviours in children and their carer(s), as identified by Pederson (1994). They can help to provide an environment in which healing can be enhanced. To apply complementary therapies effectively, sound education and skills acquisition through accredited organisations are required, together with access to supervision by experienced practitioners. Children's health and well-being can be enhanced and greater choices made available. For CCNs and the children and families for whom they care, the use of complementary therapies encourages opportunities for collaboration, evaluation and advanced child care.

FURTHER READING

Field T, Schanberg S M, Scafidi M S, Bauer C R, Vega-Lahr Ngarcia B S, Nyström J & Kuhn C M 1986 Tactile/kinesthetic stimulation effects on pre-term neonates. Pediatrics 7(5):654–658

This paper is a study on the beneficial effects of massage on preterm infants and has implications for both the babies and the appropriately qualified staff in the neonatal unit. Field has written other papers on the use and benefits of massage for children and mothers in different situations, which may be worth acquiring.

Howard J 1994 Growing up with Bach flower remedies – a guide to the use of the remedies during childhood and adolescence. C W Daniel, Saffron Walden, UK

This book gives useful and practical guidance on how to tailor the remedies to the unique qualities of the child in terms of personality and character.

Williams D G 1997 The chemistry of essential oils. Micelle Press, Weymouth, UK

Full of useful information, this text is about the chemistry and safe application of essential oils. It is reasonably straightforward to understand if the reader is prepared to spend a little time over it.

USEFUL ADDRESSES

Aromatherapy Organisations Council (AOC), 3 Latymer Close, Braybrooke, Market Harborough LE16 8LL Tel: (01455) 615 466

Association of Reflexologists, 27 Old Gloucester Street, London WC1 3XX Tel: (020) 7237 5623

Bach Flower Remedies, Mount Vernon, Sotwell, Wallingford, Oxon OX10 0PZ

British Holistic Medical Association (BHMA), 179 Gloucester Place, London NW1 6DX Tel: (020) 7262 5299

Council for Complementary and Alternative Medicine (CCAM), 179 Gloucester Place, London NW1 6DX

Department of Complementary Medicine, School of Postgraduate Medicine and Health Sciences, University of Exeter, 25 Victoria Park Road, Exeter EX2 4NY Tel: (01342) 424872

Institute for Complementary Medicine (ICM), PO Box 194, London SE16 1QZ

International Federation of Aromatherapists (IFA), Department of Continuing Education, Royal Masonic Hospital, London W6 0TN Tel: (020) 8846 8066

Natural Medicines Society (NMS), Edith Lewis House, Ilkeston, Derbyshire DE7 8EJ

Research Council for Complementary Medicine (RCCM), 60 Great Ormond Street, London WCIN 3JF Tel: (020) 7833 8897

REFERENCES

Acolet D, Modi N, Giannakoulopoulos X, Bond C, Weg W, Clow A & Glover V 1993 Changes in plasma cortisol and catecholamine concentrations in response to massage in preterm infants. Archives of Disease in Childhood 68(suppl 1):29–31

Barnes J & Ernst E 1997 Complementary medicine. British Journal of General Practice 47(418):329

Bayly D 1982 Reflexology today – the stimulation of the body's healing forces through foot massage. Thorsons, Wellingborough

Buckle J 1997 Clinical aromatherapy in nursing. Arnold, London

Bullock E A & Shaddy R E 1993 Relaxation and imagery techniques without sedation during right ventricular endomyocardial biopsy in pediatric heart transplant patients. Journal of Heart and Lung Transplantation 39:215–217

Challoner P M 1990 Illustrated handbook of the Bach flower remedies. C W Daniel, Saffron Walden, UK

Decker T W & Cline-Elsen J 1992 Relaxation therapy as an adjunct in radiation oncology. Journal of Clinical Psychology 48:388–393

Emly M 1993 Abdominal massage. Nursing Times 89(3):34–36

Estabrooks C A 1992 Toward a theory of touch: the touching process and acquiring a touching style. Journal of Advanced Nursing 17:448–456

Fowler P & Wall M 1997 COSHH and CHIPS: ensuring the safety of aromatherapy. Complementary Therapies in Medicine 5:112–115

Fritz S 1995 Fundamentals of therapeutic massage. Mosby Lifeline, New York

Grant B 1993 A–Z of natural healthcare. Optima Books, Little, Brown, London

Griffiths P 1995 Reflexology. In: Rankin-Box D (ed) The nurses' handbook of complementary therapies. Churchill Livingstone, Edinburgh, p 133

Harrison J 1995 An introduction to aromatherapy for people with learning disabilities. British Journal of Learning Disabilities 23:37–40

Health Committee 1997 House of Commons Health Select Committee. Health services for children and young people: home and school. Third report. The Stationery Office, London

Horgan M, Choonara I, Al-Waidh, M, Sambrooks J & Ashby D 1996 Measuring pain in neonates: an objective score. Paediatric Nursing 8(10):24–27

HRH The Prince of Wales 1998 Integrated healthcare: a way forward for the next five years. Royal Society of Medicine Press, London

McCormack C 1991 Massage, relaxation and touch: a review of 14 research studies on the relaxation effects of massage, with a discussion on the therapeutic role of touch. Research Unit, Marylebone Centre Trust, London

Nicoll L 1995 Complementary therapies and nurse education – the need for specialist teachers. Complementary Therapies in Nursing and Midwifery 1(3):60–72

Null G 1997 The clinician's handbook of natural healing: the first comprehensive guide to scientific review studies of natural supplements and their proven treatment values. Kensington Books, New York

Ott M J 1996 Imagine the possibilities! Guided imagery with toddlers and pre-schoolers. Paediatric Nursing 22(1):34–38

Paterson L 1990 Baby massage in the neonatal unit. Nursing 4(23):19–21

Pederson C 1994 Ways to feel comfortable: teaching aids to promote children's comfort. Issues in Comprehensive Pediatric Nursing 17:37–46

Pert C 1998 Molecules of emotion. Simon & Schuster, London

Price S & Price L 1995 Aromatherapy for health professionals. Churchill Livingstone, Edinburgh

Rankin-Box D (ed) 1995 The nurses' handbook of complementary therapies. Churchill Livingstone, London

Ryman L 1995 Relaxation and visualisation. In: Rankin-Box D (ed) The nurses' handbook of complementary therapies. Churchill Livingstone, Edinburgh, p 141

Shenton D 1996 Does aromatherapy provide an holistic approach to palliative care? International Journal of Palliative Nursing 2(4)

Stone J & Matthews J 1996 Complementary medicine and the law. Oxford University Press, Oxford

Tisserand R & Balacs T 1995 Essential oil safety – a guide for health care professionals. Churchill Livingstone, London

UK Central Council 1992 The code of professional conduct. UKCC, London

UK Central Council 1996 Guidelines for professional practice. UKCC, London

UK Central Council 1997 Position statement on complementary and alternative therapies. UKCC, London

32 Creating an effective community children's nursing service

Brian Samwell

KEY ISSUES

- The diversity of community children's nursing
- Practical relationship between effectiveness, care outcomes and care organisation
- Planning community children's nursing services as part of the total child healthcare resource

INTRODUCTION

For those of us immersed in the day-to-day reality of community children's nursing, it seems obvious that we provide an essential service. Our perception is reinforced by feedback from families who appreciate the difference that skilled nursing support can make. We can give examples of that difference, perhaps in a child able to come home after months in hospital or parents making choices and taking control in extreme situations. Such anecdotal proof of our worth is important, yet it does not give the hard evidence of effectiveness that is demanded by those who plan and commission services. Increasingly, as providers, we are forced to identify and quantify the value of our services. This chapter explores the difficulties faced by community children's nurses (CCNs) in finding that evidence. It does not aim to give any easy answers but focuses on identifying some of the key questions that we should ask of ourselves if we are to justify our share of healthcare resources.

Clinical effectiveness has been defined as the 'extent to which specific clinical interventions when deployed in the field for a particular patient or population do what they are intended to do – i.e. maintain and improve health and secure the greatest possible health gain from the available resources' (National Health Service Executive 1996). Any examination of effectiveness has to be concerned with the outcomes of care. In turn, the achievement of outcomes is directly related to care organisation and the efficient use of healthcare resources. As the above definition suggests, effectiveness can be examined at individual and population levels. While it is vital for CCNs to have a sound research base for their clinical practice, it is equally important that they consider the place of their speciality in the total picture of child health provision.

Within community children's nursing, like nursing in general, outcomes may be difficult to identify. Many will be qualitative in nature or change may become apparent only over long periods of time. Nurses work with the world of human problems, which are complex, subjective and multifactorial. We can only rarely climb on to the high ground of scientific detachment, where variables can be controlled and relationships simplified. Our clients are concerned with all aspects of the care process. Defining the outcome of care is a challenge, but it is a challenge that CCNs must meet if they are to develop services in a coherent and rational fashion.

COMMUNITY CHILDREN'S NURSING: ONE SERVICE OR MANY?

Community children's nursing services in the UK are diverse. They may be managed from acute or community trusts, or be part of an integrated children's service. They may have a generic or a specialist focus, or mix a variety of generic and specialist roles within the one team (Winter & Teare 1997). Parts of services may even be funded from different sources, with specialist team members commonly supported by charities or research funds. Evaluations of community children's nursing teams do exist, but it is only recently that researchers have started to compare different service models (Procter et al 1998). It is significant that the Health Committee (1997) noted in its third report that there was no proven research-based model of service delivery.

The variety and complexity of a service clearly pose problems in evaluating its effectiveness. For community children's nursing there are many complicating factors:

- Clients may be spread over a wide geographical area and may not form a community in any accepted sense.
- Medical diagnosis is commonly used to identify client groups yet has real limitations in predicting the need of children and families (Eiser 1990).
- Users may be targeted by source of referral, yet any one source, particularly a regional or national hospital, may generate a wide range of nursing demands, ranging from brief clinical interventions, to complex discharge planning and long-term support for children with chronic conditions.
- Ethical problems may be created by targeting the client group, for example having to deny a service to a family who attend the regional rather than the local hospital.

Clearly CCNs do not stand alone in the service they provide for families. They have to define a unique role within the complex web of community health and welfare services, while at the same time exploiting opportunities for collaborative working arrangements that make the most efficient use of resources.

DEFINING THE CLIENT GROUP

CCNs see a variety of differing demands generated by the needs of actual or potential service users. While we often propose a uniform service for all children, it is possible to relate different care outcomes and models of care organisation to different client groups. What follows is a tentative attempt to

BOX 32.1 *Children with a chronic or serious illness or condition*

Defining issues	■ The numbers of children are small ■ Dependence on services and resource demand is high ■ Nursing input is long term with variations in intensity ■ There is emphasis on empowerment and self-efficacy of child and family
Care model	■ Key worker coordinates a multidisciplinary package of care, working in partnership with child and family.
Outcomes of care	■ To minimise the physical, social and psychological impact of illness or condition on child and family ■ To increase independence and self-determination of child and family ■ Parent satisfaction with coherent service delivery ■ To minimise need for hospital care

analyse the variety that may exist within a CCN's caseload. This simple model proposes broad groupings which relate to diagnosis, referral source, and the type of care resource that children might need. The needs of children in each of the groups described below pose a distinct type of challenge, in terms of assessing effectiveness, for the community children's nursing team.

CHILDREN WITH A CHRONIC OR SERIOUS CONDITION

For many teams this client group (see Box 32.1), with conditions that have a low prevalence but high severity, is the main focus of activity. From a pragmatic point of view the group can be defined by the need for an exceptional degree of nursing care, well beyond that seen as a usual part of child-rearing. To keep these children safe and well, to ensure they grow and participate in social life, may demand exceptional skills and specialist resources. Care is often intense and technically demanding, and may place families under extreme physical and psychological pressure. While the numbers of such children are relatively small, they require complex care packages with input from a large multidisciplinary team. For many families, the complexity and coordination of care is itself a major source of stress (Action for Sick Children 1993).

The Department of Health (1989) has defined community care as 'providing the right level of intervention and support to enable people to achieve maximum independence and control over their own lives.' There are two major implications for the CCN:

1. The effect of the service cannot be measured by satisfaction with the nursing service alone, but must encompass the whole package of care provided for child and family. This may include hospital care, housing, education, respite, and even such mundane but important items as nappy supplies, waste disposal and car parking permits. Commonly the CCN accepts a role

as key worker and care coordinator, but in doing so must see the service as part of the complete package and use a client-focused evaluative framework that can address the experience and satisfaction of children and families.

2. Judging 'the right level of intervention and support' at an individual level can be problematic. Effective care demands that the relationship with families has direction and purpose, that there is evidence of a health gain. The existence of a close supportive relationship with needy families is vital, but does not justify the service. The CCN must be concerned to move child and family towards increasing self-efficacy and independence. A model of the nursing relationship that describes the progression of the interaction over time, from introduction to closure, will help to create a measure of service effectiveness (Peplau 1988).

The community children's nursing service for this group of children is usually provided by small numbers of highly skilled nurses. Most of the workload can be undertaken within the working day, Monday to Friday, although the ability to offer a service outside these hours is vital for some families.

CHILDREN WITH COMMON CHRONIC CONDITIONS

The prevalence of common chronic conditions such as asthma and diabetes demands a different model of care (see Box 32.2) to that described above. Not only will the numbers overwhelm a small team but there is also potential for role conflict with community nurses and general practitioners (GPs). If we

BOX 32.2 ***Children with a common chronic condition such as asthma, diabetes or epilepsy***

Defining features

- The conditions are common
- Potentially well children who readily access mainstream facilities
- Care is focused on a specific health issue
- Input is intensive at first but decreases

Care model

- Transitional care between hospital and community
- High level of specific nursing expertise so as to act as resource and facilitator for hospital and primary care staff
- Focus on education and self-care of child and family
- Care pathway can be used to give continuity between primary and secondary care

Outcomes of care

- Good symptom control and minimal disability
- Child and family confident in managing condition
- Access to community facilities (e.g. school) is safe and well supported
- Care managed within the community setting with minimal use of hospital facilities
- Families perceive continuity of care between hospital and community

accept that the majority of children with common chronic conditions will have their care managed within the community, then the role of the CCN can be seen to include three important functions:

1. To provide a specialist resource, available in hospital and community, to support nursing and medical staff in their management of these conditions. Commonly community children's nursing teams have a member who takes on a specialist role and develops expertise in depth, but it is vital that this person focuses on education and the devolution of essential skills.
2. To oversee the transition from hospital to community care, ensuring there is continuity of support for child and family. This may require an involvement in standard setting or, increasingly, the development of care pathways that set a consensus on standards, outcomes and processes (Morris 1997).
3. To maintain a role in directly managing those children whose level of need is exceptional, perhaps on diagnosis, or children whose condition is unstable and disabling.

Effective care in this context is clearly collaborative yet it does not demand that the CCN take on a long-term key-worker role. Rather, this role should be devolved to health visitors, school nurses and practice nurses who have an existing remit to work with such children. The effective CCN becomes a facilitator with the expertise and clinical overview to ensure high standards of care are maintained across all healthcare settings.

CHILDREN DISCHARGED FROM HOSPITAL AFTER AN ACUTE INTERVENTION

For the previous two client groups it is conceivable for a relatively small number of highly skilled nurses to provide appropriate care. However, care for this third group (see Box 32.3) presumes a substantial increase in nurse availability

BOX 32.3 ***Children discharged from hospital after surgery or an acute intervention***

Defining features	■ Large numbers of referrals ■ Input is intensive but short term; need for increased availability of service ■ Emphasis on practical and technical nursing; generic nursing expertise ■ Clinical direction largely from hospital
Care model	■ Nursing support as part of an integrated care pathway giving seamless transition from hospital to home care ■ Ambulatory care
Outcomes of care	■ Shorter hospital stays, earlier discharge ■ Faster recovery; reduced incidence of hospital-acquired infection ■ Families feel well supported throughout the care process

to cope with large numbers of visits, and to provide cover throughout the week, including weekends. The management of this client group may also increase demand for skill-mix since specialist expertise in complex care management is not always a necessity.

This part of the CCN's workload demands careful management, simply because large numbers of referrals can force out other care activities. The team has to be concerned with the whole process of discharge assessment and referral, and work with hospital staff to agree referral guidelines. Without such agreement it is easy for hospital staff to generate routine referrals which add little value to the child's care package. In some cases it may excuse sloppy discharge planning by a hospital team that has the reassurance of knowing a community nurse can deliver the forgotten medicines or teddy bear. CCNs have to uphold the value of their service by insisting that ward staff plan an appropriate after-care package for each child, referring to the community team only if necessary. For many families, high-quality information, an informed GP, and the possibility of telephone support will be all that is needed.

AVOIDING HOSPITAL ADMISSION

The final group in this simple model of the CCN's caseload are children for whom hospital admission during acute illness can be avoided if they have access to nursing support in the home (Box 32.4). Perhaps this can be seen as the ultimate contribution of community children's nursing to the Government's vision of a primary care-led National Health Service (Department of Health 1997, Scottish Office 1997). However, realisation of this vision does depend on a significant investment. Of all the service patterns discussed so far, 'avoiding admission' will demand the largest nursing resource. Twenty-four-hour availability will be needed to support families throughout the evening and night when the stress of caring for an ill child is amplified. During these hours, nurse safety becomes an increased concern, particularly for those working in inner-city areas. Nurses may need to work in pairs and will depend on a reliable effective communication system. Families will also demand a nursing service that can deliver prompt support, to ensure that home care is no less safe than that in hospital.

BOX 32.4 ***Children diagnosed with acute illness in the community***

Defining features

- Intensive short-term input
- Potentially high referral rate, yet likely to be seasonal
- Clinical direction given by GPs
- Need for an 'out of hours' service

Care model

- Integration with primary care services
- Protocols to guide referral and shared care between nurse and GP

Outcomes of care

- Families feel well supported in managing acute illness at home
- No compromise in child's safety and welfare
- Reduced hospital admission rates
- Contribute to managing demand for GP services

It remains to be seen whether this type of service development would be able to justify the substantial investment necessary to make it a safe, effective reality. There may also be questions of acceptability to GPs should there be any suspicion that hospital treatment would be harder to secure. Other forms of home support, such as telephone advice lines, might yet prove to be cheaper and more attractive.

CONCLUSION

This analysis is not intended to be definitive. It should perhaps be seen as one attempt to clear a narrow track through the jungle of information on effectiveness and evidence-based care. It is easy to think of other tracks, different models, or exceptions to this model. However, the aim has been to illustrate the complexity of community children's nursing services and the value of targeting planning for different segments of the client population. CCNs cannot be all things to all families. They have to be able to target their input so as to maximise the effectiveness of care. They also have to collaborate with other health and welfare workers to decide who can provide a service most effectively. The nurse's expertise lies not just in direct child and family care, but also in ensuring the effectiveness of the web of services that support child and family.

Whichever model of service is used by a team, it needs to consider the following key steps towards assessing effectiveness:

- Define the outcomes of care based on the assessed needs of children and families rather than the needs of service providers
- Link those outcomes to a model of care organisation that will make the most efficient use of child healthcare resources
- Develop a framework for evaluating progress towards those outcomes which is clearly client focused

The evidence base that will help us to undertake this work is small but is at last developing. Increasingly CCNs will need to participate in that research, and enter the debate on the value of qualitative evidence. If we do not become involved in the research that will underpin our services, we risk losing the argument to those who do not understand the context of care (Hobbs & Murray 1999).

The care of sick children is an emotive issue. As children's nurses we are able to create a high public profile and win resources that are denied to other segments of the population. Yet there is a limit to our ability to win resources by such means. We have to develop a more rigorous analysis of the work we do so that investment can be justified not by emotional pleading or expert opinion but by rational argument and strong evidence.

FURTHER READING

Eaton N & Thomas P 1998 Community children's nursing: an evaluative framework. Journal of Child Health 2(4):170–173

Explores the components of a comprehensive evaluation which takes into account the views and perspectives of all the key stakeholders in a service.

Jones A & McDonnell U 1993 Managing the clinical resource. Baillière Tindall, London

A broad but practical introduction to resource management with useful section on healthcare economics.

Murray P & Penman J 1996 Let our children be. Parents With Attitude, Sheffield

What is it like to be on the receiving end of health and welfare services? This little book gives valuable insight into the total experience of children and families.

REFERENCES

Action for Sick Children 1993 Caring for children in the health services – bridging the gaps. Action for Sick Children, London

Department of Health 1989 Caring for people: community care in the next decade and beyond. HMSO, London

Department of Health 1997 The new NHS. Modern, dependable. The Stationery Office, London

Eiser C 1990 Chronic childhood disease. Cambridge University Press, Cambridge

Health Committee 1997 House of Commons Health Select Committee. Health services for children and young people in the community: home and school. Third report. The Stationery Office, London

Hobbs R & Murray E 1999 Specialist nurses: evidence for their effectiveness is limited. British Medical Journal 318:683–684

Morris E 1997 Continuity of care – managing children with asthma across the health care network. In: Wilson J Integrated care management. Butterworth, Oxford, pp113–126.

National Health Service Executive 1996 Promoting clinical effectiveness. Department of Health, Leeds

Peplau H 1988 Interpersonal relations in nursing. Macmillan Education, Basingstoke

Procter S, Biott C, Campbell S, Edward S, Redpath N & Moran M 1998 Preparation for the developing role of the community children's nurse. English National Board, London

Scottish Office 1997 Designed to care. Renewing the NHS in Scotland. Department of Health, Edinburgh

Winter A & Teare J 1997 Construction and application of paediatric community nursing services. Journal of Child Health Care 1:24–29

33 Integrating and combining children's services

Helen Mehaffey

KEY ISSUES

- The impetus to develop integrated and combined services to children and their families is driven by Government policy.
- Integrated and combined services benefit staff, the overall service provision and, most importantly, children and their families.
- Strategic direction and staff collaboration is essential to its success.

INTRODUCTION

This chapter sets out to illustrate how the integration and combining of acute and community children's services facilitates a more child-centred approach in which the child is seen as a unique developing person within the context of the family. An integrated and combined service provides families with a single identifiable source for advice and treatment (if necessary) and embraces the concept of multiagency approaches to healthy lifestyle, encouraging the child to reach individual optimal potential in all aspects of development.

Integration of children's services is not a new concept. The Government report 'Fit for the future' (Department of Health 1976) gave the following recommendations:

> 'there should be one service which follows the child's development from the early pre-school years, through school and adolescence'
>
> 'services should not only be readily available to parents, but they should be easy to use'
>
> 'the child health service should be able to provide families with a single identifiable source to which they can turn for skilled advice and where necessary treatment'

Governmental thought remains unchanged on this. The fundamental principle remains in the forefront of the National Health Service (NHS) (Department of Health 1998a, Health Committee 1997, NHS Executive 1996).

Set within the political context of an increasingly centralised agenda for improving the quality of services, the integration and combining of acute and community services brings about a number of areas for consideration, as identified in Box 33.1.

BOX 33.1 *Integration and combining of acute and community services: areas for consideration*

- The strategic management approach
- Human and financial resources
- Delivering quality and cost-effective care
- Potential benefits to the child/family and staff

BOX 33.2 *Directorate services*

- Care of the newborn
- Neonatal care
- Care of the well child
- Care of the sick child

THE STRATEGIC MANAGEMENT APPROACH

Before the integration of services within Loddon Trust in the late 1980s, services for children were scattered over four different sites with different management structures within the then district health authority. For example, school health services were managed by health visitors in the community unit, learning disability services were within the adult mental health and disability service, and neonatal care was managed by the midwifery unit. Paediatricians provided the only link with the acute services. Overall, there was no cohesive strategy for children's services. This resulted in a certain amount of duplication and limited opportunities to assess for gaps in service provision or to identify the totality of resources being utilised. For children and their families, it meant fragmented care provision, with potentially suboptimal practice. These factors inhibited the health authority from having an overall view of service provision and expenditure.

Following intensive discussions, led by senior paediatricians and the acute service nurse manager with the health authority, a review of children's services was undertaken. This coincided with the introduction of Trust status and service reconfiguration. In retrospect, this was fortunate as it initiated the catalyst for change and the move of children's services in its entirety into what was to become the Community Trust. The reconfigured services are identified in Box 33.2. This reconfiguration was not without its problems, as certain professional groups were initially resistant to change. The sharing of the vision of an integrated and combined health service with the multidisciplinary team was difficult.

It was later that government policy, of integrated and combined services for children, reinforced the local view. The Audit Commission (1994) expanded on previous reports, sending a clear message to local authorities advocating collaboration between health, education and social services to plan and manage children's services. A key principle, guiding government policy and the local strategy, was the recognition that children are different to adults, with differing needs throughout their development. They are a vulnerable group and provision of effective healthcare is dependent upon understanding this. At local level these reports endorsed the strongly held belief that the health authority had embarked on the right direction for children's services.

In order to undertake this major change in the way children's services were to be delivered, it was crucial to develop a single integrated and collaborative management team. The function of this team was to define a strategy for children's services and to deliver child health services at the point of need. To achieve this, the aims were:

- Clearly to identify roles and responsibilities within the management team
- To establish effective communication pathways to facilitate collaboration between clinicians and managers

The clinical director had an overarching role in setting the strategic direction of services (Figure 33.1). The directorate manager took responsibility for delivering the agreed agenda within budget and to the highest possible standard. These roles required the support of a number of competent team leaders with demonstrable managerial skills in addition to clinical competence. A further initiative was the inclusion of a role at senior level to manage the development and business aspects of the directorate. The challenge lay in developing a two-way process of informing the strategy for children's services at Trust board level whilst devising an operational plan, to drive service delivery at directorate level. To achieve this, high levels of communication and collaboration were required to enable all multidisciplinary teams to contribute to setting and agreeing the strategic direction for the service. Clinical team participation in this, and the operational planning process, ensured that it was clinically driven with everyone involved. Central to this was to ensure that the children's management team had expertise in the needs of the area of their responsibility, together with a wider understanding of the needs of children and their families. This management structure worked well and continues to do so. It has encouraged the development of a multidisciplinary team approach, which has in turn facilitated a wider vision of the needs of children.

HUMAN AND FINANCIAL RESOURCES

This single management structure maximises the flexible use of existing resources and enables a dynamic response to changing priorities in child health and in individual children's needs. For example, the school health nursing team has prioritised the need to address the mental health and well-being of adolescents in response to the recognition of increasing mental health problems in young people. Integration and collaboration has encouraged joint-funded initiatives, in which school nurses are employed by health and education departments. This enables the nurse to participate fully in the national curriculum, with particular emphasis being placed on the health improvement programme. It is achieved in collaboration with class teachers and through the provision of 'drop-in clinics'.

A single management structure has the major advantage of pooling resources. Multidisciplinary team-working encourages the sharing of ideas and skills, and promotes a holistic approach to coordinated healthcare led by a key

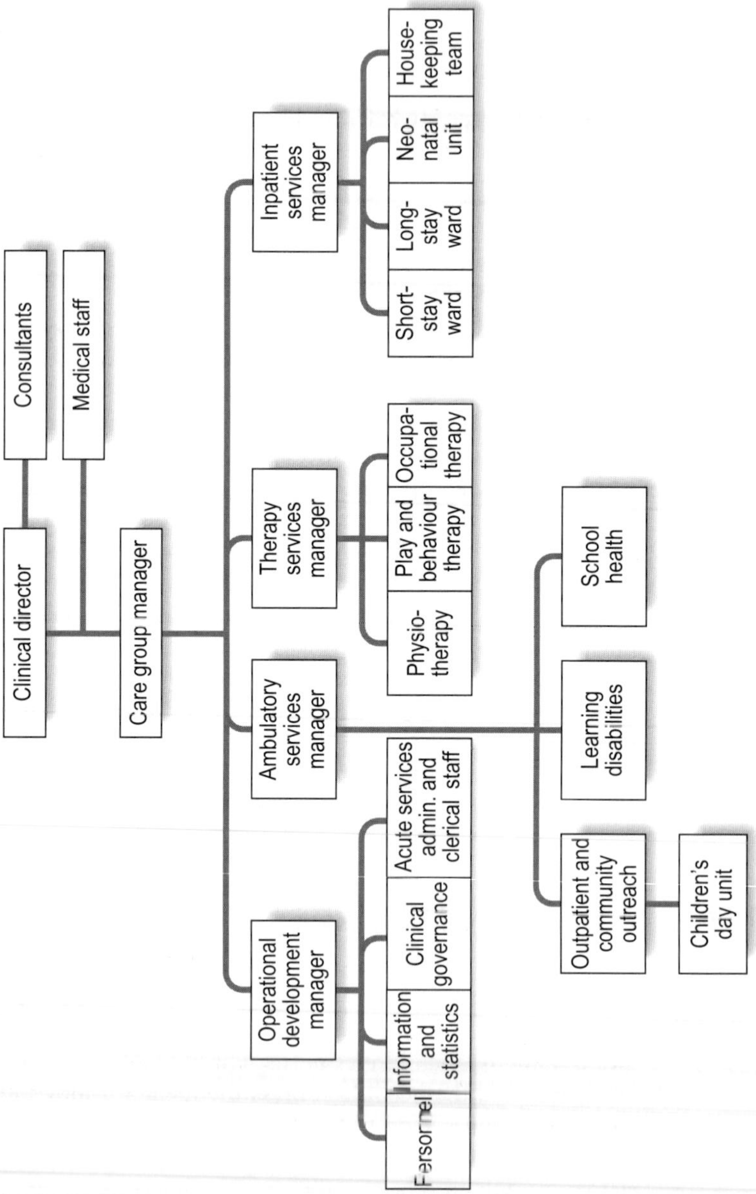

Figure 33.1 Care group structure – child health.

worker who is fully informed of available resources. This facilitates a cohesive approach to representing the health needs of the child when working within the multiagency framework. For example, geographically patched school, learning disability and community children's nurses (CCNs) work in mainstream and special schools with professionals allied to medicine (i.e. physiotherapists, speech and language and occupational therapists). In conjunction with their colleagues in education, they are able to deliver agreed care packages to a consistent standard. This ensures that a large proportion of children with chronic illness remain in the mainstream educational system, whilst those requiring education in special schools are well supported. This style of multidisciplinary working helps to foster close working relationships with colleagues from other agencies who appreciate the fact that they can access all children's services through a single point of contact.

The pooling of budgets for children's services has facilitated the management team's function of strategic planning and service delivery. Financial resources can be directed or redirected towards identified need. For example, if there is a shortfall in one area and available funds in another, team leaders can negotiate to restructure their budgets as part of the planning process. This collaborative approach is a more practical, and often quicker, way to implement change rather than waiting for funds to be available. An example of this was when the learning disabilities team identified the need for a music therapist for a fixed period. It was agreed to transfer money across teams in order to accommodate this need and to improve the quality of child health care.

The 1997 award of 'Investors in People' had a major impact on promoting the maximum potential of human resources. It facilitated the employment, retention, well-being and development of appropriately trained staff who are competent and confident practitioners, able to deliver the service objectives and meet the ever-changing needs of children and their families. It has further developed aspects of team working. For example, changes in induction programmes for new staff has meant that all staff are fully aware of the range of skills and services that their colleagues can provide, thereby avoiding duplication of effort and waste of resources. This team-working approach enabled staff to utilise the skills and/or support of others when required, irrespective of the place of care delivery.

A further consideration in human resource management is that of workforce planning, which has become a formal process since the integration of services. Education and training are key priorities within the strategic and operational plan, and a local training needs analysis is undertaken annually through the individual appraisal process. The integrated structure also facilitates multiprofessional education and skill development. It ensures that expertise is shared between professionals across the whole range of specialist areas. This has the benefit of the majority of education being delivered in-house, ensuring that the maximum number of staff can access training at a minimum cost.

DELIVERING QUALITY AND COST-EFFECTIVE CARE

The clinical governance agenda (Department of Health 1998b) calls for a unified approach to quality and performance management. The key concepts are the delivery of clinically effective care by competent and efficient staff within an effective organisation. To ensure the delivery of evidence-based practice, regular audit is undertaken by the multidisciplinary team supported by a clinical effectiveness coordinator. Several of these audits have been presented in national forums, one of which was a 3-year audit of the management of infants admitted to hospital with bronchiolitis. The results of this audit have improved the quality of care through changing practice in a cost-effective manner. Practice has altered in terms of:

- Length of stay
- Investigations undertaken
- Therapeutic intervention
- Nursing care

BENEFITS TO PATIENTS AND STAFF

Combining all aspects of community and hospital care has enabled practice to (1) be responsive to the changing agenda for children's service and (2) embrace national directives and guidance. This ensures that the service is delivered with maximum benefit to children and their families. The concept of ambulatory care has been readily absorbed. The establishment of a children's day unit helped to tackle the winter pressures agenda. It provided a fast response to the primary care team with minimal hospital admissions, whilst improving service provision to children and their families. The children's day unit is operational 7 days a week and complements outpatient and walk-in clinic facilities. It provides an environment for triage and assessment, specific investigations and observations. Children accessing the service as a result of acute referral are examined by a children's nurse and senior doctor. Following this assessment a decision is made as to whether the child requires:

1. A period of observation and treatment without accessing a hospital bed
2. Up to 48 hours of observation in a short-stay ward
3. To be admitted to the high-care ward

CCNs work closely with day-care staff and often follow up children with either a telephone call or home visit as required. They are also in attendance at the daily ward round to facilitate the early discharge of children who needed to be admitted. Preliminary evaluation of this project has shown that a large proportion of children referred to hospital do not require admission but do benefit from a period of skilled observation in a non-hospital environment before returning home.

Participation in multiagency forums has ensured that services are well placed to engage actively in planning and implementing the key principles for interagency cooperation to safeguard children. For example, the social services department and the health authority jointly agreed a policy for continuing social and health care, in line with 'NHS responsibilities for meeting continuing health care needs' (Department of Health 1995). The children's specialist learning disabilities nurse, in conjunction with a colleague in the adult services, established a criteria framework for health and social work professionals to assess the levels of care required for individual children. This assessment is undertaken by all professionals involved with the child and family, and a health and social care summary is collated. It is discussed at a multidisciplinary, multiagency meeting where a plan of care is agreed with the parents. The CCN is often identified as the key worker.

Should a child who is receiving ongoing care and support require hospital admission for an elective procedure, the key worker will arrange a pre-admission planning meeting with hospital staff, and a care plan which includes discharge information will be developed. This allows for training needs to be identified.

The benefits of an integrated service to children and their families include:

- Receiving care at the point of need by a skilled team with an identified key worker
- Being aware, at all times, of where to obtain advice and support
- The ability to participate as caregivers in the process of integrated planning and care delivery. This is especially important when the nature of illness or disability demands that a large number of multidisciplinary and multiagency professionals is involved.

CASE STUDY

Peter's story

At the age of 22 months, Peter had never been home. He had a large malignant haemangioma of the chest wall extending into the mediastinum, increased platelet consumption and hypertrophic obstructive cardiomyopathy. His care plan was agreed following a multidisciplinary assessment of needs. When the parents expressed desire to have Peter's care delivered at home, it was agreed that the community children's nursing team would take over the thrice-weekly platelet transfusions, supervised by the GP, with therapists providing advice and support to the parents on all aspects of Peter's development.

After discharge, Peter required only one emergency hospital admission. He was enrolled in his local Early Years Centre, where health staff monitored his progress. He settled well in his home environment and his health needs gradually decreased to the level that he no longer required direct nursing care. His parents were overjoyed at his progress and were convinced that, despite the risks involved, having him at home was the right thing to do.

James' story

James was born at 30 weeks with severe moulding, following loss of amniotic fluid 11 weeks into the pregnancy. James received care in the neonatal intensive care unit, during which time he was referred to the physiotherapy team for the management of positional deformities. At term, James was provided with an upright moulded insert in a specially designed chair whilst still in the neonatal unit. He was discharged home, oxygen dependent, at 18 weeks' chronological age in the care of the CCN, physiotherapist and health visitor, all of whom worked collaboratively to deliver his healthcare and monitor his development in the home. He underwent a multidisciplinary pre-school assessment at $4\frac{1}{2}$ years, which was used to inform the decision-making process for school placement. James commenced mainstream school with no specific health needs, but was kept under regular review by the school health team and therapists.

This is an excellent example of how early intervention by skilled staff, working together with parents and the primary healthcare team, can minimise problems and maximise individual potential.

CONCLUSION

The provision of an integrated and combined children's service has had the following benefits:

- Enables a more proactive approach to current challenges within the NHS
- Brings a positive approach to problem solving and breaking down existing barriers
- Allows the service to focus on the normal development and the promotion of healthy lifestyles of children and young people within the context of their family
- Develops an effective organisation which values its staff and promotes cost-effective practice

The integrated service is most appropriately sited within the community setting as it embraces the philosophy that services to children and young people should be focused on the promotion of healthy lifestyle and the prevention of ill health. It endorses the belief that children should not be admitted to hospital unless the care they require cannot successfully and safely be carried out in the community. It therefore follows that a large proportion of service strategic planning must be concentrated on continuing to develop community services and acquiring appropriately skilled staff, whilst ensuring that hospital-based staff acquire specialist training in caring for the highly dependent, acutely ill child.

The emergence of primary care groups (in England), with progression to primary care Trusts, has the potential to fragment children's services. However, integrated service provision should safeguard the rights of children and their families. It should enable access to the quality and standard of service they deserve, and form the basis of close partnership and collaboration with all agencies commissioning and providing services for children and their families.

FURTHER READING

Audit Commission 1994 Seen but not heard: co-ordinating community child health and social services for children in need. HMSO, London

This Audit Commission report details the need for the coordination of community child health and social services for children, especially those with a defined special need. It highlights the increased responsibilities of social services departments and general practitioners for safeguarding the health and development of children alongside the traditional areas of work for community child health and educational authorities.

Department of Health 1976 Report of the committee on child health services: fit for the future. HMSO, London

This was the first comprehensive report of children's services on a national basis following the reorganisation of local government and the National Health Service, which took place on 1 April 1974. Many of the recommendations have still not been fully implemented throughout the UK.

Department of Health 1991 Welfare of children in hospital. HMSO, London

This guide details three important milestones in the continuing quest to develop a quality service for children and their families. These are based on the Platt Report, the Court Report and the White Paper 'Working for patients'. It was intended to assist district health authorities to identify standards they wished providers to achieve in delivery of services.

Department of Health 1996 Child health in the community: a guide to good practice. National Health Service Executive Report, London

This guide to good practice recognises that a better appreciation of the extent to which health and lifestyle in childhood determines adult health status has given new emphasis to the importance of healthcare and health promotion for children and young people. It sets out to demonstrate how the quality and effectiveness of the children's services can be improved.

Department of Health 1999 Quality protects: transforming children's services, objectives for social services for children. DoH, London

This initiative aims to ensure that local authority social services for children who are looked after in the child protection system and other children requiring active support from social services are well managed and effective.

Department of Health 1999 Quality protects: framework for action. DoH, London.

This paper sets out the Government's objectives for children's services. It provides clarity about the work that local authority social services departments should be undertaking and how their resources should be directed.

REFERENCES

Audit Commission 1994 Seen but not heard: co-ordinating community child health and social services for children in need. HMSO, London

Department of Health 1976 Report of the committee on child health services: fit for the future. HMSO, London

Department of Health 1995 NHS responsibilities for meeting continuing health care needs. HSG(95)8LAC(95)5. HMSO, London

Department of Health 1998a Partnership in action. A discussion document. The Stationery Office, London

Department of Health 1998b A first class service. Quality in the new NHS. The Stationery Office, London

Health Committee 1997 Reports of the health committee on health services for children and young people, Session 1996–97: 'The specific health needs of children and young people' (307–1); 'Health services for children and young people in the community, home and school' (314–1); 'Hospital services for children and young people' (128–1); 'Child and adolescent mental health services' (26–1). The Stationery Office, London

National Health Service Executive 1996 Child health in the community: A guide to good practice. The Stationery Office, London

34 Economic evaluation in practice

Caroline Gould

KEY ISSUES

- Clarifying the terminology
- Examining the role of economic evaluation in community children's nursing
- Considerations for the community children's nurse

INTRODUCTION

The National Health Service (NHS) is undergoing significant change. Reconfigurations in the commissioning of healthcare in the form of primary care groups (in England), and a renewed emphasis on quality, efficiency and cost-effectiveness, are part of the Government's 10-year initiative to modernise the NHS (Department of Health 1998). The concept of clinical effectiveness aims to ensure that services are effective in terms of result and cost. Whilst there will be continuing budgetary restraints, quality is central and clinicians will be required to ensure that the services they provide are appropriate, effective, efficient and economic (Department of Health 1998).

In this political context, community children's nurses (CCNs) will need to be able to demonstrate the effectiveness and efficiency of the services they provide to children, their families and the communities in which they work. This chapter examines the ways in which economic evaluations can inform and influence nursing services for children in the community. Integral to this is the part played by the CCN, and some of the issues for these nurses will be examined.

CLARIFYING THE TERMINOLOGY

Economic evaluation is the comparative analysis of alternative courses of action in terms of both their costs and the consequences (Drummond et al 1987). Robinson (1993a) describes it as drawing up a balance sheet of the advantages (benefits) and disadvantages (costs) associated with each option so that choices can be made. Economic evaluation is only one dimension of the overall evaluation process (Coyle 1993, Robinson 1993a). Box 34.1 provides a glossary of commonly used terms.

BOX 34.1 *Glossary of terms commonly used in economic evaluation*

Costs – salaries, equipment, etc. and any deleterious effects of a programme
Effectiveness – a measure of how successfully or otherwise activities are being carried out
Efficiency – ensuring the best resource use to provide maximum benefit to the client
Cost–benefit analysis – a term often used to describe all economic evaluations. It is a method in which alternative programmes are compared and both costs and benefits are valued in monetary terms. Attributing a monetary value to healthcare outcomes is not easy and cost–effectiveness analysis is often preferred (Robinson 1993b, Wilson-Barnett & Beech 1994)
Cost–effectiveness analysis – employed when costs and consequences of alternative programmes are compared; costs are valued in money while the common effect is measured in natural units (e.g. symptom-free day or life saved)

ROLE OF ECONOMIC EVALUATION IN COMMUNITY CHILDREN'S NURSING

Effective management should ensure efficiency, quality and accessibility of the service, whilst operating within finite budgetary limits. The allocation of resources needs to be evaluated to ensure that the right service is being provided to the right people at the right cost. Often, services are measured in terms of target numbers, such as number of visits or waiting times. Whilst these may provide some measurable information, they do not fully reflect the volume or complexity of the service, nor are the quality issues addressed.

Economic evaluation may be used to assess whether the best use is being made of the resources available, for example when deciding whether to introduce a screening programme or in conjunction with clinical trials. However, the principles of an economic appraisal can be incorporated into an evaluation of a local service or team. Such studies may influence managers in their decisions to continue funding specific projects, or they may demonstrate ways in which savings can be made.

There is a need for nurses to undertake more studies to measure the impact and effectiveness of nursing care (Shamian 1997, Stone & Walker 1995). Thomas & Bond (1995) concluded that it is not acceptable to evaluate an intervention without also addressing the cost implications. More specifically the Health Committee (1997 para 49 p xix) stated:

> 'We very much regret that no research has ever been conducted into the most cost-effective way of providing the nursing service that children and their carers in the community need.'

The lack of data assessing costs, benefits and cost–effectiveness of nursing exposes the vulnerability of nurses and nursing in decisions about healthcare financing (Buchan et al 1996, International Council of Nurses 1992).

Tierney (1993) suggests that tackling the complexities of cost–effectiveness research is one of the greatest challenges for nurses. The complexities of measuring the effectiveness and the outcomes of nursing have been described (Buchan et al 1996, Lock 1996, Thomas & Bond 1995). These include distinguishing what exactly it is that nurses do, how this is separated from the input of other disciplines, and measuring the success of an intervention that may occur once client contact has ceased.

In community work, significant time is spent working in areas such as supporting families and their children, health promotion and accident prevention, the impact and long-term effects of which are particularly difficult to demonstrate (Traynor 1993, While 1991).

In community children's nursing, the psychosocial and other benefits for the child and family are well documented, but may be hard to quantify. Financial savings, by reducing numbers of hospital beds, will not be a reality in the short term (Bradley 1997, Nathwani & Davey 1996), and the establishment of schemes is more likely to increase expenditure initially (Royal College of Nursing 1994, While 1991).

Although the scheme evaluated by While (1991) increased the cost of paediatric care because the inpatient bed complement remained unchanged, she was theoretically able to demonstrate cost–effectiveness. By calculating the bed nights saved (reported to be 573) and comparing hospital costs with the costs of community nurse visits, she proposed that substantial savings could be made. This contrasts with the service evaluated by Jennings (1994), where bed numbers were reduced at the team's inception, thereby reducing costs. Both studies demonstrated effectiveness through other important benefits, such as parental preference and reduced anxiety.

In Bradley's (1997) comprehensive review of community nursing services for children she noted that, while such services offer high-quality care, financial constraints and funding problems may be a threat. It is vital that CCNs demonstrate ways in which their services are beneficial, not only to children and families, as reported in the literature (Bishop et al 1994, Jennings 1994), but also to purchasers of services (Brocklehurst 1996, Hennessy 1993).

With the advent of primary care groups (in England) and local healthcare cooperatives, community nurses are being given enormous opportunities to influence how services are provided. CCNs must ensure the groups are knowledgeable about the services they provide. Brocklehurst (1996) and Jennings (1994) note that community children's nursing services are poorly understood; it is the responsibility of those nurses working in the speciality to articulate what it is they do, how much it costs, and how effective the service is.

Quality is high on the Government's agenda, and those interventions for which there is good evidence of clinical and cost effectiveness will be promoted (Department of Health 1998). Demonstrating effectiveness in terms of result and cost will not only help to ensure continued funding of current schemes, but act as leverage to set up new schemes. There are still many children in the UK who do not have access to a CCN, and the Government has stated that unacceptable variations in services across the country will be addressed (Department of Health 1997). Undertaking economic appraisals is one way in which CCNs can influence resource allocation and decision making. Whilst complex, there are an increasing number of people with the necessary expertise to help in undertaking such a project (Brocklehurst 1996).

Contributing to financial debates is a further way in which CCNs can impact on decision making. With their knowledge and experience, they can enhance debates by articulating the quality issues of the services they provide;

representing the viewpoints of children and families is to fulfil client-advocate responsibilities. While purchasers may wish to select the cheaper option, professional arguments in favour of the positive benefits associated with the higher costs could be made.

An appreciation of economic terminology and methodology will enable nurses to recognise whether studies are valid and will increase confidence for participating in debates and for undertaking their own studies. Continuing education opportunities will empower nurses to contribute to this aspect of evaluation (International Council of Nurses 1992, Shamian 1997).

EXAMPLES FROM PRACTICE

Two examples are offered from the author's own previous practice experience. In the first example, the community children's nursing team demonstrated cost–effectiveness by calculating the number of inpatient bed-nights saved for children who were discharged early to complete their course of intravenous antibiotics at home. The one major dimension for the measurement of success, which Drummond et al (1987) suggest is necessary for a cost–effectiveness analysis, is 'bed-nights saved'.

The cost of the inpatient night was compared to the cost of visits by CCNs. The main motive for community intravenous therapy should be better care, not simply a reduction in costs (Nathwani & Davey 1996). The provision of the community children's nursing service improved care by facilitating earlier discharge, and for some children on long-term medication this enabled a return to school.

The conclusion was that the service was cost-effective: there were substantial savings to the hospitals, particularly where children were prescribed once- or twice-daily drugs. In addition, the earlier discharge allowed increased bed usage. Clinical effectiveness was demonstrated in terms of both result (early discharge) and cost (savings to hospitals).

These findings seem to support those of While (1991). However, because of the influence of local factors upon cost–effectiveness, generalisation should be cautionary. The wide variation of visiting costs reported by Jennings (1994), from £6.94 to £50.27, illustrates how great local variations can be.

In this second example, the CCNs planned to introduce geographical caseloads. There had been no specific division to date but, as the team grew, it was agreed that the change might offer a more efficient service, in terms of reducing travelling time and improving links with primary healthcare teams.

Mooney (1992) suggests that cost–effectiveness analysis can demonstrate how best to deploy a given budget to meet a particular objective. Whilst the principal aim was not to reduce expenditure, the team's travel budget needed to be used to best effect. The measurements used in the evaluation were:

- mileage claims
- travelling times
- numbers of children visited before and after the change

Whilst numbers of children do not encompass quality, they are a measurable indicator and one that was dictated by the purchasers. A review of the literature to identify previous studies that had examined caseload organisation in community nursing teams revealed little evidence of this type of evaluation. Savings of £50 000 in travelling expenses were cited in one area when nurses began working in defined boundaries (Wilson & Brown 1989). Economic evaluations are specific to a population or location (Edwardson 1992, Muir Gray 1997) and, whilst other studies may have been useful, they would not necessarily have related to this team.

This study did show that the travel budget could be used more effectively; both mileage claims and travelling times were lower. Since less time was spent travelling, there was more time available for client contact. The numbers of visits continued to meet contract requirements. Additional effectiveness indicators included an increase in referrals from primary healthcare teams, suggesting improved links and better knowledge of the service, and nurses' knowledge of the local areas improved. The study was limited, in that consideration was not given to other organisational styles, such as the nurses holding specialist caseloads.

Both of these studies formed part of a larger evaluative review of a community children's nursing team. They have been summarised here and serve to demonstrate how the principles of economic evaluation can be useful to support developments in practice.

CONCLUSION

Economic evaluation is just one aspect of the evaluation process, and one that has not been widely undertaken in relation to nursing services in this country. High quality and cost–effectiveness are central to the Government's 'new NHS' (Department of Health 1997) and nurses will increasingly be required to articulate arguments and proposals in economic as well as professional terms.

For community children's nursing to continue to develop and progress, practitioners should include an economic perspective in service evaluations. This will help to ensure that:

- Benefits and outcomes are considered in relation to costs
- Services are adequately resourced
- Economic evaluation is part of the decision-making process when services are being planned and reviewed
- A knowledge base about the value of nursing emerges

Some of the difficulties include:

- Measuring and quantifying nursing outcomes
- Generalisability
- Financial data may not demonstrate cost–effectiveness, but the supportive evidence relating to benefits should override this

Implications for community children's nurses

- Development of an understanding of the terminology to enable participation in the process
- Critical analysis of economic evaluations

- Application of the principles to practice
- The need to demonstrate and articulate the effectiveness and efficiency of the quality services being provided through (1) research studies, (2) service evaluations, (3) contributions to debates and (4) participation in decisions about resource allocation

> 'We recommend that the Department of Health should monitor for effectiveness and cost-effectiveness the various local models and structures which currently exist, so that improved advice and guidance can be given to purchasers and providers.' (Health Committee 1997 para 49 p xix)

Given recommendations such as this, it is necessary for CCNs to evaluate the services they are providing and demonstrate clinical effectiveness in terms of both outcomes and cost.

FURTHER READING

Drummond M F, Stoddart G L & Torrance G W 1987 (reprinted 1995) Methods for the economic evaluation of health care programmes. Oxford University Press, Oxford

This book provides comprehensive information and examples on cost-minimisation, cost–effectiveness, cost–benefit and cost–utility evaluations. The authors also provide a useful 10-point checklist for assessing economic evaluations.

Jones A & McDonnell U 1993 Managing the clinical resource. Baillière Tindall, London

Chapter 2 introduces the concept of healthcare economics and examines its developing role in healthcare.

Muir Gray J A 1997 Evidence-based healthcare. Churchill Livingstone, New York

This book provides clearly signposted sections on finding, appraising and using evidence to increase evidence-based decision making in healthcare, and on the implementation of evidence-based practice.

Royal College of Nursing 1998 Marketing community and specialist nursing services – an RCN guide. Royal College of Nursing, London

This guide contains useful information and case examples on marketing, analysing services and demonstrating the cost–effectiveness of nursing.

REFERENCES

Bishop J, Anderson A & McCulloch J 1994 Hospital-at-home: a critical analysis. Paediatric Nursing 6(6):12–15

Bradley S F 1997 Better late than never? An evaluation of community nursing services for children in the UK. Journal of Clinical Nursing 6:411–418

Brocklehurst N 1996 Selling children's community nursing. Paediatric Nursing 8(9):6–7

Buchan J, Seccombe I & Ball J 1996 Caring costs revisited. Institute for Employment Studies, Brighton, UK

Coyle D 1993 Increasing the impact of economic evaluations on health-care decision-making. Discussion Paper 108. University of York, York

Department of Health 1997 The new NHS. Modern, dependable. The Stationery Office, London

Department of Health 1998 A first class service: quality in the new NHS. The Stationery Office, London

Drummond M F, Stoddart G L & Torrance G W 1987 (reprinted 1995) Methods for the economic evaluation of health care programmes. Oxford University Press, Oxford

Edwardson S R 1992 Costs and benefits of clinical nurse specialists. Clinical Nurse Specialist 6(3):163–167

Health Committee 1997 House of Commons Select Committee. Health services for children and young people in the community:

home and school. Third report. The Stationery Office, London

Hennessy D 1993 Purchasing community nursing care. Paediatric Nursing 5(2):10–12

International Council of Nurses 1992 Costing nursing services. Report of the ICN Task Force on Costing of Nursing Services. ICN, London

Jennings P 1994 Learning through experience: an evaluation of hospital at home. Journal of Advanced Nursing 19:905–911

Lock K 1996 The changing organisation of health care: setting the scene. In: Twinn S, Roberts B & Andrews S (eds) Community health care nursing: principles for practice. Butterworth Heinemann, Oxford, ch 2, p 30

Mooney G 1992 Economics, medicine and health care, 2nd edn. Harvester Wheatsheaf, London

Muir Gray J A 1997 Evidence-based healthcare. Churchill Livingstone, New York

Nathwani D & Davey P 1996 Intravenous antimicrobial therapy in the community: underused, inadequately resourced, or irrelevant to health care in Britain? British Medical Journal 313:1541–1543

Robinson R 1993a Economic evaluation and health care: what does it mean? British Medical Journal 307:670–673

Robinson R 1993b Cost–benefit analysis. British Medical Journal 307:924–926

Royal College of Nursing 1994 Wise decisions: developing paediatric home care teams. RCN Paediatric Community Nurses' Forum, London

Shamian J 1997 How nursing contributes towards quality and cost-effective health care. International Nursing Review 44(3):79–84, 90

Stone P W & Walker P H 1995 Cost-effectiveness analysis: birth center vs. hospital care. Nursing Economics 13(5):299–307

Thomas L H & Bond S 1995 The effectiveness of nursing: a review. Journal of Clinical Nursing 4:143–151

Tierney A 1993 Quality, costs and nursing. Journal of Clinical Nursing 2:123–124

Traynor M 1993 Health visitors' perceptions of their role. Health Visitor 66(1):14–16

While A E 1991 An evaluation of a paediatric home care scheme. Journal of Advanced Nursing 16:1413–1421

Wilson A & Brown P 1989 Health care units and neighbourhood nursing. In: Hughes J (ed) The future of community health services. King's Fund Centre, Primary Health Care Group, London, p 21

Wilson-Barnett J & Beech S 1994 Evaluating the clinical nurse specialist: a review. International Journal of Nursing Studies 31(6):561–571

35 Launching further research in community children's nursing

Steve Campbell & Susan Procter

KEY ISSUES

- The current research foundation in community children's nursing
- Analysis of specific research studies and their relative findings
- Indications for future research opportunities in community children's nursing

INTRODUCTION

Like the practice of community children's nurses (CCNs), the research of their practice is a relatively new phenomenon. Research that has been undertaken has tended not to include the children themselves. This is a challenge that all children's nursing researchers need to take on if the practice of children's nursing is to develop: balancing the needs of children with those of their primary carer(s). Broome (1998 p 305) commented recently in a Nursing Research editorial:

> 'Investigators who study children must assemble a team of investigators who are experts in child development and the study of children, who are familiar with methodological limitations of some methods with children, and who know how to protect children from undue burden. Society has much to gain from new research conducted with children.'

Children's nursing research in the UK has developed along family-centred lines. This tends to mean the involvement of parents and prime carers; however, future studies need to be balanced with a children's focus.

The content of this chapter is influenced by a nationally funded, English National Board for Nursing, Midwifery and Health Visiting (ENB) research study carried out between 1997 and 1998, of which the two present authors were project managers (Procter et al 1998a,b, 1999). The themes that were evident to this research team, and continue to be the source of inspiration for further research, are 'Burden of care', 'Guiding principles of care' and 'Forms of service'. These themes are presented as the structure to this chapter. To provide some clarity and order to these themes, a brief description of the research study (Procter et al 1998a,b, 1999) will be presented before addressing the themes.

BRIEF OUTLINE OF THE ENB RESEARCH STUDY

The study was designed to elicit a training needs analysis for CCNs based on an analysis of the needs of families caring for sick children at home. The research used a variety of methods to (Procter et al 1998b):

- Map existing service provision nationally (England)
- Select six sites providing community children's nursing services (these were purposively sampled from all available National Health Service Trusts on the basis of a series of variables identified by an expert group) and undertake interviews with CCNs, their managers and professional colleagues
- Undertake interviews with families receiving care from each of the services used in the research
- Conduct three focus groups – a multiprofessional group, a group of nurse educationalists providing courses for CCNs, and a group of representatives from children's charities with an interest in sick children being cared for at home

The data were analysed qualitatively. Themes relating to service provision from a management, organisational and practitioner perspective were derived from the interviews with professional staff. The data from families drew on a theoretical analysis of need within a framework of health promotion–disease prevention. These were the families of a sample of children who could be characterised as largely having problems associated with chronic illness. A process model for service and curriculum development was produced, centred on a set of guiding principles and based on an analysis of the needs of families caring for sick children at home (Procter et al 1998b).

The process of this research and outcomes of the study have left the authors with a number of key issues that remain largely unresolved nationally and need to be the focus of further research. These issues will be exposed within the following themes.

BURDEN OF CARE

In reading the transcripts of the interviews with parents, the vast majority being mothers of chronically ill children, there was an impression of the enormous burden of care that parents and, in particular, mothers were obliged to take on. This burden was tempered, if not balanced, by the pride these parents took in being able to care for their child and the improvements they saw in their child. The obligation that these parents feel to care for their child at home is natural, but we are not yet clear as to how far we (or their sick children) can or should push parents into providing this care at home. The resources of the parents and the capacity of that family to care for the child are currently assessed by the multidisciplinary team involved. However, this assessment may be influenced by two conflicting perspectives: whilst getting the child home is philosophically the right thing to do, it also saves hospital funds. The multidisciplinary team assessment tends to focus on the child and the prime carer(s) rather than the total family, because those involved are most aware and most specifically concerned with the dynamic of the relationship between these two. There is a need to examine the evidence and research base on which children, particularly those with complex needs, are discharged into the care of their family, with or without the support of a CCN. The current approach to assessing the family would seem, in the main, to be too narrow. This approach fails to draw on the potential of the whole family, their ability to problem solve and utilise their full resources.

The CCN appears to be in a key position to assess the needs of the whole family that takes on the care of the sick child at home. This is perhaps best exemplified by the position of many mothers, who find themselves providing the majority of the care to the chronically ill child. Baldwin and Twigg (1991) discuss the notion of delegating care to families, but caution that this should not prevent them leading 'relatively ordinary lives'. Systematic strategies for CCNs to help the members of families to lead relatively ordinary lives have not been explored to any great extent in practice, let alone through research.

The potential use of McCubbin and McCubbin's (1993) model of family resiliency has great potential as a focus for helping CCNs to find these new ways of working. The model can be regarded as outlining the process by which families adjust and adapt to illness. By allowing objectification of a family's collective reaction to a child's illness, the model affords the CCN the opportunity to find ways of intervening in the process of adaptation, so that there is greater opportunity for all members of the family to lead relatively ordinary lives. It has been commented that such a role would be better carried out by a social worker rather than a CCN, the justification being the social basis of this intervention and the social worker's potential knowledge of family therapy. However, such an approach is not family therapy, and when challenging a focus group of special interest groups (Procter et al 1998a, 1999) with this proposition, the group was unanimous that this role needed to be carried out by CCNs because it was they who had the knowledge and credibility with the family. Such an approach would form an exciting action research project (Whyte et al 1998).

GUIDING PRINCIPLES OF CARE

Procter et al (1998a,b) suggested 17 guiding principles for community children's nursing practice (Box 35.1). Many of these principles are fundamental to the nature of good children's nursing in any setting, including hospital. Therefore, there is a need to identify those principles that are peculiar to the practice of a CCN and those that have been built up through practice in other fields of children's nursing, or even from nursing in general. Further work needs to be done to establish whether these 17 principles are exhaustive (i.e. whether there are further principles). This is especially pertinent, since the majority of the sample in this study were children with a chronic illness (Procter et al 1998a,b). The nursing of children in the community with an acute illness might well elicit different guiding principles and is an area yet to be studied. Further to this, there would appear to be relationships between some of these 17 principles. This raises the issue of whether there is a need for *all* of these principles, or whether some could be conflated. Such a study could be carried out by

BOX 35.1 ***Guiding principles of community children's nursing practice (Procter et al 1998a,b)***

1. Promoting family-centred care rather than child-centred care
2. Maintaining or improving the quality of life of the family, rather than focusing on medical needs
3. Minimising stressful events rather than giving routinised care
4. Fostering family empowerment rather than learned helplessness/dependency on professionals' solving abilities
5. Having an approach of partnership rather than the imposition of professional expertise
6. Appreciating the complexity of a problem rather than oversimplifying it
7. Solving or re-framing problems rather than avoiding them
8. Recognising the boundaries of your own expertise and knowing where to turn for appropriate help, rather than trying to solve all problems yourself
9. Establishing credibility with paediatric and primary healthcare colleagues through working together openly rather than having an insular approach
10. Having a flexible, organic, responsive role, rather than a formally directed set of functions
11. Having knowledge gained through experience rather than procedures
12. Having the knowledge to anticipate and plan for future directions in the care needs of the child, rather than reacting to crisis
13. Being available (light touch) for the family when the family wants it, rather than when it is most convenient to services
14. Promoting the health of families rather than focusing solely on tertiary interventions
15. Lightening the burden through manner of approach, rather than getting caught up in the anxieties of the situation and reinforcing the burden
16. Enabling children and families to lead ordinary lives, rather than this being regarded as secondary to biomedical interventions
17. Listening and discovering rather than imposing ready-made solutions from elsewhere

identifying the major theme areas underlying these principles and grouping them together.

Given that these principles were derived from interviews with the families involved in the study (Procter et al 1998a,b, 1999), it would be possible to construct some form of evaluation tool based upon the ways that families with a chronically ill child would like CCNs to behave. As an evaluative instrument, such as a linear analogue (Burns 1979, Cella & Perry 1986), this could then be completed by the families. Such an evaluation tool would be useful for many community children's nursing services. In the process of the ENB study, many managers of community children's nursing services indicated that they were struggling to provide data to support their practice. Specialist services, such as paediatric oncology, may be able to provide data such as morbidity and mortality statistics to justify their practice. However, generalist community children's nursing practice may be concerned much more with the quality of life of the child and family, but these issues are more challenging to evaluate. Assessing the extent to which each family believes their CCN to have worked to the principles may well help to provide some meaningful data for managers of these services.

FORMS OF SERVICE

Since the publication of the 'Wise decisions' document (Royal College of Nursing 1994), there has been a preoccupation with the different models of community children's nursing services based upon need. More recently, Eaton & Thomas (1998) characterised six models of service provision with clear relationships between each of these. It may be possible, with further analysis, to identify a continuum of their characteristics and to also identify the different forms of service, with these six models as important areas of activity on that continuum.

CCNs will be required now and in the future to be sure of where their practice needs to be placed; further work should be undertaken to establish the nature and form of this need. In particular, this work should be influenced by key authors in this area, such as Bradshaw (1972) and his form of need: normative, relative, felt and expressed. There are challenging questions to be answered with respect to how it is possible to articulate a notion of need in relation to a family.

The nature of 'good' community children's nursing services is linked to the guiding principles laid out in Box 35.1 (Procter et al 1998a,b). Is this a function of the people involved in the service, or is it derived from the nature of the form of the service? Eaton & Thomas (1998) have identified evaluative criteria derived from quality management theoretical material. These criteria have a relationship with the guiding principles, although they focus on the service itself. The criteria identified by Eaton & Thomas (1998) assist in answering important questions about what part of the organisation of the service lends itself to promotion of this 'good' community children's nursing service. However, if the success of a service is derived from the people concerned, from where did they gain these qualities? Were they innate, or taught to them in practice or in their nurse training, or learned in other forms of practice or from role models? All of these questions represent lines of enquiry in the practice of a CCN.

CONCLUSION

In this chapter it has been possible only to hint at aspects of the potential for research building on the currently limited foundations available. These foundations are strong, but need to be developed and to be a balance of family-focused and child-focused research, as discussed at the beginning of the chapter.

FURTHER READING

Eaton N & Thomas P 1998 Community children's nursing: an evaluative framework. Journal of Child Health Care 2(4):170–173

Explores the components of a comprehensive evaluation which considers the views and perspectives of all the key stakeholders in a community children's nursing service.

Procter S, Biott C, Campbell S, Edward S, Redpath N & Moran M 1998a Preparation for the developing role of the community children's nurse. English National Board for Nursing, Midwifery and Health Visiting, London

This comprehensive study offers a training needs analysis for CCNs based on an analysis of the needs of families caring for sick children at home.

REFERENCES

Baldwin S & Twigg J 1991 Women and community care – reflections on debate. In: Maclean M & Groves D (eds) Women's issues in social policy. Routledge, London, pp 117–135

Bradshaw J 1972 The concept of social need. New Society 30:640–643

Broome M E 1998 Researching the world of children. Nursing Research 47(6):305–306

Burns R E 1979 The use of visual analogue mood and alert scales in diagnosing hospitalised affective psychosis. Psychological Medicine 9:155–164

Cella D F & Perry S W 1986 Reliability and validity of three visual analogue mood scales. Psychological Reports 59:827–830

Eaton N & Thomas P 1998 Community children's nursing: an evaluative framework. Journal of Child Health Care 2(4):170–173

McCubbin M A & McCubbin H I 1993 Families coping with illness: the resiliency model of family stress, adjustment and adaptation. In: Danielson C B, Hamel-Bissell B & Winstead-Fry P (eds) Families, health and illness. Mosby, St Louis

Procter S, Biott C, Campbell S, Edward S, Redpath N & Moran M 1998a Preparation for the developing role of the community children's nurse. English National Board for Nursing, Midwifery and Health Visiting, London

Procter S, Biott C, Campbell S, Edward S, Redpath N & Moran M 1998b Preparation for the developing role of the community children's nurse. Research Highlights, no. 32. English National Board for Nursing, Midwifery and Health Visiting, London

Procter S, Biott C, Campbell S, Edward S, Redpath N & Moran M 1999 Preparation for the developing role of the community children's nurse. Researching professional education: Research Report Series, no. 11. English National Board for Nursing, Midwifery and Health Visiting, London

Royal College of Nursing 1994 Wise decisions. Developing paediatric home care teams. RCN Paediatric Community Nurses' Forum, London

Whyte D, Barton M E, Lamb A et al 1998 Clinical effectiveness in community children's nursing. Clinical Effectiveness in Nursing 2:139–144

Index